EAT FAT
LOOK
THIN

A SAFE AND NATURAL WAY
TO LOSE WEIGHT
PERMANENTLY

BRUCE FIFE, N.D.

HealthWise

Colorado Springs, Colorado

HealthWise Publications is an imprint of:
Piccadilly Books, Ltd.
P.O. Box 25203
Colorado Springs, CO 80936, USA

International sales and inquires contact:
EPS
20 Park Drive
Romford Essex RM1 4LH, UK
or
EPS
P.O. Box 1344
Studio City, CA 91614, USA

Library of Congress cataloging-in-Publication Data
Fife, Bruce, 1952-
    Eat fat, look thin : a safe and natural way to lose weight permanently
    / Bruce Fife.
        p. cm.
    Includes bibliographical references and index.
    ISBN 0-941599-52-3
        1. Reducing diets. 2. Coconut oil--Health aspects. 3. Sugar-free diet.
    4. Lipids in human nutrition. I. Title.

RM222.2.F443 202
613.2'5--dc21

                                                                    2002027376

Simultaneously Published in Australia, UK, and USA
Printed in Canada

CONTENTS ▬

Chapter 1   Eat Fat and Lose Weight 5

Chapter 2   Big Fat Lies 18

Chapter 3   Are You In Need of An Oil Change? 30

Chapter 4   What You Should Know
             About Cholesterol 47

Chapter 5   The Truth About Saturated Fat 69

Chapter 6   Carbohydrates: Friend or Foe? 82

Chapter 7   Calories and Appetite 101

Chapter 8   Malnutrition Can Make You Fat 109

Chapter 9   How to Supercharge Your Metabolism 126

Chapter 10   Satisfy Your Hunger Longer 159

Chapter 11   Drink More, Weigh Less 168

Chapter 12   Step Toward A New You 189

Chapter 13   The Healthy Lifestyle Plan 203

Chapter 14   The Low-Carbohydrate Coconut Diet 222

Chapter 15   The Raw-Foods Coconut Diet 241

Chapter 16   Recipes 251

Appendix 270

References 273

Index 284

Chapter 1

EAT FAT AND
LOSE WEIGHT ■

EAT FAT AND LOSE WEIGHT; IS IT POSSIBLE?

Leah, 42, came to me complaining of a variety of problems: frequent migraine headaches, constipation, mood swings, irritability, depression, irregular menstruation, fatigue, and recurring yeast infections. Although she didn't mention it, Leah was overweight. She stood 5'5" and weighed 180 pounds—typical for many middle-age women in America nowadays.

She'd become frustrated with doctors and medications and decided to seek help from someone experienced in alternative or natural medicine. As a nutritionist and naturopathic physician, my focus is helping people overcome health problems using safe, natural means, such as diet and nutrition.

Leah indicated that she ate many refined white flour products (e.g., bread, rolls, pastry, crackers, etc.), breakfast cereals, and frozen and prepared foods, and snacked on sweets and chips. She assured me she ate healthfully because she avoided fat, drinking skim milk and eating low-fat foods; she chose lean cuts of meat and removed all visible fat. She avoided butter like the plague, using margarine in its place, and prepared meals with what she termed "healthy" vegetable oils and margarine. Although the prepared convenience foods she used often included small portions of vegetables, she rarely ate fresh fruits and vegetables and almost no whole grains. Leah's diet was typical of most people in our modern society—nutrient deficient and weight promoting.

The first thing I did was to change her diet. I told her, "Don't eat anything that says low-fat or low-calorie, and get off the sweets and junk

5

foods. Eat whole foods with butter and coconut oil and don't be afraid of the fat in meats. Eat full-fat cheese, cream, and other dairy products. Eat fresh fruits and vegetables and whole grains. Eat as much as much as you want, just don't overeat, and enjoy your new diet."

She was surprised. "Won't all this fat and rich food make me gain weight?" she asked.

"No. You don't have to worry about your weight."

"Well I do worry, I try to watch my calories and limit my fat intake."

"What I'm giving you is a way of eating that will improve your health. It provides your body with all the nutrients it needs to overcome the health problems you mentioned. And as you become more healthy, you will also lose excess body fat."

"You mean I can eat delicious foods, gain better health, and lose weight at the same time?"

"Yes," I told her.

She returned for follow-up visits over the next several months. Each time she told me she was doing better and losing weight. She couldn't believe it. She was eating more rich, fatty foods than she ever had and was dropping pounds. In time, she reported that all of her symptoms had improved, and to her pleasant surprise, she lost 45 pounds dropping to a slim 135 pounds. Now, two years later, she continues to follow my dietary recommendations and still maintains her slim figure.

When people come to see me, they usually are concerned with chronic health problems like Crohn's disease, diabetes, and arthritis. While treatment varies for each individual, the diet I recommend is basically the same. I've had a great deal of success, especially with my diabetic patients. They are able to live normal lives without relying on medications and daily insulin injections.

Patients frequently comment, with delight, that they lose weight on my program. My main focus is to help people regain their health; losing weight is a natural consequence of that process. Losing weight is so common that I pay little attention to it. I consider it a fringe benefit from eating right and becoming healthier.

I believe that most chronic health problems are reversible. The body was designed or programmed to be healthy. I believe the body can overcome just about any natural health problem including being overweight if given the chance. My philosophy is that if you give the body all the nutrients it needs to be healthy and remove health-destroying influences, it can overcome chronic health problems. As the body becomes healthier, weight problems go away.

LOW-FAT DIETS MAY KILL YOU

"I hate diets. None of them have ever worked for me. I tried. I watched what I ate, cutting out all of my favorite foods and reducing calories. I felt deprived. I hated it. I was hungry all the time and felt miserable. I only lost a few pounds. It wasn't worth all the misery I went through. And once I stopped dieting, the weight came right back."

Does this sound familiar to you? It should. Most of us have tried dieting at least once in our lives. Why? Because most of us are overweight. Sixty percent of Americans are overweight; 30% are obese. One third of our children are now overweight. These figures are rapidly increasing. Fifty years ago overweight was a problem with which only a small percentage of the population were troubled. Now it's an epidemic. We're not alone. The same thing is occurring in Canada, Europe, and elsewhere.

You may ask why? Why are we gaining so much weight? We aren't eating that much more than we used to. In fact, we eat less fat now than ever before. Our grandparents got about 40% of their daily calories from fat. Today we are averaging about 32%. We've significantly cut down on our fat consumption. When you go to the grocery store, you're bombarded from every side with labels that read: "Low-fat," "Non-fat," and "Low calorie." When you go to a restaurant, you can get diet soda and low-calorie or reduced-fat meals. Everything nowadays seems to be low- or non-fat. We've cut our fat consumption down significantly from what it used to be. We've replaced saturated fats with polyunsaturated fats and fake fats. Sugar is being replaced by artificial sweeteners. We eat more low-fat, low-calorie foods now than ever before, yet we are fatter now than ever before. Why is that?

The simple answer is that low-fat diets don't work! They're not natural, they're not healthy, and they promote weight *gain* not weight loss.

Research confirms this fact. The longest running and one of the largest studies ever made on the relationship between diet and health is the Framingham study. The study began in 1948, was set up to continue throughout the lifetime of the volunteers, and is still going on today. The study included almost the entire population of Framingham, Massachusetts (population 5,127). After more than 40 years of research, the director of the study, Dr. William Castelli, admitted: "In Framingham, Mass., the more saturated fat one ate, the more cholesterol one ate, the more calories one ate, the lower the person's serum cholesterol... We found that the people who ate the most cholesterol, ate the most saturated fat, ate the most calories, weighed the least."[1] You would expect that the people who eat the least amount of saturated fat, cholesterol, and calories to weigh the least, but they don't, as illustrated the Framingham study.

It appears that if you want to lose weight, you need to avoid low-fat dieting. Trying to lose weight on a low-fat diet is a nightmare of deprivation and starvation. Many of us would rather die than go through the pain. There is a better way.

THE COCONUT DIET

When I first began showing people how to improve their health though diet and nutrition, I believed in the low-fat philosophy. I believed that restricting calories was the only way to lose weight and that eliminating as much fat as possible from the diet was the best approach. This is what I was taught in school. Meat and fat were something to avoid. Saturated fat and cholesterol were considered dietary villains capable of causing just about every ill from heart disease and obesity to athlete's foot and hangnails, or so it seemed by the way animal fats were criticized. We were led to believe that vegetable oils and margarine were much healthier. I ate what I thought was a healthy diet and recommended it to my patients. Many people improved with the low-fat diet I recommended and they overcame their health problems, but for many others progress was slow. At times it was frustrating because some people would not progress or they would get better for some time and then digress.

The first clue that I needed to change my thinking about fats came when I attended a meeting with a group of nutritionists. During the meeting one member of the group stated that coconut oil was healthy and that we should all be using it. We were all dumbfounded by the comment. Coconut oil is a highly saturated fat, and saturated fat was considered unhealthy because it was believed to increase blood cholesterol, which in turn, was believed to promote heart disease.

We respected this member of our group so we listened to what she had to say. She backed up her statement by citing several studies published in the medical literature. Studies showed that lab animals given coconut oil lived longer and developed fewer diseases than those given soybean, corn, or other vegetable oils. I also learned that coconut oil, in one form or another, had been used successfully to treat seriously ill patients and speed recovery. Coconut oil also possessed superior nutritional qualities over other oils and when added to baby formula, it increases the survival rate of premature infants. For these reasons, it is commonly used in hospital intravenous solutions and commercial baby formulas.

When I left that meeting, I was curious; no it was more powerful than that, I was determined—determined to find the truth. Maybe my thinking about fats, and particularly saturated fats, was all wrong. At that point, I

8

made a commitment to find the answer. I began researching the medical literature, reading everything I could on coconut oil, saturated fat, cholesterol, and vegetable oil. What I found was remarkable. Over the next several years, I began incorporating more saturated fats into my dietary program, especially coconut oil, and less and less vegetable oils. I started to see dramatic changes in patients that others had given up on. One of the biggest improvements was the loss in weight. People would add more fat, particularly saturated fat from coconut, into their diets and *lose* weight. I saw, just as the Framingham study demonstrated, that diets containing adequate fats, including saturated fat, produced better results than low-fat diets. When I say better results, I mean everything improved, not only did people lose excess weight, but their overall health improved. Health problems they had before they changed to a higher fat diet got better afterwards.

People were losing weight without even trying. For some, all they did was substitute coconut oil for other oils they had been using and the pounds began melting off. They ate basically the same foods they had before but just made a simple oil change. That's exactly what happened to me.

Over the years, like most everyone else, I had been putting on extra weight. I ate what was considered a healthy, balanced diet. I used margarine and polyunsaturated vegetable oils instead of butter and natural saturated fats.

I was a bit overweight. I tried dieting. It was frustrating. It got to the point where I gave up hope of ever losing my spare tire and just accepted the fact I was overweight and I was going to stay that way. Clothes I had outgrown, but kept around for when I lost weight, were finally tossed out. "I'll never fit into those again," I said to myself.

That was before I learned about coconut oil. When I substituted coconut oil for all the vegetable oils I had been using, I began to lose weight. The weight came off slowly but steadily, and after about 6 months, I had lost 20 pounds! I didn't change my diet, only the oils that I used. And the weight has stayed off. It's been off for many years now. I am at my ideal weight for my height and bone structure. I did this by eating more fat than I ever did before.

I started allowing patients to eat more meat and dairy. When I had people eat healthy foods and use the right types of oils, excess weight seemed to melt off without them even trying to lose weight. I began to focus on developing a diet designed specifically to help people lose excess weight as well as improve overall health. That is what this book is all about.

From this discovery came a system of weight loss like none other. For lack of a better name, I call it *The Healthy Lifestyle Plan*. Some people affectionately call it The Coconut Diet. I don't really like calling it a "diet" because it's more than that. It's a lifestyle change. It's not a temporary diet you go on just to lose a few pounds; it's a program you stick with for life.

In fact, some people don't even consider it a diet at all, at least not like the typical calorie-restricted, low-fat diets. The eating guidelines in this program allow you to eat until you're satisfied. And it's not all rabbit food either. You get to eat a variety of delicious foods—steaks, shrimp, pork, eggs, cream, cheese, creamy sauces and gravies, and of course, coconut. You don't starve. That's one of the big advantages of this program. You eat foods that fill you up and keep you satisfied until your next meal. It's almost like an "undiet." You get to enjoy eating and you lose weight—permanently!

The primary advantage of this program is not the weight loss, but the improvement in overall health. Many weight loss programs are unhealthy. They may help you lose weight, but they are nutritionally unbalanced, setting the stage for new health problems in the future. The risks are too high. But with this program, you can enjoy food, lose excess weight, and gain better health. I've had a great deal of success with this program in helping people reverse the effects of diabetes, relieve various digestive disorders, clear up nagging skin problems, overcome chronic fatigue, stop recurrent candida infections, stabilize blood sugar, and bring relief from numerous other conditions.

The Healthy Lifestyle Plan is just as much a health-restoring program as it is a weight-loss program. So be prepared to notice some remarkable changes in your life.

If you are troubled by any of the following conditions, this program may help you:

allergies	high blood pressure
arthritis	hypoglycemia
asthma	hypothyroidism
candida	kidney disease
constipation	migraine headaches
diabetes	menstrual irregularity
digestive problems	nervousness/irritability
fatigue/lack of energy	osteoporosis
frequent infections	overweight/obesity
gout	reproductive problems
gum disease	skin disorders/dermatitis
heart/circulatory problems	

THE ROAD TO SUCCESSFUL WEIGHT LOSS

What causes overweight? The most simplistic answer is that we eat too much—we consume more calories than we burn. This is the most obvious answer and the basis for all low-fat and low-calorie diets. It, however, is not the only way in which we add on excess pounds. Any diet that focuses only on calorie restriction is painfully torturous and ineffective.

There are several mechanisms that contribute to overweight. We have some degree of control over most of them. If you manipulate those mechanisms that you have control over, it can offset a great deal those that you do not. The factors that contribute to overweight which you have some level of control include:

Calorie consumption
Behavior and attitude
Metabolism
Malnutrition/food cravings
Satiety and hunger
Hydration (water consumption)
Physical activity

By controlling the above factors, you can lose excess weight and keep it off permanently. Each of these topics is discussed in detail in Chapters 7 through 11. Chapters 2 through 5 dispel many of the common myths and misconceptions about fats. Chapter 6 explains the critical role carbohydrates play in weight management.

One of the main reasons people gain unwanted weight is because they eat the wrong types of food. Consumption of unhealthy foods encourages weight problems. This is one reason why being overweight is a risk factor for many health problems. In Chapter 13 my Healthy Lifestyle Plan and dietary recommendations are outlined. Chapters 14 and 15 describe representative diets that are successful with this program. Chapter 16 contains sample recipes to get you started. In order to completely understand The Healthy Lifestyle Plan, I recommend you read each chapter in order, as the information in one chapter often contributes to the understanding of the next.

The most unique element of the weight loss system presented in this book is the use of coconut and, in particular, coconut oil. In this book you will learn about this remarkable food and how to use it to overcome weight and health problems. All statements in this book regarding the health aspects of coconut oil are fully documented in the medical literature. For those readers who want to read the medical research themselves, references are provided at the end of this book.

WHY COCONUT?

At this point you may be wondering why does this program include the use of coconut? The reason is because coconut is one of the world's healthiest foods. For thousands of years people in Asia, Africa, Central America, and the Pacific Islands have relied on coconut as a major source of food. This is particularly true in the Pacific Islands where other foods can be scarce. On some islands, the only foods available are coconuts, taro root, and fish. Since the time the early explorers first landed on these islands, they noted that the Islanders were of exquisite physical stature and possessed superb health—far better than their own. Only after colonization by Europeans and the adoption of modern foods did conditions like obesity, cancer, heart disease, diabetes, arthritis, and others appear.

The primary nutrient in coconut that makes it different from any other food, and makes it such a marvelous health food, is the oil. This oil contains the secret to losing excess weight as well as gaining better health. Coconut oil has been described as the "World's Healthiest Dietary Oil." There is a mountain of historical evidence and medical research to verify this fact. I've documented this evidence in an easy-to-understand book titled *The Healing Miracles of Coconut Oil*. This book summarizes historical, epidemiological, and medical research on the nutritional and medicinal aspects of coconut oil. It also clearly refutes the negative publicity ill-informed writers have perpetuated.

Modern dietary studies on isolated island populations who maintaine their traditional coconut-based diets have a complete absence of degenerative disease. Some island populations consume massive amounts of coconut and coconut oil and are the picture of health.[2] In fact, many of these cultures regard coconut oil as a medicine and refer to the coconut palm as "The Tree of Life."

Once considered to be bad for the heart because of its saturated fat content, we now know that coconut oil is comprised of a special type of fat which actually helps to *prevent* heart disease. Yes, the fat in coconut oil can help protect you from heart disease. (This fact is fully documented in *The Healing Miracles of Coconut Oil*, so I will not devote much space to it here.) If you don't believe me, go to Sri Lanka which has one of the highest rates of coconut consumption in the world. People there eat it daily and use coconut oil in all their cooking. Each person consumes the equivalent of 120 coconuts a year. How many coconuts do you eat a year? The national average in most Western countries would probably be a little more than none. How does the heart disease rate in Sri Lanka compare with those of the US? If coconut oil caused or even remotely contributed to heart disease, it would clearly be evident in the mortality rates of the people. In

Sri Lanka, only one or two deaths out of 1,000 are from heart disease. Contrast that with the US where heart disease, stroke, and hardening of the arteries account for nearly half of all deaths.

This isn't an isolated example. Go to any of the countries that rely heavily on coconut—Thailand, the Philippines, the islands of the Pacific. Wherever you find people using coconut oil for everyday cooking, you will find heart disease to be rare compared to those in the US, who eat very little coconut.

In the coconut-growing regions of India, heart disease is almost unheard of. When the people there were told that coconut oil was bad for them, they began switching to soybean and other vegetable oils. As a result, in just a few years, their rate of heart disease tripled! Likewise, obesity and diabetes are on the rise. When people remained on their traditional coconut-based diets, they were protected from many of the so-called diseases of modern civilization.

A major study was done on two remote Pacific Islands—Pukapuka and Tokelau. The entire populations of the islands took part in the study. Coconut provided the main source of food for these people. They derived up to 60 percent of their daily calories from fat, mostly from coconut oil. The American Heart Association recommends no more than 30% of calories should come from fat and no more than 10% saturated. Yet these people were consuming over 50% of their calories as saturated fat from coconuts. Despite eating all this fat, there was absolutely no evidence of heart disease, diabetes, cancer, or any other degenerative disease common in Western societies. Only when Islanders abandon their traditional coconut-based diet and take on the eating habits of Western countries do they begin to develop the diseases of modern society.

Dozens of studies have shown that natural coconut oil (non-hydrogenated) has no adverse effects on blood cholesterol. When you hear about a study that claims that coconut oil does raise blood cholesterol, it's because the researchers used hydrogenated coconut oil, and *all* hydrogenated oils, including polyunsaturated vegetable oils, raise cholesterol.

So, if you stop for a moment, think about it, and use a little common sense, you will realize how silly it is to think of coconut oil as unhealthy. People have been using coconut oil as their major dietary oil for thousands of years; if it caused heart disease, or any other disease for that matter, it would be clearly evident in those populations, but it's not. Common sense would tell us coconut oil is not harmful.

Unfortunately, because coconut oil has received a lot of bad publicity in the past, some misinformed writers and health care professionals still ignorantly criticize it as containing artery-clogging saturated fat. Such people are woefully behind the times and are parroting only what other misinformed writers have said. They need to read the new research, which now has been available for several years. If you hear anybody criticize coconut oil nowadays as being unhealthy, and some still do, realize they are still in the dark ages of nutritional knowledge. Have them read *The Healing Miracles of Coconut Oil*. It is fully documented with references to the medical literature proving beyond doubt the many health benefits of this most remarkable food.

One of the unique characteristics about coconut oil is that, unlike other fats, it is not stored to any appreciable extent in the body as fat. It is metabolized completely differently from the fats in meats and vegetables. When we eat coconut oil, rather than being stored as fat, it is converted into energy. It increases energy and perks up the metabolism, which causes the body to burn up more calories. Yes, eating coconut oil can help you lose weight because it promotes the burning of calories. It not only burns up the calories it supplies itself, but those of other foods as well. For this reason, it is appropriately called the world's only low-calorie fat! I discuss this topic more fully in a later chapter.

Research has now confirmed that coconut oil is, without question, one of the most nutritious and healthful foods. That is why I instruct all my patients to incorporate it into their diets. I've seen amazing results, not just in weight loss, but in overcoming many health problems.

Here are a few comments from some of those who have experienced incredible changes in their health simply by adding coconut to their existing diets:

"I have been using coconut oil for one month now; I use it to fry vegetables, also use a tablespoon or so when reheating brown rice. In the month of March, I have lost 12 pounds."
— Kitty

"I have lost over 20 pounds just using coconut oil. I dropped about a pound a week."
— Sally Werner

"I have more energy; I suddenly stopped drinking, have been exercising more, and have lost about 15 pounds. The only thing I've done differently is add coconut oil and grated coconut to my diet."
— Ken A.

14

"I've been taking about 1 or 2 tablespoons of virgin coconut oil per day for about 4 months now. I definitely notice a difference in my energy. It's steady through the day. No longer have the surges of ups and downs, especially that sleepy feeling after a meal. Obviously, my blood sugar must be steady."
— Marty Ohlson

"I have been on a low-carbohydrate diet for the last 20 months and I have lost 52 pounds. I have about 10 pounds to go. I came across a statement in one book advocating a sugar-free lifestyle, and it said that coconut will help one get into ketosis. I was intrigued by that statement and so I purchased some coconut cream and oil and began to use them. I lost 2 pounds in a week (having lost only 4 pounds in the last six months, I was quite impressed). I shared this information with the low-carb newsgroup that I am on, and many of those members began to use the product and also lost weight; some of them had been on plateaus for a long time... Some also noticed an increase in energy as well as burning sensations that would indicate that their metabolism was up. Personally I get a sensation that I can only compare to a caffeine rush, although I haven't been a caffeine user for many years. The discussion on this low-carb group about coconut has been incredible."
— Gail Butler

"I was diagnosed with hypothyroidism... When I read your email about taking 3 teaspoons all at once, I decided it was worth a try. That was about 2:00 pm. About 20 minutes later, I went for a one-hour walk on very hilly terrain, and I could not help noticing how much energy I had, compared to three weeks ago, which was the last time I took that walk... At approximately 7:15 (some five hours after taking the 3 teaspoons of coconut oil), I took my temperature and to my amazement, it was 98.6. This is the first time in at least 15 years that my body temperature has been normal, unless I have the flu or some other illness. I cannot recall the last time that I have felt as good as I do right now. Thank you. I have renewed hope that I will be successful in losing the excess weight that has been preventing me from doing the many things that I love."
— Rhea Lust

"My daily consumption is 4 tablespoons and I use it a thousand different ways. My breakfast this morning is 2 tablespoons in my pinto beans and rice dish. For dinner, I'll use the other 2 tablespoons on my salad.

It helps me get warm and I've lost 10 pounds since I started using it a couple months ago!"
— Linda Passarelli

"It takes 3 teaspoons all at once to raise my body temperature. I usually run 97.1 during the day. My new nut-balls recipe seems to be working too... These walnut-disappearing nut balls are delicious and they give me tons of energy. (I ate about 4 one-inch nut balls on an empty stomach as a snack.) Wondering where all this energy came from, I had a notion to take my temperature—98.6! Not only that, I have repeated the experiment several times this week and it works every time."
— Marilyn Jarzembski

"I am a diabetic and I have taken myself off the meds the doctor wants me to take because I do not feel they are good for me long term. Last night I indulged myself with the coconut milk. I drank the whole can before bed. The amount of carbos was not real high, but it was an indulgence, so I was expecting my morning blood sugar to be somewhat high. What to my surprise, my morning blood sugars were much lower than normal. I try for fasting blood sugars of 110-120, but lately they have been around 140. This morning, they were 109. I am pleasantly surprised."
— Alobar

"I have been on virgin coconut oil for the past two months (4 tablespoons daily) and feel better than I have in a long time! My energy levels are up and my weight is down. I am never hungry any more, and have incorporated a daily exercise routine, and have lost 20 pounds."
— Paula Yfraimov

"I did not experience any weight loss until I started cooking with coconut oil daily... After two weeks of this I started to lose fat on a daily basis. I lost about 20 pounds in about 3 weeks. I wasn't doing any exercise and was eating just the same."
— Janet

"I have lost a lot of weight recently (36 pounds in 5 months) and I use coconut and olive oil exclusively... I changed my diet to a low-carbo program (nothing but meat, eggs, seafood, nonstarchy vegetables, fruit, nuts, and anything derived from these items, including coconut products). I do believe that coconut oil is part of the success because there have been

16

times when I run out and will use only olive oil. During those times, I lose little or no weight."
— Ann

"There are a few things I eat that boost my metabolism and many things that drain it. Coconut oil definitely boosts it. Taking a tablespoon of coconut oil is the quickest way I know of raising my temperature a whole degree within 45 minutes. It is really amazing."
— Marilyn

"I am writing to express to you how happy I am with the use of coconut oil. I have been using it for all my cooking needs and have also been eating it by the spoonful. I also put it on my hair and use it in place of most hand and body creams. I am a 50-year-old overweight woman with chronic degenerative collagen vascular disorders. My energy level is improving. I am losing weight. My chronic pain is reducing. My skin and hair look much better and people are commenting on it. I can't thank you enough for telling the truth about coconut oil... Again thank you profusely!"
—Janice W.

These are just a few of the many testimonials I've read regarding the remarkable effects of adding coconut to the diet. The results are even more incredible when combined with a sensible eating plan, as you will learn in this book. Are you ready to lose excess weight and experience improved health and well-being? The following chapters will show you how.

Chapter 2

BIG FAT LIES_____ ∎

LOW-FAT DIETS MAKE YOU FAT

When people hear me say you need to eat more fat to lose weight and to achieve better health, they look at me like I'm a nut. "Why, fat is bad for you," they say. "It makes you fat." Then when I tell them that the fat they should eat is predominately saturated, they gasp in horror. "Saturated fat causes heart disease!" I have to explain to them that over the years advances in nutritional science have gone beyond the simple recommendations regarding saturated and unsaturated fats that we so commonly hear in the popular press. Popular diet books and the news media are usually years behind the advances made in science. Many of the things we believed in a few years ago have been proven wrong. One of these is the misconception that fat is unhealthy and should be avoided.

We now know that fat is a vital nutrient and must be present in the diet to maintain good health. That's why all major health organizations like the National Institutes of Health, The American Heart Association, and others recommend that we get 30% of our calories from fat rather than 20 or 10% as some extremists advocate.

Saturated fat, in particular, has received a lot of bad press in the past. What most people, including many health care professionals, don't understand is that there are many different types of saturated fat and they don't all act alike. There are at least a half dozen different saturated fats commonly found in our foods. Only a couple of them have the ability to raise blood cholesterol, which is considered a risk factor for heart disease. Believe it or not, most of them don't raise blood cholesterol and are *good* for you. In fact, we need saturated fat in our diet to maintain good health. That is why health organizations don't say eliminate *all* saturated fat from your diet.

Eating fat, particularly saturated fat, is thought to be one of the ten deadly sins. Much of this misconception is fueled by the low-fat marketing efforts of the food industry. If a food is low in fat it means customers can eat more, without guilt. The more we eat the more we buy. The more we buy, the bigger the profits for manufacturers. The bigger the profits, the happier the food industry is. It's about money, not health. The low-calorie food craze hasn't accomplished a thing, except to make food producers rich and us fat. Yes, fat! People weigh more now than ever before.

In the United States, 60% of the population is overweight; one in four adults is not just overweight but considered obese. A person is considered obese if weight is 20% or more than the maximum desirable weight for his or her height. According to the Centers for Disease Control and Prevention (CDC) the number of obese people in the US has exploded over the past decade from 12% of the total population to about 30% now. Even our kids are becoming fatter. As much as 25% of all teenagers are overweight. The number of overweight children has more than doubled in the past 30 years.

Over the past decade, during a time when the low-fat craze was in full swing, for those people aged 18—29, obesity has increased by 70%. For those 30—39 years of age, it has increased 50%. All other age groups have likewise experienced a dramatic increase in weight.

We eat more low-fat foods but we keep getting fatter and fatter. Low-fat diets don't work! Eating fat doesn't make you fat.

LOW-FAT LIES

If you are one of the millions of people who have tried to lose weight on a low-fat diet and failed, don't blame yourself; give credit to the diet. Low-fat diets don't work. The whole theory behind them is flawed. Low-fat dieting requires radical and unpalatable changes that make it almost impossible for most people to stay with for any length of time. For 30 years we have been cutting back on fat. The percentage of fat in the diet has dropped from about 40% to around 32%, yet we continue to gain weight. If you have tried to lose weight by removing fat from your diet, you have been a victim of a low-fat lie.

On the surface, the low-fat theory sounds logical. Of the three energy producing nutrients—fat, protein, carbohydrate—fat supplies the most calories. Gram for gram, fat contains twice as many calories as either

19

protein or carbohydrate. Therefore, if you replace protein or carbohydrate for fat in a meal, you can reduce the total number of calories while consuming basically the same volume of food. This much is true.

Unfortunately, it has led to the belief that the more fat you can eliminate, the fewer calories you eat, and the fewer calories you consume the better. Weight loss is looked at as simply a problem of calorie consumption. That's why so many people, including health care professionals, have been misled.

The truth is, it just doesn't work that way. Common sense would tell you differently. Have you ever seen a large person eat salad every day and still gain weight? Or have you seen a thin person who eats fatty meats, gravies, and desserts and doesn't gain an ounce? Obviously, there is more to it than just calories. Other factors such as metabolism, nutritional status, and satiety are affected by the types of foods we eat and, consequently, influence our body weight. Losing or gaining weight is not simply a matter of calorie consumption.

The food industry would have you believe that body weight is simply a result of consuming too many calories. They promote this philosophy very aggressively. They sponsor studies, distribute educational materials to schools and health care professionals, write and publish articles, and send out news releases all aimed at supporting their view. You can't pick up a general interest or health-oriented magazine nowadays without seeing articles on low-fat dieting. It's a popular subject on radio and television. Books on the topic abound. The answer to our overweight problem, we are led to believe, is conveniently provided by the food industry—eat less fat. They encourage us to buy leaner (more expensive) cuts of meat and low-fat, non-fat, and diet foods of every make and fashion. Their marketing strategy has worked. Grocery store shelves are jam packed with such items. It's a very profitable multi-billion dollar business.

Leaner cuts of meat cost us more. Low-fat convenience foods are more expensive than natural foods like fresh fruits and vegetables. Sweets—cookies, cakes, pies, candy, ice cream—which common sense tells us are not exactly health or diet foods, are all too enticing. If they are low in fat, common sense goes out the window and we are given a license to eat without guilt. The consequence to all this is higher profits for the food industry and larger waistlines for us.

People won't keep eating foods they don't like. Fat gives food flavor. Low-fat foods lack flavor, so in order to make them more enticing to customers, manufactures must add more sugar, MSG, and other flavor enhancers. The result is a product that may have more total calories than the full-fat version and contain numerous chemical additives; both of these can have adverse affects on health and weight. While promoted as "healthy" alternatives to full-fat foods, in reality they are just the opposite.

We have been inundated with the low-fat mantra for so long that we equate "low-fat" with "healthy." Fat is treated as if it were a poison. We buy the leanest cuts of meat and trim off every ounce of fat. Our preferences are low- and non-fat foods in everything we buy. Our dinner plates are piled with sugar and starch, but heaven forbid if there is just the tiniest morsel of fat!

After years of being fed low-fat propaganda, we are led to believe that if a low-fat diet is good, a very-low fat diet must be better, and a no-fat diet must be best of all. Many diet gurus such as Dr. Dean Ornish, Nathan Pritikin, and others have built empires off the low-fat hysteria. The low-fat myth extends through all corners of our society. Even our kids are brainwashed. In a poll conducted among schoolchildren, an incredible 81% thought that the healthiest diet possible was one that eliminated all dietary fat. Such a diet, however, would be a nutritional disaster.

As far back as the 1950s researchers learned that high-protein and especially high-fat diets promote weight loss better than high-carbohydrate diets. Researchers Alan Kekwick and Gaston Pawan found that when obese subjects were given diets that consisted of the same number of calories but differed in the amount of fat, protein, and carbohydrate, that those with the fat- or protein-rich diets lost weight while those on the carbohydrate-rich diets didn't.[1]

In a follow-up study Kekwick and Pawan compared the weight loss of obese subjects on a high-carbohydrate diet with a high-fat diet. Subjects on a high-carbohydrate, 2000-calorie diet failed to lose weight. The same subjects on a high-fat diet not only lost weight at 2000 calories but lost weight even when calorie consumption increased to 2600![2] A typical example of the subjects in this study was BJ. After eight days on the high-carbohydrate, 2000-calorie diet, BJ didn't lose an ounce, but lost 9 pounds in 3 weeks on the 2600-calorie, high-fat diet.

Over the years other researchers have had similar results. Most of these studies were generally ignored because they didn't fit the low-fat theory that has dominated nutritional science. Researchers and health care professionals are now finally recognizing that low-fat dieting doesn't work. In 1998 Dr. Walter Willet, Chairman of the Department of Nutrition at the Harvard School of Public Health, surveyed the scientific literature on dietary fat and obesity. His conclusion: "Diets high in fat do not appear to be the primary cause of the high prevalence of excess body fat in our society, and *reductions in fat will not be a solution.*"

Kevin Vigilante, M.D., co-author of *Low-Fat Lies*, says, "Low-fat diets as commonly conceived do not work, can be medically harmful, and do not represent the best diet for many people—especially if they want to lose weight and keep it off."

Dr. Vigilante confesses that physicians in general know very little about nutrition. "So like most Americans I was a low-fat fanatic for years," he says. "I preached it to my overweight patients, and I tried to practice it myself. But I had a hard time sticking to the program. Either I hated the food or I was hungry all the time."

Nevertheless, he kept exhorting his patients to avoid fat.

He then had an experience that changed the way he looked at diets. He went on vacation to Italy. While there, he lifted his barrier to fatty foods and ate for the sheer enjoyment of it without regard to fat. "Everything I ate was awash in olive oil," he said. All foods were full of fats—cheese, cream, sauces—nothing was made with low-fat ingredients. Judging by the foods he was eating he expected an increase in his waistline, but when he returned home, "I felt my clothes were looser. Then I got on the scale. I had lost almost five pounds!"

He mentioned this unusual experience to a nutritionist friend, Dr. Mary Flynn. She wasn't surprised. "Sure, a little fat helps you lose weight."

He was shocked. "It seemed too good to be true," he said. "I just couldn't accept the notion that you could lose weight without immense suffering."

"I don't believe in low-fat diets," Dr. Flynn said. "They just don't work. Fat makes food taste good, and it makes you feel full. Without a little fat you're always going to be hungry."

The key she said was to eat the right kind of fat, in the right amounts. Dr. Vigilante was so impressed with this information he teamed up with Dr. Flynn and wrote a book exposing the low-fat myth titled *Low-Fat Lies*.[3]

When you include adequate amounts of fat in your diet, you can lose weight and keep it off because foods taste better and satisfy longer. Diets that include fat are more enjoyable and are easier to maintain and, therefore, are more effective. In addition, if you choose the right type of fat, you can lose weight faster. Moreover, once you lose weight, you can keep it off because the foods you eat are healthier and more enjoyable than the sugar-packed, chemical-laced, low-fat alternatives.

The body needs fat. If it is not supplied in the diet, it will make its own. If you don't eat enough fat, the body, sensing fat deprivation, increases the production of fat-making enzymes. People on very-low-fat diets manufacture fat at a dramatically increased rate. So eating less fat actually can cause your body to make and store more.

Researchers at the University of Colorado found that when people go on low-fat diets, a fat-storage enzyme called lipoprotein lipase becomes more active, causing the small amount of fat you eat to be stored more easily, thus increasing fat storage in the body.[4] It's ironic that we avoid eating fat to lose weight, but end up gaining more body fat in the process.

The less fat you eat, the more fat your body tries to make and pack away into storage. No wonder low-fat dieting doesn't work! A recent study clearly demonstrated this fact. This study was conducted by researchers at Brigham and Women's Hospital and Harvard Medical School. They showed that subjects on a moderate-fat diet lost weight more effectively than those on a low-fat diet, even though they consumed the same number of calories. Those on the low-fat diet consumed no more than 20% of their daily calories as fat. The moderate-fat diet included 35% of daily calories as fat. Keep in mind that the current recommendations for fat consumption by The American Heart Association and others are no more than 30% of calories and many recommend no more than 20%, so the 35% fat used in this study could even be considered a high-fat diet in comparison. Those subjects on the moderate-fat diet lost an average of nine pounds, while the low-fat participants *gained* an average of 6.3 pounds![5] Both groups ate the same number of calories, yet the high-fat group lost weight while the low-fat group gained. It appears that if you want to *pack on extra weight,* you should *reduce* the amount of fat you eat!

You can lose weight on a low-fat diet, but it's a struggle. You feel deprived and miserable the whole time. However, by adding fat into the diet, you will enjoy the food more, feel satisfied, and lose weight! People tell me all the time that when they added fat into their diet they lost weight even though they weren't dieting or hadn't changed their eating patterns. The addition of the fat was all that was needed to bring about a loss in weight.

FAT IS GOOD FOR YOU
Building Blocks

If you removed all the fat from your body you would have a lean, beautiful body, right?... Wrong! You would be reduced to a shapeless mass of protein and water lying in a puddle on the floor. You would resemble the Wicked Witch of the East after Dorothy doused her with a bucket of water.

Fat comprises a major structural component of every cell in your body. Fats make up the cell membrane—the skin that holds the cells together.

23

Without fats, your cells would become shapeless puddles of water mixed with miscellaneous cellular debris. The cells in your heart, lungs, kidneys, and every other organ are dependent on fat to hold them together. Your brain is composed of 60% fat and cholesterol. To put it bluntly, a healthy, intelligent brain is full of fat.

Dietary fats are used not only to make structural components of cells, but also to make hormones and prostaglandins that control and regulate bodily functions. Vitamin D, estrogen, progesterone, testosterone, DHEA, and many other hormones are constructed out of cholesterol. Even cholesterol is made from fat.

Hormones are the main regulators of metabolism, growth and development, reproduction, and many other processes. They play important roles in maintaining chemical balances within the body. Fat and cholesterol are used as building blocks for many hormones. If we had no cholesterol, we would have no sex hormones and, consequently, would be sexless. That is, there would be no male or female differentiation and reproduction would be impossible.

Likewise, prostaglandins, which are hormone-like substances made from fat, influence blood lipid concentrations, blood clot formation, blood pressure, immune response, and inflammation response to injury and infection.

A diet lacking in fat can seriously reduce the efficiency of your immune system and thus make you more susceptible to disease. The immune system not only protects us from infectious illnesses but from many degenerative conditions as well. Cancer, for example, is controlled by the immune system. Every one of us has cancerous cells in our bodies— yes, you, me, everybody. It's just a part of living. We all don't develop cancer, however, because our immune systems protect us. White blood cells roaming throughout our bodies attack and destroy cancer cells, at least as long as the immune system is functioning properly. If the immune system is depressed due to a lack of dietary fat or other nutrient deficiency, cancer is allowed to develop.

Without fat and cholesterol not only would you be a shapeless mass on the floor, and totally incapable of reproduction, you would be vulnerable to cancer and all manner of disease, and worst of all, you would be dead. Life would be impossible without fat. It is essential to life.

Energy Source

Fat is fuel. Gasoline powers cars; fat powers our bodies. Fat is one of the three energy-producing nutrients. The other two are protein and carbohydrate. Our bodies use fat as a source of energy to power metabolic processes and maintain life. At least 60% of the body's energy needs are supplied by fat.

Every cell in our bodies must have a continual source of energy to function properly and maintain life. The body's first choice of fuel is carbohydrate. When there is adequate carbohydrate in the diet to meet energy needs, fat is put into storage inside fat cells. Excess carbohydrate and protein is converted into fat and also packed away into fat cells for use later. Between meals or during times of low food intake, fat is pulled out of storage and used to supply the body's ongoing energy needs.

Fat has more calories per gram than either carbohydrate or protein because it is a compact energy source that can be stored away and used later. Energy is measured in terms of calories. The body can store more calories (i.e., energy) as fat than it could as carbohydrate or protein. If the body stored protein instead of fat, you would look like a bloated pork sausage because your fat storage cells would double in size. So be thankful you store fat and not protein.

If you didn't have fat or adequate amounts of fat stored in fat cells, between meals and during prolonged periods of fasting your body would resort to using protein, such as muscle tissue, for energy. Your body would literally consume itself to get the energy it needed to stay alive.

When you diet it is important that you include fat in your meals, because if you don't your body will break down its own protein to supply its energy needs. You lose muscle mass. In extreme cases where starvation occurs, organs will be cannibalized to supply energy needs which may cause permanent damage. Organ failure is the cause of death as a consequence of starvation.

Nutritional Source

It's a mistake to think of fat as a poison. On the contrary, it is a necessary nutrient. Fat is an essential nutrient just as much as protein, vitamin C, or calcium. We need fat in our diet to maintain proper health. Without fat in our diet we would all sicken and die from nutrient deficiency.

Fats are composed of individual fat molecules called fatty acids. Two families of fat, known as omega-3 and omega-6 fatty acids, are considered absolutely necessary for good health. They are termed essential fatty acids. They are essential in that we must have them in the diet because the body cannot make them from other nutrients. These essential fatty acids are found in varying amounts in all foods, meat, fish, vegetables, as well as vegetable oils and animal fats. Avoiding fats or removing them from foods decreases these essential fatty acids.

Without these fats the body suffers from deficiency disease symptoms which include skin lesions, neurological and visual problems, growth retardation, reproductive failure, skin abnormalities, and kidney and liver disorders.

Fat is also necessary for the digestion and absorption of many other essential nutrients. For example, it is through the fatty portion of foods that we get our fat-soluble vitamins such as vitamins A, D, E, and K, as well as other important nutrients such as beta-carotene. These nutrients cannot be absorbed without adequate fat in the diet.

One of the major problems with low-fat foods and low-fat diets is that they can create a nutrient deficiency. In order for your body to assimilate the fat-soluble vitamins, you need to have fat in your foods. If you don't eat enough fat, the vitamins pass right though the digestive tract without doing you a bit of good. For this reason, low-fat diets are dangerous.

Many of the fat-soluble vitamins function as antioxidants that protect you from free-radical damage. Free-radical chemical reactions within our bodies cause the destruction of cells and their DNA. Free radicals, which are highly reactive molecules that are continually being formed inside our bodies, are implicated as the cause or at least a contributing factor in most every known degenerative disease, including heart disease, cancer, and Alzheimer's. Many researchers believe that free-radical reactions are a primary cause of aging. The more free-radical damage your body undergoes the faster you age. By reducing the amount of fat in your diet, you limit the amount of protective antioxidant nutrients available to protect you from destructive free-radical reactions. Low-fat diets speed the process of degeneration and aging. This may be one of the reasons why those people who stay on very low-fat diets for any length of time often look pale and sickly.

Carotenoids are fat-soluble nutrients found in fruits and vegetables. The best known is beta-carotene. All of the carotenoids are known for their antioxidant capability. Many studies have shown them and other fat-soluble antioxidants such as vitamins A and E to provide protection from degenerative conditions and to support immune system function.

Vegetables like broccoli and carrots have beta-carotene, but if you don't eat any oil with them you won't get the full benefit of the fat-soluble vitamins they contain. If you eat a salad with low-fat dressing you lose a good deal of the vitamins present in the vegetables. I often use a vinegar and water dressing. There is no fat in the dressing, but I always include nuts, avocado, cheese, eggs, or other fat-containing foods. The fats in these foods allow me to get the full benefit of the fat-soluble vitamins contained in the salad vegetables.

Another important nutrient that needs fat for proper absorption is calcium. How many people are deficient in calcium?... Lots. How many suffer with osteoporosis?... Lots. How many of these people eat low-fat foods?... Lots. You can drink loads of non-fat milk and low-fat cheese and shovel down calcium supplements but still develop osteoporosis. Why? Because calcium needs fat to be absorbed. If you drink non-fat milk for the calcium, you are wasting your money. You need whole milk and full-fat cheese and other full fat foods in order to absorb the calcium. Likewise, many vegetables are good sources of calcium. But in order to take advantage of that calcium, you need to eat them with butter and cream or other foods that contain fat.

Even your heart needs fat. This was shown in a study conducted by nutritionist Mary Flynn, Ph.D. Twenty subjects were given a diet with 37% of the calories from fat, and she measured their cholesterol and triglyceride levels. She then gave the same group a diet with less fat—25% of calories, but kept the total number of calories exactly the same by increasing carbohydrates. She found that the low-fat diet lowered levels of good HDL cholesterol (considered bad for the heart and circulatory system), raised triglyceride levels (also considered bad), and basically left the levels of bad LDL cholesterol unchanged (neither good or bad).[6] The overall effect was bad for the heart. You combine this with the fact that fat-soluble vitamins, such as vitamin E and beta-carotene which help to protect against heart disease, are reduced in a low-fat diet, and you see that low-fat diets may actually promote heart disease—just the opposite from what we are led to believe.

This is why many people who go on very low-fat diets become sick or develop intense food cravings. They need fat.

Nathan Pritikin advocated a very low-fat diet. Pritikin was a fanatic about keeping fat out of the diet. He claimed there was enough fat in lettuce and other vegetables to meet our body's needs. His diet limited fat consumption to a mere 10% of total calories. This is much less than The American Heart Association's recommendation of 30%. People lost weight, but they also developed health problems as a result of *too little* fat in their diet. Charles T. McGee, M.D. in his book *Heart Frauds* describes patients who tried the Pritikin low-fat diet. "Pritikin Program patients become deficient in essential fatty acids after they have been on the diet about two years. These people entered the office looking gaunt, with skin that was dry, droopy, pale, gray, and flaky. Fortunately this complication was seldom seen because most people find it difficult to keep fat intake down to the 10% level without cheating."

Protection from Infectious Disease

What do surgeons do just before performing an operation? Before touching a single thing in the operating room they first thoroughly wash their hands. Why? To kill germs. We wash our hands several times a day for the same reason. If we get a cut, one of the first things we are advised to do is wash the injury with soap and water.

Why is soap used? The reason is that it kills germs. Soap is a very effective germ fighter. Soap, in one form or another, can be gentle enough to use on a baby's skin yet tough enough to scrub the bathroom floor.

What is it that gives soap its remarkable germ-killing power? The answer may surprise you. It's fat. Yes, ordinary fat. Soap is made from fat. In the old days people used beef and pig fat. But it can be made from any type of fat or oil. Fatty acids, the individual fat molecules, are deadly to germs.

There are dozens of different types of fatty acids. Some fatty acids are more effective at killing certain types of germs than others. Some kill bacteria like E. coli, others kill streptococcus and staphylococcus, and still others yeasts and viruses. Natural fats contain a mixture of several different types of fatty acids so they are effective against a wide variety of germs.

When eaten, our bodies break fat down into individual fatty acids during the digestive process. These free fatty acids go to work immediately killing germs in the digestive tract. All animals and humans benefit from the germ-fighting character of fatty acids.[7] For example, it is primarily the fatty acids in human breast milk that protects newborns from infectious disease while their immune systems are still underdeveloped and incapable of fighting off serious infections. It's the fatty acids in natural body oils (sebum) that help protect us from infections and establishes a protective environment on the surface of our skin.

Germs are everywhere. No matter how hard you clean your dishes or wash your food, germs are always present. Acids in our stomach kill most germs, but some manage to slip by to cause illness. The fats in our foods act as a secondary means of protection. In the digestive tract they destroy disease-causing organisms on contact. Unlike antibiotics which kill all types of bacteria, fatty acids are selective. They are harmless to "friendly" bacteria that live in the digestive tract.

So when you eat a meal containing fat, you are eating food that will protect you from many forms of food poisoning and infectious disease. If, on the other hand, you avoid fat and eat low-fat foods you are making it easier for germs to survive in your digestive tract and cause trouble. A healthy diet always includes ample amounts of fat.

Avoiding infectious illnesses is yet, another reason to add fat into your diet and avoid low-fat foods.

Other Benefits

Fat has many important functions in the body. I have not mentioned all of them, just enough to show you how important they are in the diet. Researchers are discovering more benefits of dietary fat all the time. For example, in a study done at the University of Buffalo in 1999, female soccer players were able to perform longer at a higher intensity on a diet composed of 35% fat than on diets of 27% or 24% fat. This study showed that higher-fat diets boost athletic performance.

Fat also helps regulate digestion and absorption of blood sugar, thus helping to prevent insulin resistance and diabetes. Without adequate amounts of fat in the diet, blood sugar levels can go out of control after eating a carbohydrate-rich meal.

Fat helps satisfy hunger longer so you don't eat as often, thus helping you to eat fewer calories. So eating fat helps you *lose* weight.

As you see, fat is a very important component of our food. It is involved in a variety of functions throughout the body, many of which science has yet to fully understand.

Dietary fats, however, are not all alike. There are many different types of fats and each has a different effect on the body. Modern processing and food manufacturing have created some fats that are detrimental to your health and contribute to weight problems. So you must choose your fats wisely. In general, the more processing a fat or oil has undergone to reach the grocery store shelf, the unhealthier it is. Fake fats like olestra and semi-fake fats like margarine and other hydrogenated vegetable oils are the most processed and the least healthy. Natural fats and oils—those that are easily extracted from their source with even primitive methods—such as olive oil, coconut oil, butter, and animal fats are the most beneficial. Vegetable oils that have undergone extensive extraction and chemical processing proce-dures are in-between.

I know this goes against popular opinion, but just because most people believe in something that is false, doesn't make it true. Popular opinions are often wrong. Look at low-fat diets, they are still loudly proclaimed as the *only* way to lose weight, yet we know for a fact that they don't work.

Chapter 3

ARE YOU IN NEED OF AN OIL CHANGE? ____ ∎

A LITTLE ABOUT FATS AND OILS

Fat—the word conjures up images of grotesque, greasy tissue hanging off of a slab of meat. Meat isn't the only place we find fat. All living organisms have it. Animals have it, people have it, plants have it, even the tiniest organisms like protozoa and bacteria have it. Fat is an essential tissue to life. For this reason, fat in one form or another is found in all of our foods. And although most people like to eliminate it as much as possible, it constitutes an important part of our diet.

The terms fat and oil are often used interchangeably. Generally speaking, fats are considered solid at room temperature while oils remain liquid. You will often hear the term "lipid" in reference to fats and oils. Lipid is a general term that includes several fat-like compounds in the body. By far the most abundant and the most important of the lipids are the triglycerides. When we speak of fats and oils we are usually referring to triglycerides. Two other lipids—phospholipids and sterols (which includes cholesterol)—technically are not fats because they are not triglycerides. But they have similar characteristics and are often loosely referred to as fats.

When you cut into a beefsteak, the white fatty tissue you see is composed of triglycerides. Cholesterol is also present but it is intermingled within the meat fibers and undetectable with the naked eye. The fat that is a nuisance to us, the type that hangs on our arms, looks like jelly on our thighs, and makes our stomachs look like spare tires, is composed of triglycerides. The triglycerides make up our body fat and the fat we see and eat in animal foods. About 95% of the lipids in our diet from both plant and animal sources are triglycerides.

30

Triglycerides are comprised of individual fat molecules called *fatty acids*. The three general categories of fatty acids are saturated, monounsaturated, and polyunsaturated. All oils and animal fats consist of a mixture of these three fatty acids. To say an oil is saturated or monounsaturated is grossly oversimplifying. No oil is purely saturated or polyunsaturated. Olive oil, for example, is often called "monounsaturated" because it is *predominantly* monounsaturated, but like all vegetable oils, it also contains some polyunsaturated and saturated fat as well. Lard, as well, contains saturated, monounsaturated, and polyunsaturated fatty acids. In fact, lard has a higher percentage of monounsaturated fat (47%) than saturated fat (41%). It is more accurate to refer to lard as a monounsaturated fat than as a saturated one.

Animal fats come from the flesh of animals and from milk. The vast majority of our vegetable oils come from seeds such as cottonseed, sunflower seeds, safflower seeds, and rapeseed (canola), but even grains (e.g., corn), legumes (e.g., soybeans and peanuts), and nuts (e.g., almonds, walnuts, coconuts) are seeds. Some oils come from fruits (e.g., olive and avocado).

Fats and oils found naturally in foods support good health and provide many essential nutrients. Not all fats, however, are of equal value in terms of weight management or health benefits. A healthy weight-loss diet must includes an adequate amount of fat, and it must be the right kind of fat.

If you were asked which oils are the healthiest and which ones aren't, what would be your answer? If you responded to that question like most people, you would have said that polyunsaturated vegetable oils are the best and saturated fats are the worst. If this was your answer then you have been deceived, just as I was at one time and just as most people are. Contrary to what the vegetable oil industry has had us believe, polyunsaturated oils carry far more health risks than do monounsaturated fats, saturated fats, or cholesterol. If you are currently eating mostly polyunsaturated vegetable oils in your diet, you are in need of an oil change. In this chapter you will find out why.

THE VEGETABLE OIL SAGA
Traditional Oils

Over the past century we have been in the mist of a revolution—a dietary revolution. Foods our ancestors have eaten, even thrived on for generations, have been pushed aside to make way for new, technologically-advanced foods. One of the biggest changes that has taken place during this time is the type of oils we consume. Butter, lard, coconut oil, and other

31

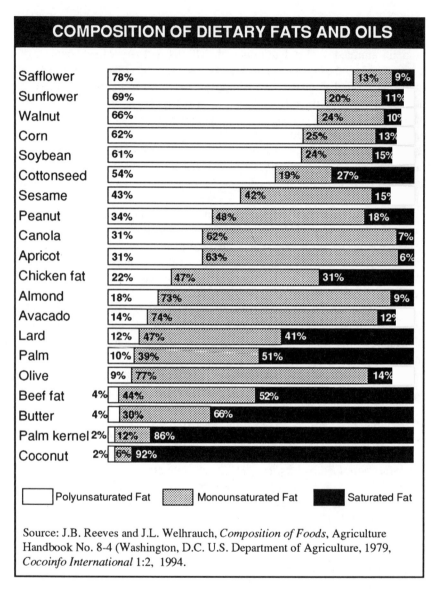

COMPOSITION OF DIETARY FATS AND OILS

	Polyunsaturated Fat	Monounsaturated Fat	Saturated Fat
Safflower	78%	13%	9%
Sunflower	69%	20%	11%
Walnut	66%	24%	10%
Corn	62%	25%	13%
Soybean	61%	24%	15%
Cottonseed	54%	19%	27%
Sesame	43%	42%	15%
Peanut	34%	48%	18%
Canola	31%	62%	7%
Apricot	31%	63%	6%
Chicken fat	22%	47%	31%
Almond	18%	73%	9%
Avacado	14%	74%	12%
Lard	12%	47%	41%
Palm	10%	39%	51%
Olive	9%	77%	14%
Beef fat	4%	44%	52%
Butter	4%	30%	66%
Palm kernel	2%	12%	86%
Coconut	2%	6%	92%

Source: J.B. Reeves and J.L. Welhrauch, *Composition of Foods*, Agriculture Handbook No. 8-4 (Washington, D.C. U.S. Department of Agriculture, 1979, *Cocoinfo International* 1:2, 1994.

Fats and oils contain a mixture of saturated, monounsaturated, and polyunsaturated fatty acids. Vegetable oils contain the highest percentage of polyunsaturated oils.

traditional fats have been usurped by highly refined, purified, and even chemically altered vegetable oils.

If you traveled to the mountains of northern Pakistan to visit the Hunza, you would find a people who relish butter and goat fat. If you went to rural China you would find lard to be the dietary fat of choice. In Thailand coconut oil is used in all cooking. In India ghee (butter) and coconut oil are traditionally the preferred choices. In Italy and Greece olive oil reigns supreme. Wherever traditional fats and oils are used you will find them eating primarily saturated and monounsaturated oils of one type or another. What you won't find much of is polyunsaturated vegetable oils.

Oils have constituted an important part of the diet for generations. Those that were most popular were relatively easy to obtain using primitive methods of extraction. Animal fat was simply cut off the meat and rendered into oil by cooking. Butter was made from churning milk. Olive oil was squeezed out of the fruit by screw-type presses or pounded out using a wooden funnel and hammer. Vegetable oils from nuts and seeds were produced by the crushing action of wooden presses or stone rollers.

By far the most common oils used throughout history were animal fats, butter, coconut and palm oils, and olive oil. Some populations used vegetable oils more than others, but because of the difficulty of extraction, vegetable seed oils were not widely used and never contributed significantly to the human diet.[1]

An Industrial Oil Becomes a Food

One of the drawbacks with using polyunsaturated vegetable oils for food is that they oxidize (go rancid) very quickly. Therefore, they could not be stored for more than a few days. Crude extraction methods leave a high percentage of impurities in the oil which produces an awful smell and flavor when the oil begins to spoil.

The fact that polyunsaturated oils oxidize quickly proved to be advantageous for industrial use. When oils oxidize they harden. A thin layer of oil could harden into a tough impervious shell. The first paints and varnishes were made out of vegetable oils. A number of industrial products were created from these oils—paint thinner, lacquer, linoleum, ink, etc. With the invention of the modern hydraulic press and the development of chemical extraction methods vegetable oil production rapidly increased during the first half of the 20th century. Before the Second World War soybean and other polyunsaturated oils were used almost exclusively for industrial purposes. When chemists learned how to make cheaper oil-based paint from petroleum, the seed oil industry found itself facing a dwindling market.

At this same time, farmers were experimenting with different ways to make their animals fatter on less expensive feed. Dietary fats and oils seemed to show promise. Fat contains twice as many calories as carbohydrate or protein, and a high-fat diet encourages weight gain. By increasing the fat content of the animals' feed they would gain more weight and bring bigger profits with lesser expense. The seed oil industries began marketing their products as an additive to animal feed.

Farmers discovered that corn and soybean oil not only added more calories but also had an antithyroid effect that caused the animals to be fattened at a much lower cost. The only problem was that the animals also developed tumors and other degenerative health problems. Since diseased cattle have severe economic consequences, the cattle industry stopped using vegetable oils.

The vegetable oil producers, confronted with dwindling sales and the rejection from the farming industry, began a new marketing strategy. They started to focus more heavily on selling their products for human consumption. At this time saturated fats were being criticized as possibly contributing to heart disease because they increased blood cholesterol. Polyunsaturated oils didn't raise blood cholesterol levels. The vegetable oil industry jumped on this and began promoting their products as heart healthy and as a healthy alternative to animal fats. The vegetable oil industry spearheaded an aggressive campaign to discredit saturated fats and promote polyunsaturated vegetable oils. They funded studies, sponsored educational seminars for health professionals, and flooded the media with news promoting the use of vegetable oils. As a result, vegetable oil use increased and animal fat consumption declined.

A problem we now face is that vegetable oils are doing the same thing to us as they did to the farm animals—making us fat and sick! Thousands of years of eating saturated fats have had no harmful effects, but as soon as we replaced them with polyunsaturated vegetable oils waistlines began expanding and cancer, diabetes, and other degenerative conditions have shot through the roof. Look at the ingredient labels in the foods you buy. Consider the amount of cooking oil, shortening, and margarine you use. Vegetable oils are in almost all our foods nowadays. We consume them for breakfast, lunch, and dinner, every day, day in and day out. If the farm animals became fat and developed hideous degenerative diseases eating this stuff, what do you expect it to do to you?

Refined and Unrefined Vegetable Oils

Fats and oils have nourished mankind for generations. But the types of oils we consume now are much different than those that nourished our great-grandparents. We have moved away from using unrefined oils to highly refined and purified polyunsaturated oils.

In the refining process, the oil is separated from its source with heat and hydraulic pressure. After the first pressing, the remaining pulp is treated further with additional heat, pressure, and petroleum solvents. The oil is then boiled to evaporate the toxic solvents. The oil is refined, bleached, and deodorized involving heating to temperatures of about 400° F (200° C). Chemical preservatives are frequently added to retard oxidation. Modern processing removes all of the non-oil components of the seed, making the oil essentially colorless, tasteless, odorless, and completely lacking in nutrients. What you are left with is a highly refined and purified fat. These oils provide lots of calories but little nutrition. Almost all of the vegetable oils sold in stores today are of this type.

Traditional methods of extraction produces a very impure oil—an oil with a rich flavor and aroma and filled with vitamins, minerals, and other nutrients. Many oils are still produced using methods similar to those that have existed for centuries. Modern methods of cold extraction use heavy stone or steel rollers to crush seeds and nuts. Vegetable oils extracted by mechanical pressure and without the use of chemicals are referred to as "expeller pressed" or "cold pressed." These oils generally contain no colorings, preservatives, or chemical additives.

The term "cold pressed" is somewhat deceptive because heat is involved in the processing. During the extraction process, heat is generated but temperatures are lower—160° F (70° C) as opposed to temperatures up to 400° F (200° C). So in comparison to conventionally processed oils they are cold pressed. However, most of these so-called cold-pressed oils are then further refined by heating to drive off impurities and remove their natural flavor and aroma. So in the end they are not much better than their highly refined cousins.

There are some vegetable oils that are produced using age-old traditional methods, without chemicals or high heat. The most popular is extra virgin olive oil. It retains its full flavor, color, aroma, and all its natural vitamins and minerals. Coconut oil is often produced by traditional methods or modern true cold-processing methods without the use of chemicals. It is sometimes referred to as *virgin* coconut oil to distinguish it from more refined oils; it retains a delightful coconut flavor and aroma. You can also find sesame, almond, and other oils produced in a similar manner. The secret to identifying truly "natural" or unrefined oil is by taste and smell. The more an oil is processed and refined, the less flavor and aroma it retains. If it is clear and tastes and smells bland, you can bet all the natural nutrients have been removed leaving a dead, lifeless oil. Use oils that taste and smell like the foods from which they came. Olive oil should taste like fresh olives and almond oil should taste like almonds.

Many oils have a very disagreeable flavor and must be deodorized to make them palatable. Soybean oil, for example, is one of these. Unprocessed soybean oil has a horrible taste and must undergo harsh extraction and chemical treatments to remove its displeasing flavor and is, therefore, always highly processed and unfit to eat.

HYDROGENATED VEGETABLE OILS

The process of hydrogenation was developed by the Proctor & Gamble company in 1907. Hydrogenation was an innovative new process that could transform a liquid vegetable oil into a solid fat that resembled lard. The first use of hydrogenation was to transform cheap cottonseed oil into a solid fat that could be used in place of lard and tallow in the making of soap and candles.

The success of their cheap imitation lard boosted company profits. It wasn't long before they reasoned that since hydrogenated cottonseed oil resembled lard, why not sell it as a food. So in 1911 they introduced Crisco shortening. The name Crisco was derived from the words *CRYSt*alized *C*ottonseed *O*il. In order to encourage women to switch from using butter and lard to shortening they distributed a cookbook and began publishing ads portraying Crisco as a more economical and healthier alternative to animal fats. The transformation away from animal fats and toward vegetable oils had begun. Before long margarine, an imitation butter, was made available. Margarine was simply hydrogenated cottonseed oil mixed with flavoring and dye so as to resemble butter. Sales were modest at first but picked up during the Great Depression of the 1930s when people switched from using lard and butter to the cheaper shortening and margarine. Sales again made an upswing in the 1950s and 1960s as people suddenly became aware of the presumed dangers of animal fats. By 1957 more people were buying margarine than butter.

It is interesting to note that Proctor & Gamble and other vegetable oil companies sponsored much of the research which supposedly linked saturated fat and cholesterol with heart disease. In fact, Dr. Fred Mattson, one of scientists who worked for P&G, was instrumental in persuading The American Heart Association to accept the cholesterol theory of heart disease and was active in influencing governmental policy concerning dietary fats.

The process of hydrogenation begins with a refined vegetable oil. Nowadays most hydrogenated oils are made from soybean oil. The oil is mixed with tiny metal particles—usually nickel oxide, which is very toxic

36

and impossible to completely remove—to act as a chemical catalyst. Under high pressures and temperatures hydrogen gas is squeezed into the oil and chemically bonded to the fat molecules. Emulsifiers and starch are then forced into the mixture to give it a better consistency. The mixture is again subjected to high temperatures in a steam-cleaning process to remove its horrible odor. The hydrogenation process is now complete, but the resulting oil is a disgusting gray color, more like what you would expect to see in a jar of axle grease, so it is bleached to give it a more appetizing white appearance. The final result is hydrogenated vegetable oil or, as we see it on the store shelves, shortening. To make margarine, coal-tar dyes and chemical flavorings are added. This mixture is compressed and packaged in blocks or tubs, ready to be enjoyed on a slice of bread. Just knowing how margarine and shortening are made is enough to keep me from eating them.

In the process of hydrogenation, liquid vegetable oils become solid fats. Another thing happens that has significant health implications. A new fatty acid, unlike those normally found in nature, is created. This is called the *trans* fatty acid. This toxic fatty acid is foreign to our bodies and can create all sorts of trouble.

"These are probably the most toxic fats ever known," says Walter Willett, M.D., professor of epidemiology and nutrition at Harvard School of Public Health. Willett, who has researched the effects of trans fats on the body, disagrees with those who say that the hydrogenated fats found in margarine or shortening are less likely to raise cholesterol than the saturated fats found in butter: "It looks like trans fatty acids are two to three times as bad as saturated fats in terms of what they do to blood lipids."[2]

Studies now clearly show that trans fatty acids can contribute to atherosclerosis (hardening of the arteries) and heart disease. For example, swine fed a diet containing trans fatty acids developed more extensive atherosclerotic damage than those fed other types of fats.[3] In humans trans fatty acids increase blood LDL (bad cholesterol) and lower the HDL (good cholesterol), both regarded to be undesirable changes.[4] Trans fatty acids have been shown to raise blood cholesterol levels even more than saturated fat.[5] Since it also lowers the good HDL cholesterol, unlike saturated fat, researchers now believe it has a greater influence on the risk of cardiovascular disease than any other dietary fat.[6]

The *New England Journal of Medicine* reported the results of a 14-year study of more than 80,000 nurses (*New England Journal of Medicine* November 20, 1997). The research documented 939 heart attacks among the participants. Among the women who consumed the largest amounts of trans fats, the chance of suffering a heart attack was 53% higher than among those at the low end of trans fat consumption.

Another interesting fact uncovered by this study was that total fat intake had little effect on the rate of heart attack. Women in the group with the largest consumption of total fat (46% of calories) had no greater risk of heart attack than those in the group with the lowest consumption of total fat (29% of calories).

The researchers, from the Harvard School of Public Health and Brigham and Women's Hospital in Boston who conducted the study, said this suggested that limiting consumption of trans fats would be more effective in avoiding heart attacks than reducing overall fat intake. About 10% of the fat in the typical Western diet is trans fat.

Trans fatty acids affect more than just our cardiovascular health. According to a study reported by Mary Enig, Ph.D., when monkeys were fed trans fat-containing margarine in their diets, their red blood cells did not bind insulin as well as when they were not fed trans.[7] This suggests a link with diabetes. Trans fatty acids have been linked with a variety of adverse health effects which include: cancer, ischemic heart disease, multiple sclerosis, diverticulitis, diabetes, and other degenerative conditions.[8]

Hydrogenated oil is a product of technology and may be the most destructive food additive currently in common use. If you eat margarine, shortening, hydrogenated or partially hydrogenated oils (common food additives), then you are consuming trans fatty acids.

Many of the foods you buy in the store and in restaurants are prepared with or cooked in hydrogenated oil. Fried foods sold in grocery stores and restaurants are usually cooked in hydrogenated oil because it makes foods crispy and is more resistant to spoilage than ordinary vegetable oils. Many frozen, processed foods are cooked or prepared in hydrogenated oils. Hydrogenated oils are used in making french fries, biscuits, cookies, crackers, chips, frozen pies, pizzas, peanut butter, cake frosting, and ice cream substitutes such as mellorine.

The liquid vegetable oils you buy in the store aren't much better. The heat used in the extraction and refining process also creates trans fatty acids. So that bottle of corn or safflower oil you have on the kitchen shelf contains trans fatty acids even though it has not been hydrogenated. Unless the vegetable oil has been "cold pressed" or "expeller pressed," it contains trans fatty acids. Most all of the common brands of vegetable oil and salad dressings contain trans fatty acids.

Liquid vegetable oils contain an average of 15% trans fatty acids. In comparison, margarine and shortening average about 35%, but some brands may run as high as 48%.

When monounsaturated and polyunsaturated oils are used in cooking, especially at high temperatures, trans fatty acids are formed. So even if you use cold pressed oil from the health food store, if you use it in your cooking, you are creating unhealthy trans fatty acids.

You might ask: does the amount of trans fatty acids that are produced when you heat oils at home pose any real danger? Studies show diets containing heat-treated liquid corn oil were found to produce more atherosclerosis than those containing unheated corn oil.[9] So, *yes any unsaturated vegetable oil becomes toxic when heated.* And even a small amount, especially if eaten frequently over time, will affect your health.

Saturated fats, from any source, are much more resistant to temperatures used in cooking, do not form trans fatty acids, and therefore, make much better cooking oils. Saturated fats are the safest to use in cooking. In an effort to create a cheap source of oil from polyunsaturated vegetable sources modern technology has created a major health problem.

After a detailed review of all the research done with trans fatty acids, the Institute of Medicine recently declared that no level of trans fat is safe to consume. Under pressure from many health organizations and the public, the Food and Drug Administration (FDA) proposed a regulation that would require food manufactures to include the amount of trans fatty acids on the package labels. Before taking such a step, however, they waited three years for the Institute of Medicine to study the issue.

What surprised everyone was that the Institute of Medicine didn't give a recommendation as to what percentage of trans fats were safe to consume, as is often done with food additives, but flatly stated that no level of trans fats is safe. If you see a packaged food that contains hydrogenated oil, margarine, or shortening, don't touch it. If you eat out, ask the restaurant manager what type of oil they use to cook their food. If they say "vegetable oil," it almost definitely is hydrogenated vegetable oil: avoid it. The reason you can safely count on it being hydrogenated vegetable oil is because regular vegetable oil breaks down too quickly and becomes rancid. Restaurants like to reuse their oils as long as possible before they have to be tossed out. Ordinary vegetable oils have too short a life span.

FAKE FATS

Turning on the evening news, Jean, a 49-year-old, sat down to enjoy a bag of potato chips before going to bed. These chips weren't the ordinary type she'd eaten before, but a new brand made with the fat substitute olestra. At the time, this product was recently introduced on the market and heavily promoted as a "healthy" alternative to those made with ordinary fat. It was touted as a way to help reduce fat calories and cut risk of heart disease.

"Normally I can eat anything without becoming sick," she says. An hour after going to bed she suffered gas pains "so sharp and of such a magnitude that I would say it was almost like the beginning of labor." As the pains began to subside she was hit with repeated waves of diarrhea. The rest of the night was spent in torment. Jean is just one of thousands who have had messy run-ins with olestra.

Olestra (also known by the trade name Olean) is a fat substitute made from sugar and soybean oil. It is designed to have the taste and texture of fat, but because its molecules are too large for the body to digest, it generally passes through the digestive tract unabsorbed. The advantage to a fat that passes through the body without being digested is obvious—no calories! The makers of olestra have promoted products made with this new fat as safe and healthy, cheerfully trumpeting that you can "eat like a kid again," snacking on junk foods without guilt. Olestra was created for use in snack foods and Frito-Lay has developed an entire line of WOW! potato and corn chips made with the artificial fat.

Regular chips deliver 150 calories and 10 grams of fat per serving, while the WOW! chips deliver only 75 calories and 0 grams of fat. It sounds like a junk food junkie's dream, but watch out. This fake fat can have serious health consequences. Because it is not digested well, it can have a laxative effect, especially if eaten in large quantities. This is what Jean discovered after her late evening snack. Olean's manufacturer, Procter & Gamble, received more than 13,000 reports of adverse reactions from customers when Frito-Lay started test-marketing olestra-containing chips in select cities. Complaints ranged from mild stomach upset to cramps so severe that in scores of cases the victims needed to be hospitalized. While most people may not experience any immediate problems, especially if they only eat the chips occasionally, repeated use may cause some serious problems down the line.

An even bigger danger than abdominal cramping and loose stools is the fact that olestra inhibits the absorption of important fat-soluble vitamins (A, D, E, and K). Each of these vitamins are essential to health. Since olestra is pushed through the digestive tract without being absorbed, it pulls these vitamins out along with it. So even if you eat vegetables containing these vitamins with an olestra-containing food, these vitamins will do you no good. Also, eating foods containing olestra means that other foods containing vitamins are eaten less. All of this combined can lead to serious vitamin deficiencies. Because of these potential health problems, the FDA has required all products made with this artificial fat to carry warning labels which read: "This Product Contains Olestra. Olestra may cause abdominal cramping and loose stools. Olestra inhibits the absorption of some vitamins and other nutrients."

To compensate for the loss of these nutrients, products containing olestra are required to add four fat-soluble vitamins. However, manufacturers are not required to add beta-carotene or other carotenoids—another group of fat-soluble nutrients. The carotenoids are potent antioxidants which have been shown to offer significant protection against cancer, heart disease, and macular degeneration—the leading cause of blindness in the elderly.

You may some day see potato chips being sold that say "Vitamin Enriched." Sounds a lot like white bread doesn't it? It's the same old marketing tactic, add a few vitamins to a nutritionally poor food and call it "enriched" or "fortified" to make it appear healthy.

While olestra is portrayed as a natural product, because it is made from sugar and soybean oil, it is as synthetic as rubber and even more unnatural than the trans fatty acids found in hydrogenated oils. Olestra is completely unlike any substance found in nature and our bodies have no way of handling it. Because of this, the National Advertising Division of the Council of Better Business Bureaus ruled the Procter & Gamble's ads were inaccurate when they portrayed olestra as a natural product that looks like vegetable oil.

Olestra is only the first of many artificial fats that are now beginning to come onto the market and are finding their way into a variety of foods. Foods you're eating now may be made with one of these synthetic substitutes. Salatrim (also called Benefat) is Nabisco's answer to olestra. Salatrim is used in "Fat-Free" cookies, chocolate chips, and other foods. Like olestra, products containing salatrim can also cause nausea and cramps. But, unlike olestra, products with salatrim are not required to carry warning labels, so you have to carefully read the ingredients label.

Other fake fats to hit the grocery shelves include Oatrim, Z-Trim, and Nu-Trim. These fat substitutes are finding their way into cookies, cakes, brownies, ice cream, pie, and all sorts of baked goods and desserts. Because these products are low in absorbable fat and low in calories, products made with them are touted as "Low-Fat," "Non-Fat," or "Heart-Healthy." Watch out for any product with these labels! Since artificial fats are relatively new, their complete effect on health is still under question.

Food is supposed to nourish us. Products containing these fake fats are only providing empty calories that rob us of the nutrients we need to fight disease and slow down the effects of aging. It's amazing that some people will choose to eat foods simply because they are indigestible!

FREE RADICALS

Research over the past few decades has identified a key player in the cause and development of degenerative disease and aging. That player is the free radical.

Simply stated, a free radical is a renegade molecule that has lost an electron in its outer orbit, leaving an unpaired electron. This creates a highly unstable and powerful molecular entity. These radicals will quickly attack and steal an electron from a neighboring molecule. The second molecule, now with one less electron, becomes a highly reactive free radical itself and pulls an electron off yet another nearby molecule. This process continues in a destructive chain reaction that may affect hundreds and even thousands of molecules.

Once a molecule becomes a radical, its physical and chemical properties change. The normal function of such molecules is permanently disrupted, affecting the entire cell of which they are a part. A living cell attacked by free radicals degenerates and becomes dysfunctional. Free radicals can attack our cells literally ripping their protective membranes apart. Sensitive cellular components like the nucleus and DNA, which carry the genetic blueprint of the cell, can be damaged, leading to cellular mutations or death.

The more free radicals that attack our cells, the greater the damage and the greater the potential for serious destruction. If the cells that are damaged are in our heart or arteries, what happens? If they are in the brain, what happens? If they are in our joints, pancreas, intestines, liver, or kidneys, what happens? Think about it. If the cells become damaged, dysfunctional, or die, can these organs fulfill their intended purpose at optimal levels, or do they degenerate?

Free-radical damage has been linked to the loss of tissue integrity and to physical degeneration. As cells are bombarded by free radicals, the tissues become progressively impaired. Some researchers believe that free-radical destruction is the actual cause of aging.[10] The older the body gets, the more damage it sustains from a lifetime accumulation of attack from free radicals.

Today some sixty or so degenerative diseases are recognized as having free radicals involved in their cause or manifestation.[11] Additional diseases are regularly being added to this list. The research that linked the major killer diseases such as heart disease and cancer to free radicals has expanded this list to include atherosclerosis, stroke, varicose veins, hemorrhoids, hypertension, wrinkled skin, dermatitis, arthritis, digestive problems, reproductive problems, cataracts, loss of energy, diabetes, allergies, failing memory, and many other degenerative conditions.

The more exposure we receive from free radicals, the more damage occurs to our cells and tissues, which increases our chances of developing the conditions listed above. We are exposed to free radicals from the pollutants in the air we breathe and from the chemical additives and toxins in the foods we eat and drink. Some free-radical reactions occur as part of the natural process of cellular metabolism. We can't avoid all the free radicals we are exposed to in our environment, but we can limit them. Cigarette smoke, for example, causes free-radical reactions in the lungs. Certain foods and food additives also cause destructive free-radical reactions that affect our entire body. Limiting your exposure to these free-radical-causing substances will reduce your risk of developing a number of degenerative conditions. In this regard, the types of oil you use have a very pronounced effect on your health.

When unsaturated oils oxidize (go rancid) they generate free radicals. The more unsaturated an oil is, the more easily it oxidizes. Therefore, polyunsaturated oils are much more vulnerable to oxidation than monounsaturated oils, and monounsaturated oils are much more vulnerable than saturated oils.

Heat, light, and oxygen act as catalysts to promote oxidation. The longer the exposure, the greater the degree of oxidation. Polyunsaturated oils when extracted from their source and exposed to heat, light, and oxygen oxidize very rapidly. When you buy a bottle of soybean oil in the store it has already begun to oxidize and go rancid. Sitting on the store shelf exposed to light and heat (even room temperature), oxidation is occurring. Once you bring it home and open the bottle, oxidation and free-radical formation accelerate. If you use the oil in any type of cooking you greatly compound the problem by accelerating the formation of harmful free radicals. Numerous studies, in some cases published as early as the 1930s, have reported on the toxic effects of consuming heated oils.[12] For this reason, you should never use polyunsaturated oils in cooking or baking. It's ironic that some people will buy "cold pressed" vegetable oils and go home and use them in cooking. Cold pressed oils oxidize just as rapidly as refined oils.

Monounsaturated and saturated oils do not oxidize as easily as polyunsaturated oils. They are much more stable for cooking purposes. Monounsaturated oils are safe to use for low- to medium-temperature heating. Saturated fats, which are the most resistant to oxidation, can be used for all types of cooking even at high temperatures without harm.

Refined vegetable oils are deceptive. You can't tell a rogue from a saint. They all pretty much look alike. They have been purified, deodorized, and stripped of all taste and character. When the oil begins to go rancid

43

it does not affect the smell or flavor.[13] You can eat a very rancid, highly oxidized oil and not even detect any difference, especially if the oil is combined with other foods as it normally is. The only time rancid oils produce an offensive smell and flavor is when they contain impurities such a protein or phytochemicals. Free radicals attack these impurities and transform them into putrid-smelling substances. An oil that has been minimally processed and still contains some of its natural plant substances is more likely to produce an offensive smell than a highly processed and purified oil. So you can eat rancid oil without realizing it.

Unsaturated oils that retain their natural flavor and aroma may go rancid in time. If the oil begins to taste bad or bitter, throw it out. Polyunsaturated oils that have been deodorized and purified will not have any flavor or smell even when they go rancid. Don't use them. The best oils are those that have a pleasant, natural flavor.

HEALTH EFFECTS OF POLYUNSATURATED OILS

One of the effects of free radicals is cancer. When free radicals attack the DNA of a cell, they cause mutations that either kill the cell or cause it to become cancerous. Many studies have shown that polyunsaturated oils promote the growth of tumors.[14, 15] This fact is well known among researchers and is not even contested. It is interesting to note that where refined vegetable oils are routinely eaten, cancer rates are high. Where they are not normally eaten, cancer rates are usually much lower.

Consuming vegetable oils lowers our resistance to infectious disease by depressing the immune system. This fact is so well known that vegetable oil emulsions with water have been used for intravenous injection, for the purpose of suppressing immunity in patients who have had organ transplants.[16] One of the ways unsaturated fats hinder the immune system is by killing white blood cells.[17] The white blood cells, which defend us against harmful microorganisms, are the primary component of our immune system.

Unsaturated oils have been linked to numerous degenerative conditions. Some researchers feel that cancer won't even occur unless there are unsaturated oils in the diet.[18] Others claim that alcoholic cirrhosis of the liver cannot occur unless there are unsaturated oils in the diet.[19] Heart disease has also been linked to unsaturated oils. This is of particular interest because most people associate saturated fat, not vegetable oil, with heart disease. Studies have shown that heart disease can be produced by unsaturated oils and prevented by adding saturated oils to the diet.[20] Researchers are discovering that polyunsaturated oils appear to be more to blame for heart disease than saturated fat or cholesterol.

Researchers have found that the consumption of polyunsaturated oil exceeding 10% of total calories can lead to blood disease, cancer, liver damage, and vitamin deficiencies.[21] In an eight-year experiment conducted at a Los Angeles veterans' hospital, a group of patients whose diet contained four times as many polyunsaturates as a second group had 60% more cancers.

In a study done at the University of Western Ontario, ten different fats of varying degrees of saturation were used to determine which ones would produce the most cancers.[22] In general the more polyunsaturated the oil, the higher the cancer rate. Coconut oil, the highest in saturated fat in the study, appeared to have a protective effect against cancer.

In another study, the effect of the amount or degree of unsaturation of dietary fat on mortality rate for rats was demonstrated. The amount and type of fat were the only significant variables used. The types of oils included lard (saturated), olive oil (monounsaturated), corn oil (polyunsaturated), and safflower oil (very polyunsaturated), listed in order of increasing amount of unsaturation. When fat intake was low (5–10%), the degree of unsaturation did not have a significant effect on the mortality rate. However, when fat intake was moderate (20%), the mortality rates increased with the degree of unsaturation.[23] All rats in the unsaturated groups died by the 36th month. The experiment terminated at 38 months with rats still surviving in the group highest in saturated fat (lard). The oils used weren't special, but were the same kind sold in stores for human consumption.

One area in the body that free radicals have a pronounced effect on is the central nervous system—the brain and spinal cord. Free-radical destruction can age the brain faster than the body. Alzheimer's and Parkinson's diseases are examples. These conditions, once rare, have now spread like a monstrous plague. Some people believe the culprit is refined vegetable oil. Since the introduction of vegetable oil into our food system, these diseases and other nerve disorders like meningitis and multiple sclerosis have become common.

One possible means of decreasing the rate of degeneration in the central nervous system and elsewhere, would be to decrease the ingestion of vegetable oil.[24] The central nervous system is more susceptible than the rest of the body to accumulative degenerative changes that lead to dementia and other central nervous system disorders. Several studies have shown the relationship between refined vegetable oil consumption and free-radical damage to the central nervous system.

In one study, the effect of varying degrees of unsaturation on the mental ability of rats was determined by analyzing their maze-learning abilities. Different oils were added to the rats' feed. The study was initiated after rats had aged considerably, allowing enough time for the effects of the oils to become measurable. Rats were tested on the number of maze errors they made. The more errors they made, the greater the deterioration of mental function.

The test was designed to test effects of the amount of fat in the diet and the type of fat. The results clearly showed that the number of maze errors increased as the oils became more unsaturated.[25] The rats given lard retained their mental capacities the longest. The ones given polyunsaturated safflower oil lost them the quickest.

Numerous studies have shown that as unsaturation of dietary oil increases, cancer rate increases, heart disease increases, mental ability diminishes, and in fact, the entire body deteriorates from the onslaught of massive free-radical damage.

So why hasn't the public been informed about the dangers of poly-unsaturated fat? A few people have voiced concern about refined vegetable oils, but the food and drug industries have been so successful in condemning saturated fat and promoting their products as healthy alternatives that we tend to ignore information that says something different. If you tell a lie often enough and loud enough, people tend to believe it.

The fact of the matter is, researchers know about it, but the consumer doesn't. The reason is that information is disseminated by the advertising and marketing efforts of big food and drug industries. Consequently, we rarely hear about the detrimental effects of vegetable oils. Even medical doctors and other health care professionals are generally unaware because they don't have the time to search through hundreds of research journals every month to find the information. Because demands on their time are so great, they often rely on promotional material from food and drug manufacturers (a highly biased source) for their information. Many books on health are written by people who are misinformed. They've been brainwashed by the media and the marketing propaganda from the food industry.

Chapter 4

WHAT YOU SHOULD KNOW ABOUT CHOLESTEROL _____ ∎

GOOD FAT, BAD FAT

I want to take you back in time. Back long before you were born. Not too far back, however, only far enough where you could meet face to face with your great-great-grandparents. The year is 1878. Why 1878? This was the year that a strange new disease was first documented in the medical literature. Dr. Adam Hammer, a British physician, described for the first time a previously unknown condition now referred to as a heart attack. Up to that time no cases of heart attack had ever been documented in the medical literature. Dr. Hammer reported that a patient had experienced crushing chest pain, then collapsed, and died. An autopsy found that muscle tissue in the patient's heart had died resulting in heart failure and death. Nowadays, the signs of heart attack are well known and common. Thousands of people die every single day from heart disease. It is the number one killer in the industrialized world. Statistically, your chance of dying from a heart attack is about one in three.

Why was heart disease so rare back then and why is it so common now? Many heart attack victims are only in their 30s and 40s. A century ago people could live to be 60, 70, and 80 years of age without dying from heart attacks. So it is not a disease caused by age. If you asked anyone on the street what causes heart disease, the most common answer you would receive is eating too much cholesterol and saturated fat. Is that really the cause of heart disease?

Let's go back to 1878. What types of fats and oils did they eat in those days? The oils that were in common use were lard (pig fat), tallow (beef fat), butter, coconut and palm oils, and to a lessor extent olive oil.

They didn't have the technology then to produce to any great degree corn, soybean, safflower, and most other polyunsaturated oils. So our ancestors, who never heard of heart disease, ate mostly animal fats and butter, all of which are loaded with cholesterol and saturated fat. The effects on their health were clearly evident—heart disease, cancer, diabetes, obesity, and numerous other diseases of modern civilization were *rare*.

If cholesterol and saturated fat cause or even contribute to all of these health problems, as many claim, why after thousands of years in the human diet have they suddenly become toxic? Or have they? We've heard that cholesterol and saturated fat cause heart disease for so long and so often that we can repeat it in our sleep. But do they really? Both medical science and history say "no."

Dr. Paul Dudley White is known as the founder of cardiology—the study of the heart and its diseases. He graduated from medical school in 1910 and served as President Dwight D. Eisenhower's physician during his terms in office. As a young man, White wrote that he had an interest in a rare new disease that he had read about in the European medical literature. It was in 1921, 11 years after he began his practice, when he saw his first heart attack patient. At that time, heart attacks were extremely rare. By the 1950s, when he served as Eisenhower's physician, heart disease had become the nation's leading cause of death. Later in his career, and as the foremost authority in the world on cardiology and, consequently, heart disease, he was asked for his opinion about the theory that cholesterol and saturated fat caused heart disease. He stated that he couldn't support the theory because he knew it didn't fit the history of the disease.[1]

The graph on the next page illustrates why saturated fat and cholesterol can't be the cause of heart disease. The number of heart attack deaths per 100,000 people are plotted over time in comparison to cholesterol and saturated fat intake. Note that cholesterol and saturated fat levels have remained essentially constant, but heart attack deaths have skyrocketed. There is clearly no correlation between heart disease and cholesterol or saturated fat consumption.[2]

From 1910 to 1920 heart disease deaths were fairly low, affecting only about 10 out of every 100,000 people per year. By 1930 the death rate jumped to 46 per 100,000 and by 1970 the rate reached 331 per 100,000. It is interesting to note that vegetable oil consumption started to become more common at the beginning of the 20th century and has steadily increased, along with the rise in heart-disease rate. It would seem that there is a much stronger correlation between heart disease and vegetable oil consumption than with saturated fat or cholesterol.

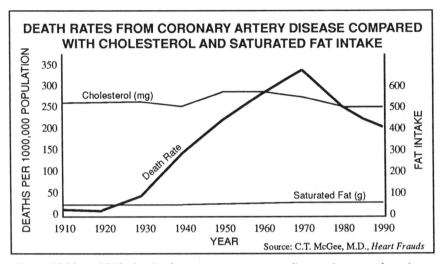

DEATH RATES FROM CORONARY ARTERY DISEASE COMPARED WITH CHOLESTEROL AND SATURATED FAT INTAKE

Source: C.T. McGee, M.D., *Heart Frauds*

From 1910 to 1970 deaths from coronary artery disease increased an incredible 3,010 percent, then began to decline. During this time cholesterol and saturated fat intake remained fairly constant, indicating little correlation between cholesterol or saturated fat with heart disease.

The food and drug industries have been very active in publicizing and promoting the theory that saturated fat and cholesterol cause heart disease. Since the 1950s they've been the primary financial sponsors in this area of study. Yet even after 50 years of research there is very little evidence to support the belief that a diet low in cholesterol and saturated fat actually reduces death from heart disease or in any way increases one's life span.

The cholesterol theory or cholesterol hypothesis implies that animal fat consumption must have increased significantly since 1920 to correlate with the rise in heart disease, but in fact the consumption of butter and animal fats in America declined steadily during that period, while use of vegetable fats increased dramatically. During the 60-year period from 1910 to 1970, the proportion of traditional animal fat in the American diet declined from 83% to 62%, and butter consumption plummeted from 17 pounds per person per year to about 4 pounds. During the past 80 years, dietary cholesterol intake has increased only 1%. During the same period the percentage of dietary vegetable fat in the form of margarine, shortening, and processed oils increased about 400%. When you look objectively at all the facts, the cholesterol hypothesis doesn't hold up.

In an attempt to scare the public and promote the increased use of vegetable oils, animal fats are blamed for every disease under the sun. It is now the politically correct thing to do, even though there is very little evidence that animal fats cause any harm. Obesity, diabetes, cancer, heart disease, you name it and someone is claiming that saturated fat or cholesterol is somehow the cause. But again, the facts don't fit the theory.

VITAMIN AND MINERAL DEFICIENCY

Despite decades of research and a significant decrease in animal fat consumption, heart disease is still our number one killer. Continuous attempts by an army of researchers over this time have failed to show a definitive link between cholesterol and heart disease. Much to the dismay of researchers and their sponsors, studies have shown only a very mild and even questionable relationship between the two.

If saturated fats and cholesterol don't cause heart disease, what does? There are a number of factors found to tie into heart disease far better than these fats.

In the 1940s and 1950s, researchers Yudkin and Lopez discovered a link between consumption of refined sugar and heart disease. Sugar consumption depresses the immune system, lowering the body's resistance to bacteria and viruses that may cause inflammation in the heart and arteries. Inflammation is one of the contributing factors in the development of arterial plaque and hardening of the arteries, which leads to heart disease.

With the use of packaged, processed foods, our vitamin and mineral intake has declined over the years. Vitamin C is one of the nutrients that is depleted in processed foods. It is necessary to maintain integrity of connective tissue including those in the arteries. One of the signs of vitamin C deficiency is atherosclerosis. The B vitamins, which have also declined in our food supply, are necessary in order to keep arteries strong and healthy. Research has shown that vitamin B deficiency is a major cause of atherosclerosis (hardening of the arteries) and heart disease.[3] Heart disease has also been correlated with mineral deficiencies. Coronary heart disease rates are lower in regions where drinking water is naturally rich in trace minerals, particularly magnesium, which acts as a natural anticoagulant and aids in potassium absorption, thereby preventing heart-rate irregularities. Vitamin D is also important in protecting the heart. It is essential for absorption of many minerals, particularly calcium and magnesium. Our bodies can manufacture vitamin D from cholesterol by the action of sunlight on the skin, but we are told to reduce our cholesterol consumption and our exposure to the sun in fear of developing skin cancer.

Excess sugar consumption also drains B vitamins needed to maintain healthy arteries. Research at the US Department of Agriculture indicates that fructose may be even more dangerous than sucrose (table sugar). Fructose, mainly in the form of high-fructose corn syrup, has become the sweetener of choice for soft drinks, snacks, and many so-called health foods.

In the 1950s, a researcher by the name of Dr. Annand discovered that heat caused a change in milk protein that encouraged the formation of blood clots. Raw milk did not have this effect. He noted that since the laws requiring milk pasteurization began in the 1920s, the heart disease rate has risen dramatically.

In 1968 the death rate from heart attacks fell for the first time in over 40 years and has continued to slowly decline ever since. By 1990 the death rate had fallen to 194 per 100,000 people (see graph below). Those who support the cholesterol hypothesis have not attempted to take credit for this decline because fat consumption has remained relatively constant the entire time. The reason why the death rate has fallen since the 1970s may be due to the increasing use of vitamin and mineral supplements. Nutritional deficiencies, which are probably a major contributor to heart disease, have lessened due to an increase use of vitamins and minerals.

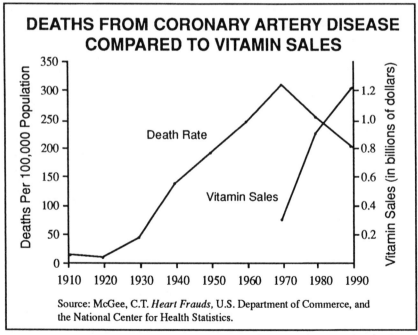

As vitamin and mineral sales have increased, heart disease deaths have decreased.

51

Refined vegetable oils contain little nutritional value other than fatty acids. They are basically empty calories. These oils not only contribute no vitamins or minerals, but actually deplete the body's nutrient reserves and thereby promote deficiency. Polyunsaturated oils are highly unstable and oxidize very easily, both inside and outside of the body. Oxidation of polyunsaturated oils creates destructive free radicals. Antioxidant nutrients such as vitamin A, vitamin E, Vitamin C, beta-carotene, zinc, selenium, and others are destroyed fighting off free radicals. In this process the body can become deficient in these essential nutrients. The result is a condition called subclinical malnutrition which can lead to physical degeneration and obesity. It is no wonder that as vitamin sales have increased, heart disease rates have declined.

Another problem with polyunsaturated vegetable oils is the fact that the primary fatty acid they contain, linoleic acid, is transformed by the body into hormone-like substances called prostaglandins. In excess, these prostaglandins can have a negative effect on health. For example, they encourage blood clotting, constriction of arteries which narrows passageways, and inflammation, all of which contribute to heart disease. In addition, the free radicals these oils generate can damage the arteries, thereby initiating plaque deposits. It's no wonder why heart disease has risen along with the increase in vegetable oil consumption.

THE CHOLESTEROL MYTH

When we hear the word "cholesterol," the first thought that comes to most people's minds is clogged arteries and heart disease. Cholesterol has almost become synonymous with heart disease. Everyone "knows" that cholesterol causes heart disease. You see it in the paper. You read about it in books. You hear it on television and the radio. They all loudly proclaim "High blood cholesterol causes heart disease." We hear it so much that it must be true. So many "experts" can't be wrong. Right?

We also know that saturated fat causes heart disease, don't we? That is what we read and that is what everyone says. Saturated fat has been labeled a villain because it can raise blood cholesterol levels too. And since saturated fat is much more abundant in our foods than cholesterol, it is considered by far the greater threat.

For years we have been told that cholesterol and saturated fat raise blood cholesterol and, therefore, cause cardiovascular disease. We hear this so often we are led to believe that there is a great deal of evidence supporting the cholesterol hypothesis. But actually, there never has been a study that demonstrated that high blood cholesterol *causes* heart disease.

Not a single one! In fact, the opposite is true. There are numerous studies that demonstrate that blood cholesterol does not cause clogged arteries or heart disease. People die of heart disease without having high blood cholesterol. Others with high blood cholesterol show no signs of cardiovascular disease—no plaque in arteries, no abnormal clotting, and blood pressure within normal ranges. If high blood cholesterol causes cardiovascular disease, then it would *have to be present in all people who die from it*. But it's not. This fact is clearly recognized.

Most cholesterol researchers will admit that high blood cholesterol does not cause heart disease. The drug industry has had a lot to do with creating a false impression because they sell billions of dollars worth of cholesterol-lowering drugs. Their cry that high blood cholesterol leads to cardiovascular disease has been so loud and so popular we've been brainwashed into believing it. Throughout history, dubious political leaders have held to the philosophy that if you tell a lie often enough and loud enough, eventually everyone will accept it as truth, no matter how preposterous it may be. That is the situation we have with cholesterol.

"The cholesterol theory is not compatible with the history of coronary artery disease," says Charles T. McGee, M.D. in his book *Heart Frauds.* "Dietary consumption of fats and cholesterol does not effect blood levels of cholesterol significantly in the vast majority of people. Many people with high blood cholesterol never experience coronary artery disease. People with low blood cholesterol can and do develop coronary artery disease. About one-third of the people who have a heart attack have a blood cholesterol level that is well within the range accepted as normal. Attempts to lower death rates from coronary artery disease with the American Heart Association diet have consistently failed. In addition, when drugs are given to try to lower blood cholesterol, overall death rates have gone *up*, not down, as anticipated."[4]

In an attempt to prove the cholesterol hypothesis, researchers have worked for over fifty years trying to demonstrate that cholesterol and saturated fat cause heart disease. No study has been able to do this and science has not gotten any closer to a solution. The Framingham Heart Study which has monitored the health of nearly 5,000 people for several decades has shown that people who eat more saturated fat do not develop heart disease any more than anyone else.[5]

Michael DeBakey, a heart surgeon, performed a study using a large number of patients at Baylor University. He found that out of 1,700 patients who had atherosclerosis, which leads to heart disease, severe enough to require hospitalization, only 1 patient out of 5 had high blood cholesterol.[6] Dr. Harlan M. Krumholz reported in the *Journal of the American Medical*

Association that people with higher cholesterol are not necessarily the most likely to have heart problems or die from heart disease. In a study, he monitored 997 people 65 years of age and older. Those with high cholesterol had about the same rates of heart attack and death as those with normal levels. You would expect that as we age, more cholesterol will build up in the arteries and thus increase the risk of heart disease. Indeed, risk of heart attack does increases with age. However, research doesn't show any correlation between age and cholesterol. For example, in a study where the mean age of the subjects was 79, the authors report there was found "no evidence that an elevated level of cholesterol increased the risk of death or heart disease among this group."[7] Paul Addis and Gregory Warner, professors in the Department of Food Science and Nutrition at the University of Minnesota state: "The prevailing opinion, that atherosclerosis is simply an accumulation of cholesterol on arteries, has clearly shown to be erroneous. Therefore, the 'lipid hypothesis' has become less well accepted by serious researchers and has been replaced by a competing hypothesis, i.e. 'response-to-injury hypothesis.'"[8] Because of the many inconsistencies with the cholesterol hypothesis, it has often been called the cholesterol myth.

In 1950, coronary artery disease became our leading cause of death, and it still is today. Avoidance of cholesterol and saturated fat, the availability of cholesterol-lowering drugs, and eating foods low in cholesterol and saturated fats have not stopped the heart-disease epidemic. It should be obvious that something else, that is generally overlooked is at the root of the problem.

CHOLESTEROL REGULATION

It is assumed that a diet high in cholesterol and saturated fat leads to high blood cholesterol. Saturated fat is included because it can be converted into cholesterol by the liver. The fat we eat, according to the cholesterol theory, is directly responsible for the amount of cholesterol in our blood. The problem with this argument is that dietary consumption of fat has only a minor affect on cholesterol levels. Why? Because the vast majority of the cholesterol in our blood does not come from the diet, but comes from our liver. More than 80% of the cholesterol in our blood is manufactured in our own bodies.

To account for this fact, it is claimed by those who believe in the cholesterol hypothesis, that the saturated fat in our diet is automatically converted into cholesterol and the more saturated fat we eat, the more cholesterol we have floating around in our bloodstream. The liver is depicted as a machine that blindly cranks out as much cholesterol as it possibly can. The more saturated fat we eat, the more cholesterol it cranks out.

Such a scenario is inconsistent with human physiology. The liver produces and carefully regulates a balance of hundreds of compounds essential for growth, digestion, and protection. Blood cholesterol is not an accident that is easily influenced by diet. The liver doesn't just crank out chemicals, like cholesterol, for the fun of it. It does it for a specific reason. And the amounts are carefully controlled and monitored to achieve and maintain homeostasis or chemical equilibrium. The liver carefully regulates the amount of cholesterol in our bodies, so it doesn't really matter how much saturated fat we eat, the liver will only manufacture the amount we need to maintain homeostasis. Everyone's bodies are different so everyone has a different level of cholesterol with which the body is happy. This level is consistent regardless of our diet and lifestyle within about 5–10%.

The liver doesn't need saturated fat to make cholesterol. It can make it from other fats and even from sugar or carbohydrates.[9] So, the claim that saturated fat raises blood cholesterol, while ignoring other fats and sugar, is illogical and inaccurate. If not enough cholesterol is eaten, the liver will make it from other dietary sources. This is why even drastic decreases in dietary cholesterol intake often produce only small drops in blood cholesterol levels.[10]

Kilmer S. McCully, M.D., a pathologist and medical researcher, has investigated the connection between diet and heart disease and cancer for over 30 years. He states: "The amount of cholesterol that is formed in the liver is carefully controlled and adjusted according to the needs of the different organs of the body. If the amount of cholesterol is increased in the diet, a healthy, well-functioning liver makes less cholesterol for the needs of the body. If the amount of cholesterol in the diet is decreased, the liver makes more cholesterol. In this way the body regulates very precisely how much cholesterol is produced for its needs."[11]

Each day the body churns out approximately 1,000 mg of cholesterol; in comparison, an average American man's daily cholesterol intake is only 327 mg and a woman's is 221 mg. Of the cholesterol we eat, only about one-third is absorbed through the intestines; the rest is excreted.

Theoretically, the dietary cholesterol that is absorbed by the body in a day would raise a man's blood cholesterol by some 163 mg/dl. However, this doesn't happen. Here's why. Instead of responding in a set way to a high-fat meal, the body has several options: the intestine can absorb large or small amounts of cholesterol; the liver can turn down its own cholesterol production; and the liver can also convert some of this cholesterol into bile acids ready for excretion. The degree to which these responses occur depends both on the cholesterol content of the meal and the genetic makeup of the person. Some people absorb more than others, but some excrete more.[12]

For most people the blood cholesterol level is determined more by heredity than it is by diet. However, drastic diets, toxins, or drugs can upset the normal cholesterol balance. Lowering cholesterol will have little, if any, effect on your overall health. Lowering it too much may even be detrimental.

GENETICS AND CARDIOVASCULAR DISEASE
Worldwide Populations

In studying populations from around the world, the cholesterol hypothesis just doesn't hold up. Studies have shown populations from such diverse places as South and Central Africa, South America, Europe, the Middle East, and Western Asia to be free of heart disease and high cholesterol despite the fact that their diets are very high in saturated fat.[13-16]

A good example of a high saturated fat and cholesterol diet is found in the Masai. The Masai are a nomadic people who live in East Kenya and Northern Tanzania. They herd cattle, goats, and sheep. Most of their diet consists of fresh, raw cow's milk. Adults consume up to five liters of milk a day. This is whole milk, not skim or low fat, so it's loaded with saturated fat and cholesterol.

About 66% of calories in their diet come in the form of saturated fat. Even with a diet high in animal fat, the blood cholesterol of the Masai runs only 135 mg/dl and they don't have heart attacks as long as they eat their traditional diet of meat and whole milk.

Cholesterol researchers traveled to Kenya to study the Masai. During the study, cholesterol in their diet was manipulated in volunteers. When fed 2,000 mg/day of cholesterol (one egg yolk contains about 300 mg) blood cholesterol averaged 135 mg/dl. When fed no cholesterol at all, blood cholesterol levels stayed the same. These people did not fit the parameters of the cholesterol hypothesis at all. In order to explain the apparent discrepancy, the researchers simply concluded that the Masai must have some genetic trait that protects them from getting high cholesterol and heart disease.[17]

Genetics has been the favorite answer in defense when those who champion the cholesterol hypothesis are faced with facts that go contrary to their beliefs. Several studies testing the genetic hypothesis have been performed and all have given similar results, much to the dismay of the cholesterol promoters.

Japanese Study

To explain the difference why some people are affected by cardiovascular disease and why others are not, even when both have high blood cholesterol levels, people have pointed to genetic differences. It's all in the genes, they say. Some people are more susceptible to heart disease than others. Perhaps those people whose ancestries were predominantly meat eaters have a higher tolerance for animal fats than those who descended from agrarian societies. We know that carnivorous animals, such as dogs and cats, can consume huge quantities of saturated fat and cholesterol without any ill effect; maybe the human population varies in its ability to handle such fats.

A study to verify this hypothesis was undertaken. Men of Japanese descent were chosen for the study because the Japanese have one of the lowest rates of cardiovascular disease and many have migrated to various parts of the world. The study analyzed the rate of heart disease and stroke of Japanese men in different countries who ate according to the local diets. The results showed that the death rate from heart disease and stroke of the Japanese men matched those of their adopted countries.[18]

This study clearly showed that heredity was not a factor. Diet and lifestyle were the essential ingredients to cardiovascular health.

Irish Study

In a classic study begun in 1963, researchers at the Harvard School of Public Health joined with scientists at Trinity College in Dublin, Ireland. At the time of the study, the heart disease rate in the United States was four times greater than in Ireland. The goal of the study was to determine why Irish immigrants who had lived in the United States for ten or more years experienced the same rate of heart disease as native-born Americans.

To eliminate genetic differences, the subjects chosen in the United States had brothers living in Ireland who also participated in the study. By comparing electrocardiograms, blood pressure readings, and cholesterol levels, the researchers discovered that the cardiovascular condition of the subjects in Ireland was far superior to that of their American brothers. Autopsies performed on subjects who died during the course of the study revealed that the hearts and arteries of the American brothers had "aged from fifteen to twenty-eight years more rapidly."[19]

Most astonishing of all, the Irish participants consumed a diet *much richer in saturated fat and cholesterol* than that of the Americans! If

57

cholesterol and saturated fat were the major factors affecting coronary health, the Irish brothers would have been less healthy. Why the difference? Several answers have been suggested. The American brothers took on the dietary habits of their adopted country which included more polyunsaturated oil and more sugar, both of which we now know to contribute to the deterioration of cardiovascular health. Another factor is that the Irish brothers generally worked at more physically demanding jobs, giving them more exercise. Both diet and physical activity probably made the difference. Exercise does help, but the biggest factor was probably diet. It is of interest to note that now in areas of the world where people still work hard physically, since they have adopted diets more like those of affluent countries, like the United States, by eating more polyunsaturated oils and sugar, their rates of cardiovascular disease has skyrocketed.[20]

OXIDIZED CHOLESTEROL

Both animal studies and human autopsies show cholesterol is found in atherosclerotic arteries. Doesn't this suggest that cholesterol plays an important role in the development of the disease? Not necessarily. Cholesterol has unjustly been accused as the primary instigator of arterial plaque. Normal cholesterol, the type used to make hormones, vitamin D, and brain tissue is guilty only by association. It's like a group of school children playing baseball and the batter hits the ball through a neighbor's window. All the kids involved in the game run for cover. The only kid that sticks around was one who was sitting watching the game and minding his own business. When the owner of the house comes out and sees only that boy, he is automatically accused as the guilty party. Cholesterol is that innocent bystander. The real troublemakers have hidden out of sight and until recently have escaped detection.

It was in the 1970s that researchers discovered that dietary cholesterol existed in two forms, oxidized and reduced. In fresh, natural foods, cholesterol and other fats occur only in the harmless reduced form. This is the normal cholesterol, the innocent bystander, the type that makes up the majority of our brain tissue or that is used as a component of cell membranes; it is *not* found in human arterial plaque. The type of cholesterol that builds up in the arteries is *oxidized* cholesterol along with oxidized fatty acids. These are the *only* types of fats found in plaque.[21]

Only the oxidized form is toxic to arteries. Dr. Ishwarlal Jialal of the University of Texas Southwestern Medical Center in Dallas states, "Fats in the bloodstream become lodged in artery walls and begin to clog arteries *only* when their transporters, the lipoproteins, have chemically combined with oxygen to turn rancid."[22] Lipoproteins are tiny bundles of protein packed with cholesterol and fatty acids (including polyunsaturated fats). The polyunsaturated fats are highly susceptible to oxidization, which causes free-radical formation. When polyunsaturated oils turn rancid, they produce free radicals that attack the cholesterol, causing it to become oxidized as well. The result is that both the cholesterol and polyunsaturated fats in the lipoprotein become oxidized.

In a series of studies of oxidized cholesterol, medical scientists at Albany Medical College showed that highly purified cholesterol, uncontaminated by polyunsaturated oils, chemically free of all traces of oxidized cholesterol, and protected from the oxygen in air, does *not* produce atherosclerosis.[23, 24] Pure unadulterated cholesterol is not harmful to the arteries and cannot initiate or promote heart disease.[25] Cholesterol *must* be oxidized before it can cling to artery walls.[26]

A very large number of research publications support the fact that oxidized fats (both cholesterol and polyunsaturated fats) are far more harmful to arterial health than native or ordinary fats. Therefore, cholesterol is now viewed as harmless unless it becomes oxidized.[27]

It is very important to understand the difference between normal (reduced) and oxidized cholesterol. Cholesterol doesn't simply come strolling freely down the artery and suddenly decide to stick somewhere. The process begins with an injury to the inner lining of the arterial wall. The injury can be caused by a virus, excessive blood pressure, or other factors, even free-radical damage. Because of a process which is still not fully understood, cells in the artery wall attract oxidized cholesterol and oxidized triglycerides (e.g., fatty acids such as those found in vegetable oil) from the blood. Only oxidized fats are involved. Other materials such as calcium and fibrous tissue also combine with fat to form plaque. As the plaque builds up within the wall of the artery, the wall bulges inward, slowly closing off the arterial opening. Over many years, the process gradually obstructs the artery, blocking the flow of blood.

Prior to the 1970s studies with rabbits given cholesterol showed that they developed plaque in their arteries. These studies provided the evidence that initiated the cholesterol hypothesis. When it was discovered that only oxidized fat is involved in the generation of arterial plaque, researchers became curious enough to repeat the original rabbit-feeding studies. They suspected that early researchers put the fat-rich food into cages and left it for the rabbits to eat throughout the day. This allowed the fat on the surface of the food to react with the oxygen in the air and become oxidized. Oxygen, sunlight, and heat (even room temperature) can initiate rancidity and free-radical reactions.

When researchers repeating these experiments made efforts to protect the fat in the food from oxidizing, the animals' arteries remained healthy. The fat content of the food was increased and the rabbits' blood cholesterol went as high as 1,500 to 2,000 mg/dl—ten times the upper limit currently considered acceptable for humans—but no fatty deposits formed! So even in vegetarian animals cholesterol is harmless.

Some researchers questioned whether the small amount of fat that would be oxidized on the surface of the food in the original studies would make any significant impact. In response, researchers designed experiments using very small quantities of oxidized fat. Rabbits fed a diet containing a mere 1% oxidized cholesterol developed extensive obstructions in their coronary arteries. In another group, rabbits ate the same amount of fat and cholesterol, which were protected from oxidation, and their arteries remained disease-free. So even a tiny amount of oxidized oil can have a very significant impact on health.[28]

Several factors affected the cholesterol in early studies to give erroneous results. If the cholesterol was mixed with vegetable oil, the oxidation process was accelerated. Vegetable oil was routinely added in many studies. Because eggs contain a high percentage of cholesterol, they were often used as the source in many studies. However, the type of eggs they used was always in dried, powdered form. Drying the eggs *oxidizes* the cholesterol in them. So the researchers were conducting tests using highly oxidized cholesterol and not the type typically found in ordinary foods.

Most of the older scientific articles don't specify the type of cholesterol used or the other oils that were combined with them. So there is no way of telling if the fats were oxidized or not. However, if not specified, it is assumed that steps were *not* taken to protect fats from oxidation, usually because researchers did not recognize the difference at the time. Because of this, most feeding studies reported over the past 80 years are worthless. The results of these flawed studies were then applied to humans in making dietary recommendations. This is why in real life doctors and researchers have failed to find a correlation between people who eat a high-cholesterol diet and heart disease.

All oxidized lipids (fats), whether they are cholesterol or polyunsaturated fatty acids, because they involve free radicals, can damage arterial walls. Studies on rabbits showed those fed oxidized cholesterol had damage, while those fed normal cholesterol didn't.[29] What we know now is that it's not the total level of fat or the LDL (so-called bad cholesterol) in the blood that's important, but the amount of *oxidized* fat and *oxidized* cholesterol that is the issue. Many people with relatively low blood fat levels develop cardiovascular disease because a large amount of this fat is oxidized. Others who have high-cholesterol readings do not experience cardiovascular disease because the fat in their blood is normal or not oxidized. LDL cholesterol can be either oxidized or normal. So you can't rely on LDL levels to predict heart disease risk.

How does the body accumulate oxidized fat? Oxidation can occur in food either before or after it's eaten. Rancid or heat-damaged oils become oxidized before eating. Once these damaged oils are consumed, through free-radical chain reactions, they can cause other oils inside the body to become oxidized. The best defense against free-radical destruction is to eat oils that are not oxidized and those that are not susceptible to oxidization. As noted the rabit studies above, even a very small amount of oxidized fat or oxidized cholesterol can have a dramatic effect on cardiovascular health.

Probably the biggest contributor to fat oxidation and free-radical formation in the body comes from eating polyunsaturated vegetable oils. Saturated fats are not a problem because they are not vulnerable to oxidation like unsaturated fats or even cholesterol. Cholesterol can be oxidized within the body, so a higher level of cholesterol in the blood can theoretically increase the risk of developing oxidized cholesterol. This is why there is a risk, howbeit very small, with elevated cholesterol levels. The vast majority of the cholesterol in our blood is made by the liver and is pure and natural, thus harmless, unless it comes in contact with rancid polyunsaturated fatty acids or other free-radical-causing substances like homocysteine (caused by a lack of certain B vitamins), xanthine oxidase (obtained from homogenized milk), or excess iron (abundant in processed cereal and grain products).

Heat is a major factor in free-radical formation, and cooking with vegetable oils causes massive free-radical generation. When you eat anything that is cooked in polyunsaturated vegetable oil, you are quite literally damaging your heart, your brain, and all other organs and tissues in your body. Any polyunsaturated oil that has been heated contains free radicals.

Cooking meat causes some fat oxidation particularly on the surface where it is exposed to oxygen. Currently, however, there is little evidence to show that cooked meat causes any significant problems from oxidization. The reason is probably because meat contains primarily saturated and monounsaturated fat, both of which are fairly stable under heat and help protect polyunsaturated fats from oxidation. You don't need to worry about the saturated fat in the meat because it is not vulnerable to oxidation and free-radical formation like unsaturated fats are. This is why our ancestors could cook their meals in lard and butter without experiencing any signs of cardiovascular disease.

Eggs have frequently been condemned because they are high in cholesterol and saturated fat. A much bigger health hazard is the vegetable oils commonly used in cooking eggs. It's safer to cook them in lard than in vegetable oil. Hard-boiled eggs are cooked at temperatures below 212° F (100° C)—the boiling point—and are not exposed to oxygen during cooking, so the cholesterol they contain is not oxidized. Despite the fact that eggs are high in cholesterol and saturated fat, when hard-boiled they do not contribute to heart disease.

Charles McGee, M.D., tells in his book, *Heart Frauds,* about an experience with one of his patients who participated in an animal-feeding study. This patient worked in a regional primate center, one of several research centers funded by the federal government. "One old baboon named George was selected to participate in the study because he had a mean disposition and none of the animal keepers liked him," relates Dr. McGee.

"The staff dreamed up an experiment in which George was given the opportunity to give his life for science and not be around to bother them any more. They fed the old baboon nothing but hard-boiled eggs for one year, then put him down (killed him) and performed an autopsy.

"Because of the propaganda about the cholesterol theory, the staff confidently expected to find massive obstructions in the old baboon's arteries. They dreamed of seeing their names in large print on the top of a published scientific paper supporting the widely accepted and popular cholesterol theory.

"But it was the old baboon who had the last laugh. Because no evidence of atherosclerosis was found in George's arteries, no paper was written. This feeding study demonstrated once again the fats and cholesterol in fresh eggs are harmless because they do not become oxidized. It also demonstrated that studies that do not support an accepted theory usually don't get published."[30]

Dr. Kilmer McCully states: "The entire history of the cholesterol/fat hypothesis explaining the cause of atherosclerosis is based on the unproved assumption that the disease is produced by overconsumption of the normal dietary constituents—cholesterol and fat. Only in the case of the oxycholesterols (oxidized cholesterol) is there compelling evidence to suggest that a trace or contaminant constituent associated with fat and cholesterol in the diet is actually injurious and capable of initiating atherosclerotic plaques."[31]

All cells in our bodies need cholesterol. It forms an integral part of the cell's membrane. It has an important structural role in the brain and in the conduction of nerve impulses. "Because cholesterol is so important physiologically," states Nicholas Sampsidis, M.S., "It is a rather foolhardy assumption that, since the dawn of mankind, the human system has been performing the suicidal experiment of becoming dependent on a biochemical which can trigger its self-destruction. The human system takes very good care of itself and it does not manufacture cholesterol in order to clog up its own arteries and start heart disease."[32]

You don't need to worry about cholesterol in natural foods. Overly processed foods, however, can contain significant amounts of oxidized cholesterol. Those that contain significant levels of oxidized cholesterol or oxidized fat and should not be eaten include: powdered/dehydrated milk, cheese, eggs, and butter; highly processed meats (baloney, pepperoni, salami, etc.); overcooked meats and dairy; and processed polyunsaturated vegetable oils.

MILK AND DAIRY PRODUCTS
Processed Milk

Your first food was milk. It was all you ate for the first few months of life. Milk is a highly nutritious food packed with essential vitamins and minerals. After all, it was specifically designed to be a complete and nourishing food for humans and other mammals. For thousands of years people have consumed dairy products and thrived, existing without degenerative disease as we see it now. But if you drink milk nowadays you're risking your life. This isn't because of the saturated fat or cholesterol content, but what we do to it.

The milk we drink nowadays is far different from the milk the Masai of Africa drink or that even our grandparents and great-grandparents drank. Modern milk isn't the natural food it once was, but is now a man-made version of the original. Milk contains contaminants just like meat, so it is full of antibiotics, hormones, and pesticides. If that wasn't bad enough, it is chemically altered into a substance unfit to drink.

When you go to the store you can buy whole milk, reduced fat (2%), low-fat (1%), or nonfat (skim). How are these varieties produced? You don't get whole milk from a whole cow and nonfat from a lean one. There are no nonfat cows! All milk comes from the same source and is highly processed, involving heating, fractionalization, reconstitution, and homogenization. In the process, nutrients are lost and toxic byproducts produced.

All milk is heated or pasteurized to kill any bacteria that may have contaminated it. This is done by law in many places to prevent illness. Some localities do allow the sale of raw milk. You have to check with your area.

Fresh raw milk is full of fat, which tends to float to the top. The milk at the top is richer and creamier than the milk at the bottom. You rarely see this in milk in the stores any more because, for one reason, almost all milk is fractionalized and reconstituted to produce a product with a precise amount of fat. This involves removing all the fat from the milk. This fat can be used to make butter or cream. Some fat is added back to the watery fluid to make reduced fat and low-fat milks. In this way, milk producers can create milk products that are exactly alike.

According to the late Henry Schroeder, M.D., a prominent researcher at Dartmouth, when dairies "fractionalize" milk to remove fat, the skimmed or low-fat milk loses many essential nutrients. The only way to restore all the nutrients is to reintroduce the original butter. Nutritionists unanimously recommend whole milk for weaned toddlers, because of the essential fatty acids, vitamins, and energy not contained in skim or low-fat milk. Whole milk is also better tolerated by those who are lactose intolerant.[33]

While fresh raw milk does *not* contribute to heart disease, modern pasteurized and homogenized milk may. When whole milk is dehydrated, its fat content becomes oxidized, including the cholesterol. Powdered whole milk containing oxidized cholesterol is added back to nonfat milk to make reduced fat and low-fat milks.[34] When you drink this type of milk, you are consuming dangerous oxidized fat, and this isn't heart healthy. All varieties of milk have been homogenized and this too contributes to heart disease.

Homogenization

When you look at a container of milk, it proudly states "homogenized" as if this were something that is of benefit to the consumer. But what is homogenization and why is it done?

Milk is primarily water with various nutrients, proteins, and fats floating in it. If allowed to stand quietly for any length of time, the fat being lighter than other constituents of the milk would float to the top. To some people having the richest or creamiest part of the milk at the top is undesirable. So to make the texture of the milk uniform it is homogenized.

Homogenization was introduced in the United States in 1932. This process involves forcing the milk though tiny screens to break the fat down into minute particles. These fat particles are so small they remain suspended in the milk without floating to the top. The result is a product that has a uniform or homogenous texture. This may sound desirable, but in the process an enzyme is affected that can have a significant influence on our health.

Milk contains an enzyme called xanthine oxidase. When eaten, xanthine oxidase is completely digested by our stomach acids and digestive

64

enzymes and poses no threat. According to Dr. Kurt A. Oster, formerly Chief of Cardiology at Bridgeport's Park City Hospital, homogenization causes xanthine oxidase to become trapped within the tiny fat globules. This forms a protective layer of fat around the xanthine oxidase so it passes through the stomach and into the intestinal tract unharmed. Here it is readily absorbed through the intestinal wall and into the bloodstream where it acts as a free radical attacking the arterial wall, causing injury and contributing to the atherosclerotic process. Dr. Oster feels that this rogue enzyme is a principal player in initiating atherosclerosis and heart disease.

In support of his theory, he notes that those countries that have the highest homogenized milk consumption also have the highest atherosclerosis death rate. He noted that Finland (at the time he conducted the study, 1967) had the highest death rate, 244.7 per 100,000, and consumed 534 pounds of homogenized milk per person.[35] Sweden, Finland's next door neighbor who shares similar genetic roots, consumes a total of 374 pounds of milk, but only 7 pounds per person is homogenized. Their death rate is only 75.9 per 100,000. They consumed lower amounts of homogenized milk and had a lower atherosclerosis death rate.

In the United States, the death rate at the time was 211.8 per 100,000, and consumed 259 pounds of homogenized milk per person. The Swedes consumed 162 pounds more milk per person than those in the U.S., but had a death rate only one third as much. But their homogenized milk consumption was far lower than Finland or the U.S. Japan, which consumed only 2 pounds of homogenized milk per person, had a death rate of only 39 per 100,000.

Raw Milk

Whenever I tell people they should switch to using raw milk they often question me, "Doesn't raw milk contain germs?" My answer, "Not any more than any other food you eat." In fact, it's much safer than most foods. Our ancestors didn't need to pasteurize their milk to kill harmful germs. They ate it straight from the cow, goat, llama, or camel as the case may be. Raw milk was never a health problem. If they didn't eat it immediately, they let it sit and ferment, transforming it into kefir or yogurt. It didn't spoil, it fermented—there is a difference.

Pasteurized milk is a product of modern technology, created to kill germs which are introduced into the milk by the complexities of mass production and sloppy handling. Milk is often contaminated by germs introduced during the extraction, transport, and storage of milk which end up in large commercial vats. In these vats the milk of 100 cows could be contaminated from the milk of a single diseased cow. Or a tiny contaminant from one incompletely washed udder could infect the milk taken from an

65

entire herd of dairy cows. Because this sort of thing happens every day in large dairy operations, it is nearly impossible to keep milk free from contamination. Thus large dairy operations have led the way in the lobbying efforts for mandatory pasteurization.

Once milk is pasteurized all bacteria is killed including the good bacteria. It's the good bacteria that allow it to ferment and even protect the milk from harmful bacteria. Pasteurized milk, as it gets old, does not ferment—it petrifies and spoils. In the past, if you wanted soured (raw) milk that you could drink and enjoy, all you had to do was leave it out on the countertop. Nowadays, if you did that you would get rotten milk with a horrible stench. The difference between the two is that raw milk is a living food; pasteurized milk is dead, and if not refrigerated, the rate at which it rots accelerates.

Raw, unpasteurized, unhomogenized milk is a healthy, nutritious food. It is a food that has nourished humans for thousands of years. Dairies that sell raw milk must follow strict sanitary practices. Animals are checked constantly to maintain good health. Since the livestock and milk are treated with greater care, raw milk is usually a little more expensive, but well worth the price. Not all areas allow the sale of raw milk so you must check your locality. The best place to look for it is in your local health food store, see also the resources in the Appendix.

All organic raw dairy products are good. So is organic butter. Butter, which is made from cream through a churning process, is mainly milkfat. It is two-thirds saturated fat with some protein, vitamins, and minerals. Cultured milk products (sour cream, cheese, cottage cheese, and yogurt) are good too, even if they've been pasteurized. The cultured or soured milks are the end products of fermentation. Fermented milk is more stable and resistant to spoilage than fresh, and can aid digestion. Fermented milk contains bacteria (some brands, however, do not; so look on the label for live cultures) that partially digest the milk, making it easier for our bodies to process, and reinforce the "good" bacteria in our intestines. Even though some nutrients in cultured milk are destroyed or killed during pasteurization, fermentation by living bacteria cultures bring it back to life.

There are alternatives to cows' milk. The most healthful natural milk is goat milk. Goat milk is the closest commercial dairy product to human milk in content and usually lacks chemical additives. Goat milk when properly handled tastes remarkably like cow's milk. If it has a strong "goaty" flavor, it has not been handled properly. You don't need to worry about homogenization with goat milk; it's not necessary. Goat milk is not homogenized because the fat globules are smaller and more evenly distributed than in cow's milk.

OXIDIZED DAIRY AND MEAT PRODUCTS

Arteriosclerosis (hardening of the arteries) can develop without eating cholesterol, because it can be caused by injury from free radicals and an unbalanced diet that lacks protective nutrients. Any oxidized cholesterol (or oxidized polyunsaturated fat) in the body is attracted to arterial plaque like a magnet and contributes to the clogging of the arteries. Oxidized fat generates free radicals that can injure arterial walls.

Food processing can oxidize the cholesterol and unsaturated fat in animal products. There are a few foods that are extremely high in oxidized cholesterol and fat and, therefore, highly dangerous to health. They constitute some of the worst foods you could possibly eat in regards to cardiovascular health. If you want to die from a heart attack or stroke, the foods that will contribute the most toward this end are: food fried in polyunsaturated vegetable oil; powdered eggs; powdered milk; dehydrated cheddar, blue, Parmesan and Romano cheese, as well as sour cream and butter powders; and freeze-dried and cured meats.[36] All of these foods contain variable but significant quantities of oxidized products capable of ripping free-radical holes through your cells, disintegrating DNA, and quickly aging your skin, liver, kidneys, and brain. No organ is immune.

Out of this list, the most troublesome are deep fried foods. Heated vegetable oils are quickly oxidized, and the more often they are heated and the higher the temperature, the worse they become. Deep fried foods cooked in vegetable oil are perhaps the worst foods on the planet to eat. Foods cooked this way constitute some of the most popular restaurant and snack foods we eat, such as French fries, onion rings, chicken and fish nuggets, donuts, potato chips, corn chips, egg rolls, fried wonton, etc. If you eat fried food it should be cooked in a saturated fat like coconut oil.

The cholesterol in fresh milk, eggs, and meat is *not* oxidized and is utilized in the body to strengthen cell membranes, synthesize vital hormones, and build brain and nerve tissue. The drying process in making powdered milk, cheese, and eggs fully oxidizes the cholesterol in these products. Once oxidized it cannot be utilized in the normal fashion to build and strengthen body tissues, but is packed away into the plaque of injured arteries. Eating such foods will surely clog your arteries faster than any other substance known on the face of the earth.

Cholesterol from fresh meat is harmless for the most part. Even when cooked intact, beef muscle contains little or no cholesterol oxides.[37] But when meat is cut, molded, cured, mixed with spices and preservatives, and rendered into hot dogs, pepperoni, baloney, and other luncheon meats, it has ample opportunity for the cholesterol and other fats to oxidize. Things that cause more oxidation in fresh meat are cutting and grinding (more fat exposed to oxygen), overcooking (heat oxidizes fat), age (the longer the meat hangs around, the more oxidation occurs), and the addition of nitrates and nitrites (used in curing meats) intensifying free-radical potential.

Dried eggs and powdered milk contain high levels of oxidized cholesterol.[38] Powdered eggs are often used as a source of oxidized cholesterol in laboratory experiments to test its detrimental effects on animals.

You may be thinking to yourself, "I don't have to worry about these foods; I don't drink powdered milk and I never eat powdered eggs. Who eats powdered eggs anyway?" Chances are you do. If you eat packaged convenience foods, you eat them all the time. Look at the ingredient labels of the foods in the stores and you will be surprised how many items have powdered milk, cheese, or eggs. They don't always say "powdered" or "dehydrated," but it is obvious that a cake mix, for example, that lists eggs in the ingredients uses *powdered* eggs. They can't very well put fresh eggs into the mix, can they?

Powdered eggs and milk are widely used in boxed cake, pancake, and muffin mixes, and by commercial bakeries to make all types of baked goods. The breads you buy at the store are often made with them. Boxed meals that contain cheese, such as macaroni and cheese, use dried cheese that comes in little packets. You would be surprised at how many packaged foods contain these powdered items. Even many frozen foods use them because it is more convenient and economical for the manufacturer to store and use dried dairy products than fresh. Food producers don't always tell you the dairy products they use are dried or powdered. But if you see eggs, milk, or cheese listed on a boxed item stored on a shelf, you know they are powdered because these items when fresh are highly perishable.

If that isn't enough, you can buy these items in powdered form yourself to add even more free radicals to your foods in the form of instant milk, grated romano and parmesan cheese, and powdered eggs. Even if the powdered milk you buy says "non-fat," it may be full of oxidized troublemakers.

Restaurants use many powdered dairy products. One particularly common item found in most fast food outlets as well as many other types of restaurants is soft-serve ice cream. This is the soft ice cream you get out of self-serve machines or that fast food chains use for ice cream cones and milk shakes. This stuff is made from powdered milk and sugar and often has hydrogenated vegetable oil added to it. So you get both oxidized cholesterol and hydrogenated oil at the same time—two of the worst oils you can put in your mouth! If you want to eat ice cream, it's better to stick to the real thing.

Chapter 5

THE TRUTH ABOUT SATURATED FAT _____ ∎

EFFECTS ON CHOLESTEROL AND HEART DISEASE

Saturated fat, like cholesterol, is often criticized as causing heart disease. The reason saturated fat is condemned is not because it clogs the arteries or harms the heart, but because it can be converted into cholesterol by the liver, thereby increasing blood cholesterol levels. According to the cholesterol theory, the higher the cholesterol level the greater the risk of heart disease. Therefore, it is not so much the saturated fat that is bad, but that it raises blood cholesterol that is considered the problem.

The error with this reasoning is that the cholesterol that is made from saturated fat is *natural* cholesterol, not oxidized cholesterol and, therefore, is completely harmless. Most people don't realize that the liver makes cholesterol out of many foods including fruits and vegetables. So why not condemn fruits and vegetables too? The reason is that these foods don't compete for customer dollars with vegetable oils like animal fats do. So those pushing for the use of vegetable oils have no reason to attack other foods.

Those industries promoting the use of vegetable oils say these oils are better because they do not raise blood cholesterol levels and, in fact, can even lower them. But we have seen that blood cholesterol level really isn't important. What is important is the amount of *oxidized* fat (triglycerides) and cholesterol in the blood.

Much is said about *blood* cholesterol, but cholesterol is in other parts of the body as well. High intakes of polyunsaturated fatty acids have been found to *increase* whole-body cholesterol, especially liver cholesterol.

Dietary changes in favor of polyunsaturated fatty acids usually lower both the so-called "bad" LDL cholesterol and the "good" HDL cholesterol. So there is no benefit.

Let me ask you a question. When polyunsaturated oils lower blood cholesterol, what happens? Where does the cholesterol go? Vegetable oil does not magically make cholesterol disappear. And cholesterol is not excreted with the consumption of vegetable oil, so how does it lower blood cholesterol levels? I'll tell you. It causes the cholesterol to migrate out of the blood and into surrounding tissues. The cholesterol is still there, but now it is in the cells and tissues rather than floating in the blood. Where else is it going to go? Some of this cholesterol becomes oxidized by the polyunsaturated oils. Where do oxidized fats end up? In the arteries, that's where. You get a lower blood cholesterol reading, but is it any healthier? No, because you'll likely have *more oxidized* cholesterol in your arteries.

The question one might ask is why does cholesterol migrate into the cells when polyunsaturated fat is eaten? The answer is that the membranes of the cells are made predominantly from fatty acids, both saturated and unsaturated. Cholesterol is also an important component of the cell membrane. Polyunsaturated fatty acids make the membrane more fluid. Saturated fat and cholesterol act as stabilizers, providing support. A balance is needed in all of them for the cells to function optimally. When the diet is rich in polyunsaturated fatty acids, more of these fats are used as building blocks for the cell membranes. As a consequence, the cells become too fluid and become leaky, resulting in a loss of function. In order to maintain optimal function, more cholesterol is extracted from passing lipoproteins (bundles of fat and cholesterol) in the blood and incorporated into the cell membrane to strengthen it. Therefore, less cholesterol is left in the blood. Eating polyunsaturated oils to reduce blood cholesterol doesn't do a bit of good for your health. Actually, it causes more harm and increases the chance of packing more oxidized cholesterol and oxidized triglycerides (fatty acids) into the arteries.

As far back as 1965, studies have shown vegetable oils contribute to cardiovascular disease. But because they could also lower cholesterol, and everyone believed that lowering cholesterol was good, the bad side effects were ignored. For example, one study was conducted where volunteers ate either a diet high in saturated fat and cholesterol (the control group) or a low-fat diet supplemented with four teaspoons of corn oil per day. After two years, blood levels of cholesterol in the corn oil group went down, but the incidence of major cardiac events doubled![1] So even though polyunsaturated oil reduced the blood cholesterol, the incidence of heart disease increased over that of the saturated-fat diet.

There have been many studies that demonstrate that saturated fat is not nearly as bad as it has been made out to be. If saturated-fat consumption caused heart disease, then eliminating it from the diet would prevent the illness. The *Lancet* reported a study of 2,000 men who went on a low-saturated-fat diet to see how that would affect cardiovascular health. The study found that those participants who went on diets low in saturated fat didn't experience any reduction in heart attack death risk over a two-year period.[2] Again, there was no benefit in using polyunsaturated fats in place of saturated fats.

In a recent study published in the *Journal of Clinical Epidemiology*, researchers analyzed all published studies on saturated fat and polyunsaturated fat in relation to heart disease. The conclusion was that there was no positive correlation between saturated fat consumption and the occurrence of heart disease. In fact, in the larger and more recent studies they found that saturated fat appeared to have a protective effect against heart disease. They also found that polyunsaturated fats do not protect against heart disease.[3]

From the evidence presented it appears that vegetable oils contribute far more to the development of atherosclerosis and heart disease than might either cholesterol or saturated fat. It's no wonder the recommendation to cut back on these two fats has not produced any improvement in cardiovascular health and why heart disease is still our number one killer. Perhaps if we cut out the processed vegetable oils and stopped worrying about how much saturated fat and cholesterol we ate, the heart disease rate would finally come back down to levels before the "age of vegetable oils."

WHY YOU NEED SATURATED FAT

Although we don't normally think of saturated fat as an essential nutrient, it is just as important to health as any other nutrient. In fact, saturated fat is an essential component of every cell in your body. Cell membranes are made of at least 50% saturated fat. This is necessary to give our cells the stiffness and integrity they need to function properly. If your cells don't get enough saturated fatty acids to maintain structural integrity, they become soft and leaky. This can lead to tissue degeneration and malfunction. Every organ in your body is made of specialized cells that are designed to perform a specific task. If the cells in any organ do not perform the function for which they were designed, the entire organ becomes dysfunctional. Kidney failure results because the cells die or fail to perform properly. Liver disease is the result of cells becoming dysfunctional. All diseases are cellular diseases. Therefore, a healthy body requires

71

healthy organs, which require healthy cells. Your cells need saturated fat to be healthy. Every cell in every organ of your body needs saturated fat— your brain, liver, kidneys, lungs, heart, etc. Your brain is especially important because it is composed of about 60% fat, much of it saturated.

Saturated fat is necessary for proper bone development and for the prevention of osteoporosis. Many people are eating low-fat diets, and especially low-saturated-fat diets, and taking huge amounts of calcium supplements, yet they still suffer from osteoporosis. For calcium to be effectively incorporated into the bones, at least 50% of the fats in the diet need to be saturated.[4] Vegetarians usually consume smaller amounts of saturated fat than nonvegetarians. The consequence is that vegetarians are at greater risk of osteoporosis. In a study of Seventh-Day Adventists, who are generally vegetarians, it was shown that they were more likely to suffer from hip fractures than nonvegetarians.[5] If you want to prevent osteoporosis you need to be eating saturated fat.

Saturated fats support the immune system and help keep you healthy.[6] It is the immune system that fights off infections and keeps you safe from cancer. Having an adequate amount of saturated fat in your diet will help protect you from these problems.[7] Saturated fats protect the liver from the toxic effects of alcohol, drugs, and other toxins.[8, 9]

Contrary to popular opinion, saturated fatty acids can protect you against heart disease. Saturated fatty acids lower Lp(a), a substance in the blood that indicates susceptibility to heart disease.[10-12]

Do you need saturated fat to be healthy? Yes, especially if you want to avoid cancer, liver disease, osteoporosis, and a myriad of other health problems. Nature recognizes the importance of saturated fats. It is so important to proper function and good health that nature has incorporated saturated fat into almost all of the foods we eat both of animal and plant origin. Even the so-called polyunsaturated oils like safflower oil and corn oil contain saturated fat. Medical science acknowledges the need for saturated fat. The World Health Organization and the American Heart Association recommend that we get saturated fat in our diet to maintain optimal health. This type of information is usually ignored because recommending saturated fat is not the politically correct thing to do right now. Why has nature considered saturated fat so important to include it in all our foods? Nature doesn't do things just for the fun of it. In nature there is always a reason for everything. Nature doesn't put saturated fat in vegetables, mother's milk, and other foods for kicks. It's there for a reason. The reason is our bodies need saturated fat.

When you look at all the evidence, you will find that saturated fat is not as bad as it has been portrayed. In fact, it provides many health benefits. One of these is to protect you from the destructive action of free radicals caused by polyunsaturated fats. Saturated fat is not vulnerable to oxidation like unsaturated fats are and actually protects you against oxidation and free-radical formation. One of the consequences of destructive free radicals on our bodies is cancer. Saturated fat in the diet helps to protect against cancer.

In the 1950s and 1960s when saturated fat was first being associated with elevated cholesterol, researchers began looking for other effects caused by saturated fat. They reasoned that if excessive consumption of saturated fat increased blood cholesterol, it may be associated with other undesirable conditions as well. Researchers began studying the link between saturated fat and cancer. What they found surprised them. It appeared that saturated fat had a protective effect against cancer rather than a causative one when compared with other oils. Polyunsaturated oils were identified as *causing* cancer and the higher the degree of unsaturation, the greater the risk.[13] Other conditions such as asthma, allergies, memory loss, and senility also showed a greater degree of occurrence with polyunsaturated oils over saturated fat. It has later been determined that free radicals are largely to blame. Free radicals have also been linked to heart and other cardiovascular diseases.

Researchers have shown that saturated fatty acids in the diet of both animals and humans help to *prevent* stroke—a cardiovascular disease. In particular, Dr. Yamori reported decreased stroke incidence among rats fed a high-fat, high-cholesterol diet.[14] In addition, Dr. Ikeda demonstrated a decreased stroke risk among rats fed a diet high in milk fat.[15] Two studies in the 1980s from Japan found correlations between increased fat intake and decreased death from ischemic stroke in humans.[16, 17]

In another study of Japanese men living in Hawaii, intake of both total fat and saturated fat was inversely associated with all stroke mortality, after adjustment for multiple risk factors.[18] These studies were generally ignored because they were contrary to the prevailing belief that saturated fat promotes ischemic stroke rather than protects us from it.

On December 24, 1997, headlines around the world proclaimed that saturated fat *lowers* rate of strokes. This pronouncement came after the publication of a 20-year study performed by Dr. Matthew Gillman and colleagues at Harvard Medical School and published in the prestigious *Journal of the American Medical Association.*[19] The study involved 832 men aged 45 through 65 years who were initially free of cardiovascular disease. The results of the study raised howls of protest from health experts who had spent years trying to teach (brainwash) us to eat less saturated fat. Yet many researchers familiar with fat metabolism and cardiovascular disease were not surprised at the results of this study.

The purpose of the Harvard study was to examine the association of stroke incidence with intake of fat and type of fat during 20 years of follow-up among middle-aged men participating in the Framingham Heart Study. In conformity with other studies performed in Japan, intakes of saturated fat were associated with *reduced* risk of ischemic stroke in men. The study also showed that the *highest* incidence of stroke was associated with the most *polyunsaturated fat* consumption.

Again, polyunsaturated oils were linked to cardiovascular disease more than saturated fat. It's ironic that the oils that are safest to eat are condemned the most, and those that cause the most problems are hailed as "healthy."

When you take into account all the above facts, saturated fat becomes a relatively harmless food if eaten in moderation. In some cases it can even promote better health.

A NEW HEALTH FOOD

If you go to your local health food store, and in some cases your grocery store, you are likely to find a new, and rather curious, product on the shelves. It is being highlighted in magazines, health newsletters, and on the Internet. This product is selling so rapidly in some areas of the country that store owners can hardly keep it in stock. This remarkable product can protect you from the effects of many degenerative diseases, aid you in losing unwanted weight, give your skin a more youthful appearance, and help you feel years younger. Technically, it really isn't new, it's been used for thousands of years in the Far East, South Pacific, and elsewhere as a food and as a medicine. While not exactly new, its health benefits have only recently been discovered by the rest of the world. What is this amazing substance? This new health food, believe it or not, is coconut oil. Yes, ordinary coconut oil, which by the way, is predominantly a saturated fat.

As food, coconuts and coconut oil have been staples in the diets for many Polynesian and Asian peoples for thousands of years. It still is a major food source in Malaysia, Polynesia, and parts of the Philippines and India. Among these people, coconut oil has served as their sole source of cooking fat. Interestingly, the people who use these products have a much lower incidence of heart decease, hypertension, atherosclerosis, stroke, and cancer than those of us who eat modern foods, in which refined vegetable oils are the predominant dietary sources for fat.

These people have been consuming coconut and palm oil products in their daily diets without any ill effects on their health. In fact, they have

74

regarded coconut products as health foods with medicinal value. In traditional medical systems, such as Ayurveda in India, coconut oil enjoys a place of importance and is essential in some of the medicinal preparations. In some parts of the world coconut oil is consumed by the glass to fight off illness. Among the Islanders in the Pacific it is considered the cure for all disease. Over thousands of years these people have learned the health benefits of using coconut oil.

In the Western world, coconut oil has been branded a villain because of its high saturated fat content (as much as 92%). To date, there has been no study that can show that unadulterated coconut oil has any adverse health effects. (Some studies cleverly use *hydrogenated* coconut oil in order to manipulate data.) To the contrary, research has turned up many beneficial effects unique to the tropical oils.

THE PUKAPUKA AND TOKELAU ISLAND STUDIES

It has long been noted that people in Polynesia and Asia who consume large quantities of coconuts and coconut oil are surprisingly free from cardiovascular disease, cancer, and other degenerative diseases. Since saturated fat has been tagged as a major culprit in the development of these diseases, it seems an enigma that people who have diets higher in saturated fat than those in North America and Europe are much less prone to degenerative disease. Coconuts are used extensively in the diets of many people around the world. *In these populations coronary heart disease is rare.*

Some of the most thorough research conducted on people who have a high-fat diet derived primarily from coconuts are the Pukapuka and Tokelau Island studies. These studies involved many researchers and extended for over a decade.

The Islands of Pukapuka and Tokelau lie near the equator in the South Pacific. Pukapuka is an atoll in the Northern Cooks Islands and Tokelau, another atoll, lies about 400 miles southeast. The populations of both islands have been relatively isolated from Western influences. Their native diet and culture remain much as it has for centuries. Pukapuka and Tokelau are among the more isolated Polynesian islands and have had relatively little interaction with non-Polynesians.

The coral sands of these atolls are porous, lack humus, and will not support the food plants that flourish on other tropical islands. Coconut palms and a few starchy tropical fruits and root vegetables supply the vast majority of their diets. Fish from the ocean, pigs, and chickens make up what little meat they eat. Some flour, rice, sugar, and canned meat are obtained from small cargo ships that occasionally visit the islands.

The standard diets on both islands are high is saturated fat derived from coconuts. The diet is high in fiber, but low in sugar. The major food source is coconuts. Every meal contains coconut in some form: the green nut provides the main beverage; the mature nut, grated or as coconut cream, is cooked with taro root, breadfruit, or rice; and small pieces of coconut meat make an important snack food. Plants and fruitfish are cooked with coconut oil. In Tokelau, coconut sap or toddy is used as a sweetener and as leavening for bread.

The studies were begun in the early 1960s and included the entire populations of both islands. This was a long-term multidisciplinary study set up to examine the physical, social, and health consequences of migration from the atolls to New Zealand which has jurisdiction over the islands. The total population of the two islands consisted of about 2,500 people.

The overall health of both groups was good. There were no signs of kidney disease nor hypothyroidism that might influence fat levels. No hypercholesterolemia (high blood cholesterol). All inhabitants were lean and healthy despite a very high saturated-fat diet. In fact, the populations as a whole had ideal weight-to-height ratios as compared to the Body Mass Index figures used by nutritionists. Digestive problems were reported to be rare. Constipation was uncommon. They averaged two or more bowel movements a day. Atherosclerosis, heart disease, colitis, colon cancer, hemorrhoids, ulcers, diverticulosis, and appendicitis are conditions with which they were generally unfamiliar.

The American Heart Association recommends that we get no more than 30% of our total calories from fat and that saturated fat should be limited to no more than 10%. The Tokelauans apparently aren't aware of these guidelines, because about 60% of their energy is derived from fat, and most all of that is saturated fat largely derived from coconuts. The fat in the Pukapukan diet is also primarily from saturated fatty acids from coconut with total energy from fat being 34%.[20] Most Americans and others who eat typical Western diets get 30–35% of their calories from fat, most of which is in the form of *unsaturated* vegetable oils. And they suffer from numerous degenerative conditions and weight problems. The islanders in this study consumed as much or more total fat and a far greater amount of saturated fat. Yet, they are relatively free from degenerative disease and are generally lean and healthy.

Ian Prior, M.D., who headed some of the studies on these two island populations, stated: "Vascular disease is uncommon in both populations and there is no evidence of the high saturated-fat intake having a harmful effect in these populations."[21]

76

The migration of Tokelau Islanders from their island atolls to the very different environment of New Zealand is associated with changes in fat intake that indicate increased risk of atherosclerosis. This is associated with an actual *decrease* in saturated fat intake from 57% to around 41% of energy, an increase in dietary cholesterol intake and an increase in carbohydrate and sugar. The *total* fat content of their diet drops, declining from 63% in Tokelau, with 80% of that from coconut oil, to around 43% in New Zealand.[22] They eat more white bread, white rice, processed vegetable oils, and other Western foods and less of their high-fiber, coconut-rich foods.

Dr. Prior says, "The more an Islander takes on the ways of the West, the more prone he is to succumb to our degenerative diseases." He states that the further the Pacific natives move away from the diet of their ancestors, "the closer they come to gout, diabetes, atherosclerosis, obesity, and hypertension."[23]

The conclusion we can make from these island studies is that a high saturated-fat diet, particularly one consisting of coconut oil, is not detrimental to health and does not contribute to atherosclerosis. A diet rich in coconut oil and other natural foods offers protection from many health problems, including obesity, that are so common in modern society. Adding coconut oil to your diet is one of the healthiest things you can do for yourself and will assist you in taking off unwanted body fat and keeping it off.

THE MIRACLES OF COCONUT OIL

So much has been said against saturated fats over the years that the idea that all saturated fats are harmful is firmly entrenched in our minds. It may come as a surprise to you to learn that saturated fats aren't that bad and at least some can promote better health. There is one unique group of saturated fats that provides health benefits far beyond those of most all other fats. This class of saturated fats is known as medium-chain fatty acids (MCFA), also called medium-chain triglycerides (MCT).

Both saturated and unsaturated fats in our foods are composed almost entirely of long-chain fatty acids (LCFA). As the name implies, LCFA form relatively long molecules. Medium-chain fatty acids (MCFA), on the other hand, are much shorter. The length is important, because our bodies metabolize fats differently depending on their size. Only a very few foods contain any appreciable amount of the medium-chain fatty acids. By far the richest source of MCFA is found in the tropical oils and particularly coconut oil.

Researchers have discovered a multitude of health benefits associated with the medium-chain saturated fatty acids in coconut oil. Of particular importance is the fact that coconut oil can help you lose excess weight and keep it off. Some of the benefits of these fatty acids are briefly summarized below:

- Protects against viruses that cause mononucleosis, influenza, hepatitis C, measles, herpes, and other illnesses[24]
- Protects against bacteria that cause pneumonia, earache, throat infections, dental cavities, food poisoning, urinary tract infections, meningitis, gonorrhea, and dozens of other diseases[25]
- Protects against fungi and yeast that cause candidiasis, jock itch, ringworm, athlete's foot, thrush, diaper rash, and other infections[26]
- Expels or kills tapeworms, lice, giardia, and other parasites[27]
- Boosts energy and endurance[28]
- Improves insulin secretion and utilization of blood glucose[29]
- Reduces symptoms associated with pancreatitis[30]
- Improves calcium and magnesium absorption and supports the development of strong bones and teeth[31]
- Relieves symptoms associated with Crohn's disease, ulcerative colitis, and stomach ulcers[32]
- Reduces chronic inflammation[33]
- Supports and aids immune system function[34]
- Helps protect the body from breast, colon, and other cancers[35-38]
- Is heart healthy; does not increase blood cholesterol or platelet stickiness[39-45]
- Helps prevent heart disease, atherosclerosis, and stroke[46, 47]
- Functions as a protective antioxidant[48-51]
- Helps relieve symptoms associated with chronic fatigue syndrome[52]
- Reduces epileptic seizures[53]
- Helps protect against kidney disease and bladder infections[54]
- Helps protect the liver[55, 56]
- Is lower in calories than all other fats[57]
- Supports thyroid function[58]
- Promotes loss of excess weight by increasing metabolic rate[59]
- Is utilized by the body to produce energy in preference to being stored as body fat like other dietary fats[60-63]
- Helps prevent obesity and overweight problems[64-66]
- Softens skin and helps relieve dryness and flaking[67]
- Does not form harmful by-products when heated to normal cooking temperatures like other vegetable oils do[68]
- Has no harmful side effects[69]

The statements listed above are documented by research published in the medical literature. Reading through this list you can see that coconut oil offers a wide variety of health benefits. All it takes for you to enjoy these benefits is to try it yourself. Once you begin using it you'll see why so many people are embracing it as the new health food of the 21st century.

Below are some comments by professionals in the medical field who are familiar with dietary fats and the benefits of coconut oil:

"I use it on all my very sick patients. All my cancer patients get coconut oil and vegetables. I have to say, my HIV patients, even the full blown AIDS patients, my Crohn's disease patients, my chronic irritable bowel patients, my lupus patients, and my rheumatoid arthritic patients, every single one of them are improving."
—Eliezer Ben Joseph, N.D.
Natural Solutions

"Coconut oil is a thyroid-stimulating oil which helps balance thyroid function and also has antiseptic and immune-stimulating properties."
—Lita Lee, Ph.D.
Author of *The Enzyme Cure*

"Coconut and olive oil are the only vegetable oils that are really safe, but butter, which is highly saturated, is generally quite safe. For those of us who use coconut oil consistently, one of the most noticeable changes is the ability to go for several hours without eating, and to feel hungry without having symptoms of hypoglycemia."
—Ray Peat, Ph.D.
Author/researcher

"Clinically, the unique occurrence of medium-chain fatty acids in coconut oil confers on it desirable properties. These properties make it less prone to be deposited as fat in the peripheral tissues. It is also the easy and rapid digestibility, together with its relatively high content of vitamin E, which makes coconut oil a useful component of diets for the treatment of malnourished children. It was found that recovery of such children was facilitated by the inclusion of coconut oil in their diet. Other studies show that coconut oil possesses anti-carcinogenic properties."
—Robert L. Wickremasinghe, M.D.
Head of Serology Division, Medical Research Institute, Sri Lanka

"Coconut eating peoples like the Polynesians and Filipinos have low cholesterol, on the average, and very low incidence of heart disease... Folkloric and Ayurvedic writing are replete with accounts of the efficacy of the coconut for many ailments, from the cure of wounds, burns, ulcers, lice infestations to dissolution of kidney stones and treatment of choleraic dysentaries. The people of South Asia and the Pacific also look to the coconut as an important provider of food, drink, and fuels, not to mention its many uses in industry. Hence, it has been called the *tree of life*."

—Conrado S. Dayrit, M.D.

Emeritus Professor of Pharmacology, University of the Philippines

Past President, Federation of Asian Scientific Academies and Societies

Past President, National Academy of Science & Technology

"Medium-chain triglycerides (MCTs) are special types of saturated fats separated out from coconut oil... MCTs are used by the body differently from the long-chain triglycerides (LCTs) which are the most abundant fats found in nature. LCTs are the storage fat for both humans and plants. This difference in length makes all the difference in how MCTs and LCTs are utilized. Unlike regular fats, MCTs do not appear to cause weight gain, they actually promote weight loss."

—Michael T. Murray, N.D.

Professor of Naturopathic Medicine, Bastyr University

"Contrary to what is generally believed by both the lay public and medical profession the saturated fats found in coconut oil are actually good for you. This should not be surprising since Nature has always provided man with agents against illness. Historically coconut oil is one of the earliest oils to be used as a food and as a pharmaceutical. Ayrvedic literature long promoted the health and cosmetic benefits of coconut oil. Even today the Asian Pacific community, which may represent half the world's population, uses coconut oil in one form or another. Studies on people who live in tropical climates and who have a diet high in coconut oil are healthier, have less heart disease, cancer, and colon and prostate problems. It is rare in the history of medicine to find substances that have such useful properties and still be without toxicity or even harmful side effects."

Jon J. Kabara, Ph.D.

Emeritus Professor of Chemistry and Pharmacology,

Michigan State University

"Coconuts play a unique role in the diets of mankind because they are the source of important physiologically functional components. These physiologically functional components are found in the fat part of whole coconut, in the fat part of desiccated coconut, and in the extracted coconut oil. Lauric acid, the major fatty acid from the fat of the coconut, has long been recognized for the unique properties that it lends to nonfood uses in the soaps and cosmetics industry. More recently, lauric acid has been recognized for its unique properties in food use, which are related to its antiviral, antibacterial, and antiprotozoal functions. Also, recently published research has shown that natural coconut fat in the diet leads to a normalization of body lipids, protects against alcohol damage to the liver, and improves the immune system's anti-inflammatory response. Clearly, there has been increasing recognition of health-supporting functions of the fatty acids found in coconut."

—Mary G. Enig, Ph.D.
Fellow of The American College of Nutrition
President of the Maryland Nutritionists Association
Author of *Know Your Fats*

To adequately explain all the health benefits of coconut oil, as well as provide testimonials and success stories would require an entire book. If you are interested in learning more about the benefits of coconut oil and how it can improve your health, I highly recommend my book, *The Healing Miracles of Coconut Oil*. In this groundbreaking book I go into detail explaining why coconut oil is heart healthy and why you should be using it to prevent heart disease as well as cancer and many other health problems.

Chapter 6

CARBOHYDRATES: FRIEND OR FOE? ▪

THE SIMPLE AND THE COMPLEX

When you look at a hamburger what do you see? What makes a hamburger a hamburger? Most of us would see a skinny little meat patty stuck inside a bun with a dab of secret sauce and, if we're lucky, a pickle, diced onions, and a slice of tomato. If you were a dietitian you would view the meal differently. You would describe it in terms of its nutritional content: how much fat, protein, and carbohydrate it contains. The meat patty would represent the majority of the protein and fat. Fat would probably be included in secret sauce, since it would be mostly egg-based mayonnaise. The bun and veggies would comprise the carbohydrate.

The majority of the fat and protein in our diet comes from animal sources. Carbohydrate on the other hand, comes from plants. The only significant animal source for carbohydrate is milk. Next to water, carbohydrate is the most abundant substance found in plants. The wall that surrounds each plant cell and gives the plant structure and strength is made of carbohydrate. Plants also store carbohydrate as a source of energy. Seeds use carbohydrate for energy during germination. While plants do contain some protein, fat, and other substances, carbohydrate, in one form or another, is by far the most abundant. Carrots are mostly carbohydrate, so are onions, potatoes, cucumbers, as well as crabgrass, oak trees, and petunias.

When you eat *any* plant food, you are really eating *sugar*. Why? Because carbohydrates are nothing more than sugar. All carbohydrates, whether they come from an artichoke, a watermelon, or a tree stump are composed of simple sugars. Yes, the tree in your front yard is composed of sugar, so is the grass in your lawn and the weeds in your yard, so are the fruits, vegetables, grains, and nuts you eat every day. They are all basically sugar.

The technical name for sugar is saccharide. Saccharides form the building blocks for all carbohydrates. Carbohydrates come in different sizes; those that consist of a single molecule of sugar are called *mono*saccharides; those with two molecules of sugar are called *di*saccharides; and those forming long chains of sugar molecules are called *poly*saccharides.

Monosaccharides and disaccharides are referred to as sugars or *simple carbohydrates*. When eaten they produce a sweet taste. Examples are glucose, fructose, and sucrose. When you eat fruit, the sweet taste comes from simple carbohydrates. Polysaccharides are called *complex carbohydrates* because they may contain hundreds or even thousands of sugar molecules linked together. Starches for example, are composed of long chains of glucose molecules. Fiber, which is another complex carbohydrate, is also made of sugar. Squash and beans don't taste sweet because most all the sugars are tied up in complex carbohydrates.

THE PROCESS OF DIGESTION

Our bodies need sugar. Sugar is what keeps us alive and ticking. Now, before you get too excited and before you get the idea that the ideal diet is loaded with sugary foods like ice cream and Twinkies, let me explain. There is a difference between the way the body processes simple and complex carbohydrates.

When we eat carbohydrates digestive enzymes break the links that hold the sugar molecules together. Individual sugars are then released. These sugars are absorbed into the bloodstream. Glucose is absorbed by our cells and used as fuel. Other sugars, such as fructose and galactose, are picked up by the liver and converted into glucose. All sugar molecules are eventually converted into glucose.

Simple carbohydrates consist of only one or two molecules of sugar. They are instantly absorbed into the bloodstream. Starches and other complex carbohydrates take a longer time to break down into individual sugars. Small starches that may contain only 100 or so sugar molecules will digest quicker than larger ones that may contain a 1000 or more. The more "complex" the carbohydrate, the longer it takes the body to convert it to sugar. Foods in their natural form, such as whole wheat, are composed of a higher percentage of large complex carbohydrates. Processed foods, such as white bread, are less complex and digest quickly.

Some forms of carbohydrate, such as fiber, are not broken down into individual sugars and provide little or no energy or calories. Our bodies do not produce the enzymes needed to break down fiber. So fiber remains intact as it travels through the stomach and small intestine. When it finally reaches the large intestine (colon), bacteria there partially digest it and use it for their own nourishment. In this process the bacteria produce some vitamins and other nutrients that are absorbed and utilized by us. In this way, we form a symbiotic relationship with the bacteria where we both live together in a mutually beneficial way. We provide the bacteria a home and food, and they produce vitamins for our use.

Fiber and complex carbohydrates slow down the digestive process. Sugars from complex carbohydrates are released over an extended length of time (2–3 hours). This allows the sugar to enter the bloodstream at a moderate and relatively even rate. Sugars from simple and processed carbohydrates (e.g., refined grains) are released very quickly. A surge of sugar is dumped almost immediately into the bloodstream. Blood sugar soars dangerously high. The body immediately kicks into a feverish level of activity to move glucose out of the blood and into the cells. This process creates a tremendous amount of stress. This stress is often manifested as a surge and then a rapid drop in energy followed by feelings of hunger. Headaches, irritability, nervousness, and depression may also occur.

If the body is continually put in a state of stress by eating lots of sweets and refined grains, something has to happen. Something is going to give. It is like trying to run a 26-mile marathon every day. Even if you are healthy and in shape you could not do it day after day. If you try, it wouldn't be long before your muscles give out, injury occurs, or you become ill.

Likewise, when you eat processed carbohydrates on a regular basis, headaches, irritability, and other symptoms mentioned above may intensify. Tissues and organs may degenerate or lose sensitivity and become less responsive, which could lead to obesity, high blood pressure, hypoglycemia, and diabetes and all the health problems associated with these conditions.

One of the most significant effects from eating refined carbohydrates is weight gain. You will gain more weight eating carbohydrates than you will fat or protein. One of the primary reasons for this is that refined carbohydrates digest very quickly, causing blood sugar to rapidly rise and drop. The drop in blood sugar sends a signal to the brain to eat, thus creating feelings of hunger. So within a couple of hours after eating, you're hungry again. You can stuff yourself silly with breads and sweets, yet in a few hours you will be starving again. We eat between meals to satisfy hunger and if we hold out until the next meal, we are so famished we overeat. In either case we consume more calories than if we ate foods rich in fat, protein, and fiber.

Our bodies were never meant to consume simple and refined carbohydrates on a daily basis. Most natural carbohydrates found in vegetables, grains, and even fruits are complex and digest slowly. Fruits which do contain some simple carbohydrates, are always accompanied by complex carbohydrates and fiber which help to slow down and modulate sugar absorption.

HEALTH BENEFITS OF WHOLE FOODS

Hardly a day goes by that I don't read how eating complex carbohydrate foods—whole grains, fruits, or vegetables—lowers the risk of some type of degenerative disease. For example, recently I read that fruits and vegetables may reduce the risk of oral precancerous lesions in tobacco users. I also read a study showing that just one additional daily serving of fruit or vegetables a day lowers the risk of heart disease, and a greater consumption affords greater protection.

In another study researchers found that the risk of stroke was 31% lower in women who consumed five or more servings of fruit and vegetables per day. In still another study, those who ate legumes at least four times a week had a 22% lower risk of heart disease over those who consumed legumes only once a week. Those who ate the most legumes also had lower blood pressure and total cholesterol, and were less likely to be diagnosed with diabetes.

The evidence is so strong that some researchers are now suggesting that we try to eat *nine* daily servings of fruits and vegetables a day. Few of us, however, eat this much produce. A recent survey reported that only 19% of men and 26% of women in the US eat *five* or more servings of fruits and vegetables a day. If people are not eating fruits and vegetables, what are they eating? Most likely lots of processed, packaged foods which have been stripped of most of their nutrients.

Why are whole grains, fruits, and vegetables so good for us? The answer is because they contain the vitamins, minerals, and phytonutrients that nourish our bodies, protect us from disease, and keep us healthy. Phytonutrients are chemicals produced in plants that have vitamin-like characteristics. One of these is beta-carotene. Beta-carotene acts as an antioxidant and helps protect us from cancer and heart disease. It can also be converted into vitamin A if the body needs it. Beta-carotene gives carrots, squash, and other vegetables their characteristic yellow and orange colors. Lycopene is another phytonutrient that has gained recognition lately for its ability to lower the risk of prostate cancer. It produces the red pigment in tomatoes, watermelon, and pink grapefruit. There are over 20,000 phytonutrients that have been identified in plant foods.

In the past, individual vitamins and minerals were thought to be adequate in curing health problems. We now know that while a single nutrient may be helpful, a variety of nutrients working together provides the greatest benefit. Nutrients work together in concert like a philharmonic orchestra producing music. All of the instruments are needed to produce the right sound. Likewise, a wide variety of nutrients is needed, in the proper proportion, like that found in whole foods, to provide the health benefits scientists see in nutritional studies.

We've been told for years to eat more calcium to protect our bones from osteoporosis. We eat more calcium than ever before, yet osteoporosis is still a growing problem. We now know that calcium alone isn't going to do it. You can eat calcium tablets until your are blue in the face and it won't have much effect on your bones unless you also include other nutrients. Researchers are now saying potassium, magnesium, boron, silicon, beta-carotene, and vitamins C, D, and K are also necessary. A deficiency in any one of these could affect bone health.

This is why it is better to eat food containing *hundreds* of phytochemicals than take a vitamin tablet which only has a dozen or so. This is why it is better to eat bread made from whole wheat flour than white flour which has had some 20 nutrients removed in the refining process.. This is why fresh fruits and vegetables are superior to processed, packaged foods containing refined carbohydrates.

SUGARS AND SWEETENERS
The Monsters Among Us

Do you remember the classic horror story of Frankenstein's monster? In this tale a scientist, Dr. Frankenstein, attempted to create a living human being from the body parts of cadavers. In his attempt to create life he went against the order of nature. He succeeded, but his creation was not a normal functional human, but a mentally distorted monster. When this monster was free to roam the countryside he began killing innocent people.

We have in the food industry a similar situation. Scientists are creating Frankenfoods. Like Dr. Frankenstein, scientists start off with real foods, strip them of nutrients and fiber, combine the lifeless residue with chemical additives, synthetic vitamins, and artificial flavors, and create foods never seen before in nature or eaten by man or beast. This new food only resembles the real thing. When sent out to retail markets throughout the land, like Frankenstein's monster, it stirs up trouble.

Frankenfoods work their mischief slowly, causing obesity, sickness, and premature death. They kill by denying people the nutrients they need to achieve and maintain good health and proper weight. The process is so gradual that many people don't recognize that what they're eating is slowly killing them.

A rule of thumb to protect you from the Frankenfoods that lurk inside grocery stores awaiting their next victim is to keep in mind that the more processing a food undergoes the less healthy it becomes. All the health benefits attributed to whole grains and vegetables are lost when foods are overly processed, refined, and manipulated. Whole wheat is turned into white flour by stripping it of most of its fiber and nutrients, leaving a nutritionally depleted starch.

Sugar is even worse. Like Frankenstein's monster who was made from real body parts, sugar comes from real food. Sugar can be made from corn, beets, rice, and other carbohydrate-rich foods. Beets, for example, start off as healthy food full of vitamins, minerals, and fiber. All of these nutrients are removed as beets are transformed into sugar. What remains when all the nutrients are removed is a white crystalline powder which acts more like a drug than it does a food. It stimulates pleasure centers in the brain, creating sugar addictions and destroying health.

Sugar by Any Other Name Is Still Sugar

The sweetener which we are all most familiar with and which serves as the standard upon which all others are compared is white or table sugar. Table sugar is 100% sucrose. It is the single most widely used sweetener. Regardless of the source, most natural and refined sweeteners are primarily sucrose. Brown sugar, corn syrup, honey, and maple syrup are all primarily sucrose.

You will often hear that natural sweeteners are better than refined. The only advantage that natural sweeteners have is that they are less processed and, therefore, retain some of their nutritional value, but it isn't much. The most commonly used natural sweeteners are: raw honey, unrefined maple syrup, sucanat (raw sugar from sugarcane), chopped dried dates, fruit juice, barley malt, brown rice syrup, and molasses. Like most sweeteners, these are made primarily of sucrose.

In addition to the sugars listed above, you may find others included on ingredient labels such as: dextrin, dextrose, fructose, glucose, and maltodextrin. Some of these sugars differ slightly from sucrose, but they are all sugars and all are empty calories.

Sugar in one form or another has found its way into a wide variety of foods. Besides the obvious candy and desserts, sugar is found hidden in many of our "non-sweet" foods. It is by far the most common food additive. You can find it in processed meats, baked goods, cereals, catsup and barbecue sauce, peanut butter, spaghetti sauce, canned goods, and frozen foods; it's even added to canned and frozen fruits. It's hard to find a packaged, prepared food which doesn't contain sugar or some other sweetener. Even nonfood items like toothpaste, mouthwash, chewing gum, and vitamins contain sweeteners.

What's so bad about sugar? After all it doesn't cause cancer or seizures like artificial sweeteners. The sugar debate has raged for years. On one hand, you have people that say there is nothing wrong with sugar; it's natural, the body converts carbohydrate and protein into sugar for use as energy. Our cells need sugar to fuel metabolism.

On the other hand, others point out that sugar is digested and pumped into the bloodstream almost immediately. This creates a drug-like reaction which stresses the hormonal system; creates dangerous swings in blood sugar levels; promotes diabetes; leads to increased feelings of hunger; depresses immune function making us more vulnerable to infection; and creates numerous distressing physical and emotional symptoms. Sugar stimulates sweet cravings and encourages overeating which contributes to overweight. Sugar drains the body of nutrients. Sugar supplies no nutritive value itself, but requires the body to use up nutrients as it is metabolized, thus depleting nutrient stores. If an adequate intake of nutrients from wholesome foods is not obtained, the body can become nutrient-deficient. So sugar contributes to nutrient deficiencies.

Many people are surprised to learn that sugar consumption dramatically inhibits immune function. The ingestion of sugar in any form—sucrose, fructose, honey, etc.—significantly reduces the ability of white blood cells to destroy bacteria. Sugar begins to suppress the immune system within thirty minutes after you eat it, and the effects last for over five hours. Impairing the activity of the immune system leaves the body vulnerable to increased chances of infection. People who eat sugary foods at mealtime and for snacks constantly keep their immune systems depressed.

Whether you eat table sugar, honey, or molasses makes little difference. Sugar by any other name is still sugar.

Fructose

If you read ingredient labels you will frequently come across the word "fructose." Fructose is found in all types of foods from "health" foods and dietary supplements to junk foods and candy. Fructose has gained a reputation as a "good" sugar primarily because it doesn't raise blood sugar and insulin levels like table sugar does. For this reason, it has been the sugar of choice for many diabetics. Another reason fructose has become popular with the public is because it is perceived to be more natural than sucrose (table sugar) and more healthy. It is often called "fruit" sugar implying that its origin is from fruit rather than sugarcane or sugar beets and, therefore, is a less processed or more natural sweetener.

Unfortunately most of this is untrue. Fructose is not, by any stretch of the imagination, a "natural" sugar, is not extracted from fruit, and is one of the last sweeteners a diabetic should ever use. The reason for much of this misinformation and its popularity is due to clever marketing tactics by the sugar industry. Fructose is preferred over sucrose as a sweetener by food producers for the simple reason that it is cheaper. Economics, not health, is at issue here. Fructose is much sweeter than sucrose and, therefore, can sweeten foods at less expense.

The biggest myth about fructose is that it is fruit sugar and comes from fruit. Fructose is not made from fruit. It comes from corn syrup, sugarcane, and sugar beets, just like any other sugar. The similarity between the names fructose and fruit helps to perpetuate this myth. I've heard many a health food and supplement salesperson claim their product was superior to others because it was made with fruit sugar, meaning fructose.

Fructose is one of the most extremely refined sugars in existence. Sucrose or table sugar is composed of equal parts fructose and glucose. In order to make fructose, you must refine sugar cane or corn, down to sucrose first. Then you must process and refine it further, splitting the sucrose molecule into fructose and glucose. Fructose is so highly refined that it cannot be reduced into a simpler sugar. It's as refined as it gets. To say that fruit contains fructose is technically true. The natural sugar in fruit is mostly sucrose, and all sucrose, whether it comes from fruit or corn syrup, is 50% fructose.

Another problem with fructose is that while it doesn't affect blood sugar and insulin levels like sucrose, it has a more detrimental effect on insulin resistance which increases the risk of a number of health problems like heart disease, high blood pressure, and diabetes. Studies on animals and humans have shown that consuming large amounts of fructose impairs the body's ability to properly handle glucose (blood sugar) which ultimately leads to hyperinsulinemia (elevated insulin levels) and the development of insulin resistance. This fact is so well established now that researchers purposely use fructose to induce insulin resistance to create high blood pressure and diabetes in laboratory animals. Some physicians are now claiming that the increased use of fructose in all our foods is largely

89

responsible for the skyrocketing incidence of diabetes we are experiencing now.

Fructose has also been shown to increase the rate at which fats in our body undergo peroxidation which produces destructive free radicals. It adversely affects blood lipids and blood pressure, increasing risk of cardiovascular disease and interfering with nutrient absorption.[1]

Nutritionists have been aware of the health problems associated with sucrose for some time. Until recently fructose was considered a much healthier alternative. As questions about the safety of fructose began to emerge, researchers wanted to know whether it was the fructose or the glucose in the sucrose that was causing the problems. An idea of just how bad fructose is was revealed by a team of USDA researchers led by Dr. Meira Field. They conducted studies with two groups of healthy rats, one given high amounts of glucose in their food and one given high amounts of fructose. Researchers found no change among the animals in the glucose group. However, in the fructose group the results were disastrous. Young male rats were unable to survive to adulthood. They suffered from anemia, high cholesterol, and heart hypertrophy (their hearts enlarged until they ruptured). They also had delayed testicular development. Dr. Field explains that fructose in combination with copper deficiency in the growing animals interfered with collagen production. Collagen provides the protein matrix upon which all organs and tissues are built. In humans copper deficiency is common among those who eat a lot of processed convenience foods, as most of us do. The rats' bodies more or less just fell apart. The females were not as severely affected, but they were unable to produce live young.

"The medical profession thinks fructose is better for diabetics than sugar," says Dr. Field, "but every cell in the body can metabolize glucose. However, all fructose must be metabolized in the liver. The livers of the rats on the high fructose diet looked like the livers of alcoholics, plugged with fat and cirrhotic."[2]

After looking at all the evidence, fructose has emerged as a much more detrimental sweetener than table sugar. It's best to stay away from it.

Artificial Sweeteners

Even after all the processing and refining sugar goes through, it still retains calories. So scientists have continued to perfect their Frankenfoods to create a sugar with fewer calories. And they have succeeded. If real sugar wasn't bad enough, we can now "enjoy" artificial sugar—aspartame, saccharin, and such. These man-made products have the sweetness of sugar yet fewer calories. Like sugar these crystalline powders are just as addictive but even more detrimental to health. Yes, they contain fewer calories than sugar, but like any drug, they have undesirable side effects that range from headaches to death.

Artificial sweeteners are the ultimate in Frankenfoods. They are created in a laboratory from components derived from a variety of sources much like Frankenstein's monster. The end product looks like sugar, tastes like sugar, and can be used to sweeten foods just like sugar, but without the calories in sugar. In fact, compared to sugar, artificial sweeteners have almost no calories. Sounds like a dieter's dream, but in reality it's a nightmare. Artificial sweeteners have a dark side much more sinister than sugar.

Sugar, even as refined as it is, is still a product the body recognizes and can process, even though the processing causes the body a great deal of stress and drains nutrients. Artificial sweeteners, on the other hand, are strange new creatures the human body has never seen before and isn't programmed to handle safely or efficiently. This creates problems. While the materials that scientists use to make artificial sweeteners may come from "natural" sources, they are combined into unique chemicals that are unnatural and cause all types of mischief.

The most widely used artificial sweetener is aspartame. Aspartame is sold under the brand names NutraSweet, Equal, Spoonful, and Equal-Measure. Discovered in 1965, it was approved for use as a food additive in the US in the early 1980s. The US Food and Drug Administration (FDA) allowed its use even under the heavy criticism by several scientists who warned of its dangers. Despite objections, approval was granted based on research funded by aspartame's manufacturer (Monsanto and its subsidiary, The NutraSweet Company).

Since its approval, aspartame has accounted for over 75% of the adverse reactions to food additives reported to the FDA. Many of these reactions have been serious enough to cause seizures and death. At least 90 different symptoms have been documented as being caused by aspartame. Some of these include: headaches/migraines, dizziness, seizures, nausea, numbness, muscle spasms, rashes, depression, fatigue, irritability, tachycardia, insomnia, vision problems, hearing loss, heart palpitations, breathing difficulties, anxiety attacks, slurred speech, loss of taste, tinnitus, vertigo, memory loss, joint pain, and, believe it or not, weight gain.[3] In addition, aspartame has triggered or worsened brain tumors, multiple sclerosis, epilepsy, chronic fatigue syndrome, Parkinson's disease, Alzheimer's disease, birth defects, fibromyalgia, and diabetes. Would any sane person knowingly eat a substance that caused or even contributed to these types of problems? The justification given to use aspartame even though it is known to cause adverse reactions is that this is a small price to pay in order to lose excess weight. The potential benefit it *might* have in helping people lose a few pounds is worth the risk, or so says the manufacturer and the doctors and researchers funded by them. Sure it's worth the risk for the people who benefit financially, but not for those people who lose their health in the process. It's interesting to note that one of the reported side effects of aspartame is weight gain! So why use it at all?

Aspartame is a relative newcomer compared to saccharin. Discovered in 1879, saccharin was the first of the artificial sweeteners. In 1937 cyclamate came on the scene. This was followed by aspartame in the 1960s and more recently acesulfame K and sucralose. These artificial sweeteners are many times sweeter than sugar. Saccharin has a sweetening power 300 times that of table sugar. Cyclamate is about 30 times as sweet as sugar and aspartame is 200 times sweeter. Gram for gram these sweeteners contain about the same number of calories as sugar, but since they are so much sweeter, only a fraction of the amount is needed for the same effect. This feature makes artificial sweeteners enticing for dieters. Their popularity has soared as waistlines have expanded.

Saccharin and cyclamate have fallen in stature since the late 1960s when it was discovered that they caused tumorous growths in laboratory animals. Cyclamate was banned in the US in 1970, although it has remained

FRANKENFOODS

Frankenfoods are those food products which are overprocessed, highly refined, or chemically altered. The most common include:

- White flour products
- Refined sugars (sucrose, fructose, corn syrup, etc.)
- Artificial sweeteners
- Artificial fats (olestra, etc.)
- Partially hydrogenated vegetable oil
- Margarine
- Shortening
- Processed, refined vegetable oils (canola, corn, soybean, safflower, etc.)
- Processed lunch meats (hot dogs, balogna, pepperoni, beef sticks, etc.)
- Powdered/dehydrated milk, eggs, cheese, and butter
- Pasteurized, homogenized milk

in limited use in the United Kingdom and Canada. In Canada it is only allowed as a tabletop sweetener on the advice of a physician and as an additive in medicines.

In 1977 a ban was also proposed for saccharin. Since it was the only remaining artificial sweetener in use at the time many people opposed the ban, claiming the action was unfair to diabetics and the overweight. In response to the public outcry the ban was put on hold. Instead of the ban, products containing saccharin are required to carry a warning which reads "use of this product may be hazardous to your health. This product contains saccharin, which has been determined to cause cancer in laboratory animals." Saccharin, however, is banned completely in Canada.

Acesulfame K which was approved by the FDA a few years ago is of the same general chemical family as saccharin. It has the same potential drawbacks as saccharin in regards to cancer. Like saccharin, it also stimulates insulin secretion which makes it less desirable for diabetes.

The newest kid on the block is sucralose known by the trade name Splenda. It has been in use in Canada for about 10 years. It is 600 times sweeter than sugar. This chemical sweetener is so alien to our bodies that the digestive system doesn't know what to do with it. It travels through the digestive tract without being absorbed. Thus it provides no calories and does not affect insulin or blood sugar levels and, therefore, is considered safe for diabetics. Sound too good to be true? Judging from the track record of all other artificial sweeteners, it is too good to be true. It is still too early yet to know of all the health problems it may cause.

The main reason people use artificial sweeteners is to reduce total calorie consumption in an effort to control weight. Some people are so desperate to reduce calories that they ignore health warnings and consume artificial sweeteners anyway. They willingly take the risk of getting cancer or suffering from any number of discomforting symptoms just so they can enjoy sweet foods. Cravings for sweets can be very powerful. So powerful, in fact, that we throw good sense out the window and gamble with our health.

Artificial sweeteners are not the answer to weight problems and do not provide any real benefit. All sweets, including artificial sweeteners, keep sweet cravings alive and desensitize our taste receptors. Both of these conditions encourage the over-consumption of sweet foods. Sweet cravings drive us to seek out and consume sweet foods whether we are hungry or not. As we eat more and more sweets our taste buds become desensitized to them. It takes a larger dose of sugar or artificial sweetener to get the same degree of sweetness. As we develop a taste for highly sweetened foods, we lose our taste for less sweet, natural foods. Natural foods lose their appeal and artificial or manufactured foods full of sweeteners and flavor enhancers are preferred. Give an average kid a choice between a fresh juicy peach and a chocolate sundae topped with whipped cream, and guess which one he will choose? Nine times out of ten it will be the ice cream. The peach isn't sweet or tasty enough. He would only eat it if there weren't another choice. We do the same thing. As adults we have a choice of the foods we eat. Yet we generally choose the highly sweetened, manufactured foods (which are generally high in calories and low in nutrition) over fresh, wholesome foods. Replacing sugar with an artificial sweetener doesn't do a thing to curb sweet cravings or to resensitize our sweet receptors.

Artificial sweeteners also give a false sense of security. We drink a diet soda and then feel it's okay to eat foods we shouldn't. The American Cancer Society has reported that people who use artificial sweeteners actually gain *more* weight than those who avoid them.[4] If you're trying to lose weight or maintain your weight, artificial sweeteners are not the way to go; they aren't effective and can cause serious harm.

If you're not convinced that artificial sweeteners are harmful, and you're using them to control your weight, I recommend that you read *Excitotoxins: The Taste That Kills* by Dr. Russell L. Blaylock, a professor of neurosurgery at the Medical University of Mississippi. This book provides details on the medical research documenting the dangers of aspartame and other food additives.

Stevia

Just when you were beginning to think that all sweeteners were probably bad, along comes stevia. Stevia is a different kind of sweetener. It's actually an herb that grows in South America. It's similar to artificial sweeteners in that it is many times sweeter than sugar with essentially no calories. Yet it is unlike other sweeteners in that it appears to have no adverse health effects and is nonaddicting. Many consider it nature's sugar substitute.

Stevia comes from a small shrub that grows in Paraguay and Brazil where it is known as the "sweet herb." Its leaves have a sweetness about 30 times sweeter than sugar. The Guarani Indians who live in the region have been using the herb for centuries. It is highly regarded among them as both a sweetener and as a medicine. It is used to sweeten beverages, to disinfect wounds, and as a tonic to improve digestion.

Ground or whole stevia leaf makes a good sweetener for herbal teas and strong beverages. Stevia used in leaf form is not practical for most other situations because it tastes too much like an herb. A more useable form is stevia extract. The extract is a concentrate of the phytochemicals (steviosides) which give the plant its sweetness. Stevia extract is 200 to 300 times sweeter than sugar and does not have a leafy taste. The extract is available in either a powder or liquid. Because of its sweetness, only a small amount is needed to sweeten foods. About $1/4$ to $1/2$ teaspoon of stevia extract can replace one cup of sugar.

Stevia extract has been used as a sweetener in Japan, Taiwan, Korea, Paraguay, Brazil, and Israel for many years. Japan has been using it since the mid-1970s. Instead of aspartame they use stevia to sweeten low-calorie foods. It's used commercially in chewing gum, candy, soft drinks, juices, frozen desserts, and baked goods. Stevia makes up 50% of the high-intensity sweeteners used in Japan.

Is it safe? It seems to be. We know that it does not have the undesirable effects that sugar has nor does it pose the same health dangers that artificial sweeteners do. Stevia has been used for centuries in South America and for the past 25 years in Japan and other countries without any noticeable harm. The Japanese consume the largest quantity of the sweetener in the world and have reported no ill effects. Extensive research and safety testing has been done on stevia. None of these tests have shown any harmful effects, even at very large doses normally given to lab animals. Few substances can make this claim. Testing so far has shown the herb and extract to be non-toxic and beneficial as a means to help reduce calorie consumption. It does not affect blood sugar or insulin levels, so is safe for diabetics. It does not feed yeast like sugar so it is a perfect sweetener for candida sufferers. In many ways it is far superior to both sugar and artificial sweeteners.

In recent years stevia has been growing in popularity in the US. The FDA, however, does not permit it to be labeled as a sweetener. Since there is no medical or scientific reason for this restriction it is believed by many that the makers of aspartame have pressured the FDA to take this action in order to prevent competition. Stevia is currently sold as a dietary supplement like any other herb or herbal extract. You can find it available at most any health food store.

It is difficult to overuse stevia. If you use too much it produces a sharp, molasses-like aftertaste. So you use just enough to sweeten your foods without getting the strong aftertaste. This takes a little practice. I suggest you learn how to use it from one of the many stevia cookbooks that are available. I list a few in the Resource section at the back of this book.

OVERCOMING SUGAR ADDICTION

Our love affair for sweets has created a society of sugaraholics. Sugar and artificial sweeteners are dangerously addicting much like narcotics. As with cocaine and other drugs they stimulate pleasure centers in the brain. The desire for this pleasurable sensation can become so intense that it controls our thoughts and actions just like cocaine controls an addict. We get sweet cravings and uncontrollable urges. We can be going along fine and then all of the sudden we get a desire to eat something sweet. It can be a candy bar, chewing gum, coffee, or a soda, anything just so long as we get a sugar fix. Because sugar stimulates feelings of pleasure, even when we are full we often continue to eat sweet foods. How many times have you been full but just had to have dessert? Or you weren't feeling hungry but couldn't resist the temptation of a sweet treat that is placed in your view? Or began eating something sweet, such as a cookie, thinking you'll only eat one or maybe two at most, but end up devouring nine or ten? No, you couldn't eat just one. The sweet taste often overpowers good intentions, sound reasoning, and the strongest will power. If you can identify with any of these situations you've become a slave to sugar.

Sweets have never been a major source of food in the human diet. In the past, fruit provided the majority of our sweets. Since fruit was only available during the summer it was only eaten a few months out of the year. The lack of refrigeration prevented the storage of fruits for long periods of time. While refined sugar has been around for a couple of centuries it never was a major part of the diet. In the 1890s the average yearly consumption of sugar was only 5 pounds per person. Since that time annual consumption of sweeteners (including artificial sweeteners) has risen to about 160 pounds per person. We eat over 30 times the amount of sweeteners as our great-grandparents did. Considering there are 365 days in a year, on average we consume nearly a *half pound* of sugar and other sweeteners each day! Can you imagine eating that much sugar? This is an average. Some people eat much more. We surely have become a society of sugaraholics. Oh, how we love that sweet taste!

One of the big problems with both sugar and artificial sweeteners is that because they stimulate pleasure centers in our brain we tend to overeat. Most sweetened foods are high in calories and low in nutrition. Therefore, we tend to fill up on nutritionally deficient, calorie-rich, artificially flavored foods, leaving little room for nutritionally dense, high-fiber, wholesome foods. When children grow up eating nutritionally poor foods, these are the foods they learn to like. Consequently, as they become adults they continue to eat these types of foods and suffer the consequences of poor health and obesity as a result. With each succeeding generation we eat more and more refined, processed foods and less and less whole, natural foods. Kids nowadays are fatter than ever before. So are adults.

Another problem with eating a lot of sweetened foods is that they desensitize our taste receptors. As a consequence, sweets don't taste as sweet. Foods don't taste as good. You might wonder why taste receptors would become desensitized to sweets. I like to explain this using an analogy with another one of our senses—smell. It's like walking into a closed room that has a bad odor. When you first enter the room the smell may be overpowering. But if you remain in the room for any length of time the receptors in your nose become less sensitive and you no longer notice the smell. The smell in the room may not have gotten any less, but your ability to detect the smell has decreased. As long as you are exposed to the odor your nose remains desensitized. If you leave the room for a while and give your nose a break, it recovers and becomes resensitized, so that if you returned to the room with the offensive odor you will again notice the smell. In like manner, the sweet receptors in our mouths become dulled or desensitized when they are constantly bathed in sugary foods. Overstimulation causes them to become less sensitive to sweets. In response, we often increase the intensity of the sweets in our foods. This desensitizes the sweet receptors even more.

Like a drug addict that needs a larger and larger dose to achieve the same effect, we need more and more sugar in our foods in order to detect the same level of sweetness or get the same amount of pleasure. After awhile, natural foods, like fresh fruits, gradually become less appealing. This is one reason why sugar is often added to frozen fruit. Fresh fruit isn't sweet enough so sugar is added to make it more appealing. Canned fruits have syrup added to sweeten them up. We've become so accustomed to sweetened fruits that natural fruits begin to taste bland.

Desensitizing taste receptors also makes vegetables and other natural foods less appealing. Kids nowadays don't like vegetables. In our great-grandparents' day kids ate their vegetables, they didn't turn up their noses to peas and broccoli like they do now. Nor did they get soda pop, candy, and sugar-coated breakfast cereal every day either. Kids don't like vegetables because their taste buds are desensitized by eating too much sugar and artificial flavor enhancers. Many adults don't care much for vegetables for the same reason. If fresh unsweetened fruits and vegetables aren't appealing to you, you're not going to eat them. Instead, what you wind up eating are less healthy foods which keep your sweet cravings alive and active.

One of the key ingredients to a successful weight loss program is gaining control over your sweet tooth. If you can harness your cravings for sweets, you will automatically eat less food. The only way to fight sweet cravings is to nip it in the bud—the taste bud that is. If you remove the desire for sweets, they lose their power and control over you. This can be done. The key is abstinence, just like for any other drug addiction. Abstain from using sweeteners or eating sweet foods for a period of time. I recommend a period of at least six weeks. Six months is better. The longer you can go without eating any foods with added sweeteners, the more your taste receptors will recover and resensitize themselves. Abstaining from sweets is like leaving a smelly room and having your sense of smell restored. When you refrain from eating sweets your taste receptors can recover.

When you do add sweeteners back into your diet you will find that you don't need as much as you did in the past. Not only will sweets taste sweeter, you will find that all foods taste better. You'll begin to appreciate the natural sweetness of peas, squash, and fresh fruits. You won't need as much sweetener as you did before in order to enjoy certain foods. In fact, commercially sweetened foods will taste too sweet. This fact was brought home to me some time ago. After not eating any sweetened foods (other than fruits occasionally) for several months my wife and I decided to reward our good efforts by buying a pint of Haagen-Dazs ice cream and splitting it. We purchased vanilla with almonds because we thought it would not be as rich as the other flavors. When we began eating we both noticed how overly sweet it tasted. We'd eaten this flavor many times before in the past, but now it seemed so sweet as to lose its appeal. Neither one of use could even finish the serving. We ended up throwing it away. Can you believe it, throwing away Haagen-Dazs ice cream? From that time on, I've had little desire to eat commercially made ice cream again. It has lost its appeal for us, for which I was happy because we are better off not eating it. On occasion we do eat homemade ice cream made with real cream, sweetened with a tiny bit of stevia, and topped with fresh fruit. It's not too sweet and tastes great.

I notice the same thing whenever I eat white bread, which isn't very often. Commercially made white bread, which almost always has added sugar, often tastes overly sweet. It's more like candy or sweet bread than just plain bread. All commercially made treats taste too sweet to me now, and they will to you too, when you break the sugar habit.

Artificial sweeteners should be completely avoided all the time. Natural sweeteners, such as raw honey and molasses, should be used in preference over the highly refined ones. As you resensitize your taste receptors you will lose your desire for sweets. You will no longer have cravings. When you come face to face with sweet treats in the course of your day, you will not be drawn in by their beckoning call. You will have the will power to resist and not feel deprived because you have full control over your actions.

Many people blame fat for making them fat. Fat isn't the culprit; sugar is a more likely candidate. Sugar is the number one cause for overweight because, like a drug, it creates addiction. If you are going to lose weight, and lose it permanently, you *must* conquer your sweet tooth. The only way to do that is through abstinence. Using so-called natural sweeteners in place of refined sugar won't do it. Switching to artificial sweeteners won't do it. Consumption of all sweets needs to be curtailed.

Once you've broken the grip sugar has over you, keep in mind that sugar addiction is like alcoholism. A recovered alcoholic can relapse with just a few drinks. Likewise, a sugaraholic can relapse with just a few sweets. Even when you break the sugar habit, sweets may always retain some allure, but they won't control you as they once did. You will be able to resist them as long as you don't fall prey to their enticements.

Does this mean you can never eat sweets again? For some people maybe so. Others may be able to handle a little sweetening or a treat now and then, but it is so easy to fall into the habit of eating sweetened foods that it is best to stay away from them as much as possible. Fruits or foods sweetened with a little whole fruit are okay. But not fruit juice. Fruit juice is too sweet and is not much different from Kool-Aid or soda. Fruit juice can easily jump-start sugar addiction. "Natural" sweeteners are not much better than any other sweetener. Sweet addictions can be kept alive and thriving on natural sweeteners just as well as any other. To keep sweet addictions away you need to refrain from all added sweetening, with the possible exception of stevia and fresh fruit.

White flour products have an addicting power similar to that of sugar and they should be avoided for the same reasons.

A LOW-SUGAR DIET

One of the primary reasons why most low-calorie, low-fat, and other reducing diets don't work is because they continue to allow sugar or other sweeteners. One of the biggest problems with most weight-reducing diets is that they do not focus in on the biggest cause for overweight—refined carbohydrates. They focus so much on calorie reduction that they miss the real troublemaker. Calorie reduction should not be a torturous affair filled with struggling and starvation. When you focus *only* on calorie reduction you are setting yourself up for disappointment. A better approach is to eliminate the *cause* for excess calorie consumption. If you eliminate the

99

desire to overeat, you automatically eat fewer calories, feel satisfied, do not feel deprived, feel good about your dietary choices, and lose weight with much less effort and pain.

Most diets allow sweets in one form or another because we have become so addicted to them that many people would be turned off by a diet that didn't have them. But what do you want? Do you want to lose weight and lose it permanently, or do you want to keep both your sweets and your body fat? The choice is yours. If you conquer your sugar addictions you will be far more successful in losing weight because you will be eating foods that are more filling and satisfying and that don't entice you to overeat. You end up eating less—by choice, not by restraint.

If your diet is going to be successful over the long run, you must gain control of your sweet tooth. I meet too many people so enslaved by sugar they won't or can't break away from it. Sugar controls their lives. They try diet after diet, but keep their sweet tooth and sugar addictions alive and their willpower under bondage to sugar cravings.

A successful weight-loss program will be one that involves a low-sugar diet. When I say sugar, I include artificial sweeteners as well. You can't break sugar addictions by substituting one drug for another. A successful diet will also limit refined grains, such as white flour and polished rice. All refined carbohydrates are addicting.

The evidence documenting the health benefits of complex-carbohydrate foods is so overwhelming it is unreasonable to eliminate them completely from a healthy diet or weight-loss program. The foods with the highest amount of beneficial fiber also happen to be the ones with the highest carbohydrate content. When you eliminate one, you eliminate the other. It's counterproductive. For this reason, I recommend what could be described as a low-refined-carbohydrate diet.

A good weight loss program, one that is healthy and can be maintained for life, will include foods with a mixture of complex carbohydrates, protein, and fat from a variety of wholesome, natural sources. These foods would be much like those typically eaten by our great-grandparents and their parents—whole milk, rich full-fat cream and butter, meat marbled with fat, fresh fruits and vegetables, and whole grains of all types. These are the foods that nourished our ancestors for thousands of years. These are the foods that nature, not some chemist, has provided for our nourishment. These are the foods that fed people in the days when heart disease was so rare doctors could work their entire careers without seeing a single case; a time when cancer, diabetes, and obesity were rarities, not the norm as they are today.

Chapter 7

CALORIES AND APPETITE _____.

WHY PEOPLE ARE OVERWEIGHT

What makes people fat? Some say it's a lack of exercise, others claim genetics or metabolism is to blame, while most people simply say it's because we eat too much. There is truth in all these statements. Many factors are involved. However, when you boil it all down what you are left with is the simple fact that being overweight is a result of consuming more calories than the body uses—input is greater than output. Regardless of whether you have a metabolic disorder or simply can't control yourself, the process is the same. If you eat more calories than your body burns, the excess is tucked away into storage.

The food we eat is converted into energy to power metabolic functions and physical activity. Any excess energy is converted into fat and packed away into fat cells producing the cellulite on our legs, the spare tire around our middle, and the oversized seat cushions on our backsides. So, the more we eat the bigger we get.

If that's all there is to it, the answer to being overweight seems obvious—eat less. This is not always a good answer or an easy one to implement. How many people have tried to diet by eating fewer calories? Probably everyone reading this book. If it worked, you wouldn't be here and I wouldn't have had to write it. While the underlying cause of overweight is taking in more calories than you expend, there are many approaches to solving this problem. In this chapter you will learn why it's not possible to lose more than about 2 pounds of fat a week, why low-calorie dieting ultimately makes you *gain* more weight, why overweight people seem to gain weight easier than thinner individuals, and why you need more than a simple low-calorie diet to lose weight permanently.

CALORIES IN, CALORIES OUT

The energy we obtain from food is measured in calories. Everybody needs a certain amount of calories to keep basic metabolic processes functioning—the heart beating, lungs expanding and contracting, stomach digesting food, and every other cellular process working that keeps the body alive.

The rate at which the body uses calories for these maintenance activities is called the basal metabolic rate (BMR). It is equivalent to the amount of calories a person would expend while lying down, completely inactive but awake. Any physical activity, no matter how simple, would require additional calories. At least two-thirds of the calories we use every day goes to fuel basic metabolic functions. Only one-third is used for physical or voluntary activity.

The BMR is different for each individual. Many factors determine our BMR and the amount of calories our bodies need and use. Young people require more calories than older ones. Physically active people use more than less active ones. People who are fasting, starving, or even dieting use less calories than ordinarily. Overweight people use fewer calories than lean people. These last two are unwelcome news to people who are overweight and dieting. It means they have to eat even less to see a change. The two most influential factors in determining body weight, with which we have control, are calorie consumption and physical activity.

Let's look at an example of how food consumption affects weight. A 150-pound man with a sedentary job, such as a computer keyboard operator, needs about 1600 calories for basic metabolic functions and another 800 calories for daily physical activities. He would need to consume a total of 2400 (1600 + 800) calories a day to maintain his body weight. If he ate less, say 2300 calories, he would lose weight, because his body requires 2400. Since his body uses 2400 calories, if he doesn't get them all from his diet, the extra 100 calories must come from the breakdown of fatty tissues. He loses fat and his weight decreases. However, if he eats more than 2400 calories, all the additional calories will be converted into fat and he gains weight.

Now let's look at an example where physical activity changes but calorie consumption remains the same. If the man in our example (consuming 2400 calories/day) becomes even less active than he already is, his body would use fewer calories. If he uses only 2300 calories, the excess 100 calories he consumes would be turned into fat and he would gain weight. If, on the other hand, he started an exercise program, the physical activity would increase his daily calorie requirement, for example say up to 2500 a day. He would lose weight because body fat (100 calories worth) would have to be used to supply his extra energy needs. This is why active people are usually much slimmer than inactive people, and why inactive people tend to gain weight.

If the man in our example had a job that required moderate activity, such as janitorial work, he would need about 2600-2800 calories a day to maintain his weight. If he had a heavy job, such as a brick layer, he would need about 2800-3200 calories a day. An average-sized person needs between 2200 to 3200 calories a day depending on physical activity. Women are generally smaller and have less muscle mass than men so they need a little less, about 200-400 fewer calories.

This is why one person can eat like a gorilla and look as skinny as a bird, while someone else can eat like a bird and still pack on weight.

HOW MUCH WEIGHT CAN YOU LOSE?

You've seen the advertisements "I lost 50 pound in 4 weeks" or "I went from a size 18 to a size 8 in 30 days!" All sorts of diets claim to "quickly" lose weight. Is it possible to lose weight this fast?

A pound of body fat stores about 3,500 calories. To lose it, you must reduce your calorie intake by 3,500. On average, a reduction of 500 calories a day (3,500/week) brings about a weight loss of one pound a week. A reduction of 1,000 calories a day equates to a loss of 2 pounds of fat a week.[1] This means that true fat loss takes time. You cannot lose 50 pounds of fat in 6 weeks. Six to 12 pounds is more realistic in this time frame.

Many people will argue with the above statement saying "I lost 10 pounds in 2 weeks." Weight loss is deceiving. A pound of body weight lost does not necessarily indicate a reduction in body fat. Quick changes in weight are *not* changes in fat, but are due primarily to a loss of water. Look at the numbers. On average a person needs about 2,500 calories a day to maintain current weight whether they are over- or underweight. This is the amount needed just to stay even. Out of this number, two-thirds or 1,667 calories are needed just to power basic metabolic processes. The remaining 833 calories are used for daily activities. A reduction of 1,000 calories a day is dramatic and borders on starvation. Even at that drastic rate a person will only lose 2 pounds of fat a week. In addition, you would be constantly hungry and fatigued due to a lack of energy. Claims in advertisements that state that somebody on a particular diet lost 10 pounds in 1 week or 40 pounds in 4 weeks or some other incredible figure may be true, but it wasn't all fat they lost, it also included muscle mass and water. In time, the water will be added back and weight will increase. If water isn't eventually replaced it could lead to very serious health problems, some of which are discussed later in Chapter 11.

If you are very overweight you can expect to lose fat at a slightly faster rate. Up to 4 or 5 pounds a week is possible. This is fat loss. Total weight loss may be greater because you lose water and muscle mass as well. If you follow the plan I outline later in this book, your water and muscle mass loss will be minimal and your weight loss will be mostly all fat.

In order to lose fat and excess weight permanently and healthfully, you need to do it slowly. The best way to lose weight is to make little adjustments in the types of food you eat, increase your actively level, and stop worrying about counting calories or denying yourself. It can be done.

DIETING MAKES YOU FAT

I overheard one man speaking to another, "Over the past several years I've lost 200 pounds. If I'd kept it all off I would weigh minus 20 pounds." I think many of us could relate to this statement.

Take Susan, for example. Susan was like many overweight people. She wanted to lose weight and worked hard at it. She tried one diet after another. Most of them seemed to work—at least at first. She would go on one diet and lose 10 pounds, but before long the weight would come right back. She would try another diet and maybe lose 20 pounds, but over time the weight would be back. Every diet she tried ended with the same results. After years of dieting not only was she still overweight, but weighed more than ever. All the dieting she did hadn't helped her lose a single pound. In fact, it seemed to make her even bigger. The truth is, dieting was part of her problem.

According to the Mayo Clinic, 95% of those people who go on weight-loss diets regain all their weight back within 5 years. Many regain more weight than they had before. Typical weight-loss diets not only don't work but often make matters worse. Yes, dieting can actually make you fat.

The problem with many weight-loss diets is that they focus *only* on calorie restriction. The reasoning is that the fewer calories you eat, the less you will weigh. While paying attention to calorie consumption is important, it is not the only factor that influences body weight. Some diets may give lip service to other factors, such as exercise, but because most people don't like to exercise it's given little attention. The sad fact is that all low-calorie diets are doomed from the start. No matter what type of foods you eat, if the diet relies solely on calorie restriction it is programmed to fail.

In addition to calories, if you are going to be successful you must consider other factors. One of these is metabolism. You can't ignore metabolism and expect to be successful. Let me explain why.

Your metabolic rate is affected by many things. One of the things that influences it is the amount of food you eat. Our bodies have a built-in mechanism that strives to maintain a balance between our metabolism and the environment. This mechanism was vital in the days of our ancestors who relied on seasonal availability of foods for survival. When food was plentiful, metabolism ran at the height of efficiency. A higher metabolism has advantages in that it improves immune system function and speeds healing and tissue growth and repair. During winter or famine when food was less plentiful metabolism slowed down. The advantage was that less energy (i.e. food) was needed to fuel metabolic processes. People were able to survive on less food during times of need.

Today with modern food preservation and delivery methods, getting enough to eat is no longer a problem for most people. Food is abundantly available all year around. However, our bodies still maintain the ability to adapt quickly to famine. If we suddenly start to eat less food, it signals to our bodies that there must be a famine and, as a means of self–preservation, our BMR decreases to conserve energy. The problem with this is that when we diet, we cut down on calorie consumption and the body thinks it's starving so it slows our metabolic rate down. Slower metabolism also means our bodies have less energy and we become fatigued more easily.

When you go on a calorie-restricted diet, your body reacts as if it were experiencing a famine. For the first few days, while your metabolism is still running at normal levels, the restriction in calories works and you lose weight. Weight loss is always greatest for the first few weeks. After awhile as your body adjusts to lower calorie consumption, metabolism slows down. Now the calories you consume are balanced with the calories you burn. Weight loss stops. You hit a plateau.

In order to lose more weight you must restrict your calorie intake even further. If you do, you will lose a few more pounds until your body adapts and your metabolism again slows down. As long as you continue to restrict calories your metabolism will drop to balance calorie intake with calorie output. Dieting becomes very restrictive and uncomfortable (some would say painful).

When you decide to end the diet, even if you still eat less than you did when you started, the extra calories start to add on weight. Your metabolism is depressed. It still thinks you're in a famine. Now when you increase calorie consumption the excess calories are packed on as fat even though you may be eating fewer calories than you did before you started the diet. By the time your metabolism has figured out that the famine is over, you've added back the weight you've lost. In addition, your body tends to add on more fat to protect itself in case of another famine. So after dieting you gradually gain back all the weight you lost and a few extra pounds as well. In the end you weigh more than when you started. This whole cycle may take only a few months or drag out for several years. The end result is the same.

The next weight-loss diet you attempt has the same outcome as does the next and the next. Each time you diet you end up weighing more than you did before. This process is termed "dieting-induced obesity" or the "yo-yo effect."

Most weight-loss diets are considered temporary dietary restrictions and as soon as the weight is lost, old eating habits are resumed. It's these habits that probably caused the weight problem in the first place. Consequently, weight comes back on. You can never stay slim by eating the way you used to. In order to lose weight permanently, you must make a permanent change. This, however, is undesirable for most people. Who in their right mind would want to remain on a weight-loss diet forever? These diets are just too restrictive and in many cases unhealthy. In order for any diet to work, it needs to be something you can do permanently. You've got to make it a permanent part of your life. So the diet you choose must be one that is satisfying, filling, and healthy. If a diet isn't satisfying, it won't last long.

Notice that I said that for a diet to be successful it must also be healthy. A diet which is lacking in nutrition, as are most all low-calorie and low-fat diets, has a negative effect on metabolism and encourages overeating as a means to prevent starvation or malnutrition. Metabolism is discussed in more detail in Chapter 9.

HUNGER AND APPETITE

Which of the following best describes you? Are you a picky eater, habitual eater, recreational eater, or professional eater? Judging by our expanding waistlines, most of us are approaching the professional ranks.

Eating in excess of one's needs is the underlying cause of overweight. While there are many factors involved, all of them ultimately influence calorie input and output. One of the factors that influences calorie intake is behavior. Behavior involves those actions that are influenced by habits, attitudes, environment, and psychological stimuli.

Behavioral influences cannot be ignored as they can play a powerful role in your success with any weight-loss program. For many people, overeating is just as much a problem as substance abuse is to a drug addict or an alcoholic. Food can exert a powerful psychological and physical influence over us that is every bit as addictive as drugs. In this section we will discuss some of the psychological or behavioral factors that make foods addicting. In the next chapter we will discuss physical addictions (food cravings) and how you can conquer them.

It isn't easy to break addictions, but it isn't impossible either. If you can make a commitment to follow a program or make a lifestyle change you can break your dependence on overeating. Let me make it clear that it is impossible to overeat without gaining weight, therefore, you must be conscious of what you eat. Often we eat whenever the desire hits, regardless of whether we are hungry or not. One of the first things you need to do is to eliminate eating simply for the sake of eating.

There are two reasons why we eat. We eat because of hunger or because of appetite. Hunger is a *physical* need to eat. Our bodies need nourishment and energy to fuel metabolism. When the body needs nourishment we get feelings of hunger. Appetite, on the other hand, is a sensation or desire to eat. Appetite may or may not accompany hunger. When we smell a fresh baked pie we have the desire to eat even though we may not be hungry. At a social gathering where a variety of snack foods are available, their presence stimulates our appetite even though we may have no need for food. Appetite is a *psychological* desire for food.

One of the main reasons why we are so overweight nowadays is because of appetite. Hunger doesn't make us fat, appetite does. Foods are so readily available and so tempting we tend to overindulge. Understanding some of the environmental stimuli that trigger appetite can help to overcome inappropriate eating habits.

Eating behavior is often triggered by external factors unrelated to feelings of hunger. We can be conditioned to automatically eat in response to certain environmental stimuli. An example is eating at predetermined times each day regardless of whether or not we are hungry. The clock says it's time to eat so we eat. Social gatherings are often times to eat and drink.

The sight and smell of food stimulate its consumption. We see food or someone eating and our appetite is triggered. In the home or workplace if food is readily available and in plain sight it's a constant reminder for you to eat. Restaurants and grocery stores know the power of smell. This is why they release the aroma of cooking foods into the path of potential customers. Haven't you ever been shopping without the faintest thought of eating and then smelled food cooking on the grill and suddenly felt hungry?

We often develop habits of eating in response to certain cues. If you eat while watching television, for example, you soon develop a habit. Watching television triggers a response to eat. Food companies know this and show enticing commercials for soft drinks, beer, and snack foods—just the type of things you might eat while watching. Walking past a refrigerator or a vending machine may be all that's needed to lure someone into eating or drinking something.

Emotional factors often affect our eating habits. Foods, especially sweets, taste good. We find comfort and pleasure in eating. Psychologists have observed that stress, anxiety, loneliness, boredom, or anger can stimulate eating. Because food gives pleasure, eating can provide emotional comfort in times of duress.

Sight, smell, thoughts, and emotions can all trigger appetite. Environmental stimuli are around us constantly, enticing us to eat. Advertisers have mastered the science of motivation and bombard us from every angle. Temptation is everywhere. If we have no set limits or guidelines to follow, these stimuli will keep our appetites active and have us continually eating and our waistlines ever expanding. One of the steps in losing excess weight and keeping it off is to understand this problem and control it. In order to control it you need a set of guidelines to follow (such as the ones given in Chapter 13). Knowing that you have a set of standards to live by will give you power to refuse temptation, control your appetite, and to a great extent, control your health.

Don't think of it as a diet that you are going on just to lose weight. The term "diet" gives a connotation of a temporary restriction on foods in order to lose weight. Once the weight is reached the diet is over. Consequently, most people eventually regain all their weight back. Instead, think of it as a health plan or lifestyle change that you will adopt for life. When you view it this way there is a greater commitment on your part to stick with the plan. Commitment is important. No diet can work if there is not a concerted commitment to follow through with it.

You need to resist environmental stimuli to eat, which we all face every day. Cultivating a positive mental attitude is important as you make dietary and lifestyle changes. Think positively about the health plan. Visualize how good you will look and feel. Avoid celebrating your success by resuming old eating habits; they should be gone forever. If you think of your new way of eating in a positive light, you will enjoy yourself more and have greater willpower and a stronger determination to stick with the program and avoid poor eating habits and choices. You will be a success.

Chapter 8

MALNUTRITION CAN MAKE YOU FAT___.

SUBCLINICAL MALNUTRITION

Are you overweight? Believe it or not, the reason you are overweight may be because you are malnourished. Yes, you read that correctly. You may be overweight because of malnutrition. When I say this, I'm not suggesting that you run out and eat *more* food. What you need to do is learn how to make wise food choices.

Malnutrition is one of the major underlying causes of obesity. How could someone who overeats be malnourished? The amount of food you eat doesn't determine your nutrient status. You could stuff yourself with 10 pounds of donuts every day and still be malnourished. Donuts are not a good source of nutrients. They provide lots of calories but little in the way of vitamins and minerals.

Most of the foods we eat nowadays are nutrient deficient. Processing and refining remove and destroy many nutrients. Sugar, for example, has a total of zero vitamins and minerals. But it does contain fattening calories. White flour, likewise, has been stripped of its vitamin and mineral rich bran and germ, leaving almost pure starch. Starch is nothing more than sugar. A molecule of starch consists of a chain of sugars attached to each other. So eating white flour products is essentially the same as eating pure sugar. When you eat products made with white flour such as bread, pasta, crackers, pancakes, rolls, cereal, sandwiches, cake, stuffing, pizza, and the like, you are eating primarily sugar, which is essentially void of any nutritional value. White rice is the same. The vitamin-rich bran is removed leaving the white starchy portion behind. Potatoes are almost all starch. The skins contain most all of the nutrients, but how many people *always* eat the skins with their potatoes?

Most all of the foods we typically eat are made from sugar, white flour, white rice, and skinless potatoes. These foods supply roughly 60% of the daily calories of most people. Another 20–30% come from fats and oils. The most popular oils are margarine, shortening, and processed vegetable oils like soybean and corn oils. Oils are often hidden in our foods. All packaged, convenience, and restaurant foods contain loads of fats, including a high percentage of hydrogenated fats. Ugh! Like sugar, processed oils contain no vitamins and minerals, only calories.

For the most part our typical diet consists of foods which are mostly empty calories—starch, sugar, oils. Few of us eat fruits and vegetables. When we do, it's generally as condiments—pickles and lettuce on a sandwich, tomato sauce and onions on a pizza. Our food is loaded with calories, but nutritionally deficient. We consume lots of calories and few nutrients. The consequence is that you can eat and eat and eat until you are overweight, yet be malnourished.

The US Department of Agriculture states that most all of us don't get enough (100% RDA) of at least 10 essential nutrients. Only 12% of the population obtain 100% of seven essential nutrients. Less than 10% of us get the recommended daily servings of fruit and vegetables. Forty percent of us eat no fruit and 20 percent no vegetables. And most of the vegetables we do get are fried potatoes (cooked in hydrogenated vegetable oil).

In November of 1993, the *Journal of the American Dietetic Association* reported a study of 1,800 second- and fifth-graders in New York State and found that on the day they were surveyed, 40% of the children did not eat any vegetables, except potatoes or tomato sauce; 20% ate no fruit, and 36% ate at least four different types of high-calorie, nutritionally poor snack foods. It's no wonder kids nowadays are getting fat.

It's bad enough that most of the foods we eat are nutritionally poor, but the problem is compounded even further by the fact that these same foods also destroy the nutrients we get from other foods. Sugar, for example, has no nutrients, but it does use up nutrients when it is metabolized. Eating sugary and starchy foods can drain the body of chromium, a mineral vital to making insulin. Without insulin, you develop blood sugar problems like a diabetic. The more processed our food is, the more nutrients we need in order to metabolize it. Polyunsaturated oils, another source of empty calories, eat up vitamins E and A, and zinc reserves; certain food additives burn up vitamin C, etc. A diet loaded with white-flour products, sugar, and vegetable oil quickly depletes nutrient reserves, pushing us further toward malnutrition.

Advanced stages of malnutrition can exhibit themselves as a number of characteristic diseases such as scurvy (vitamin C deficiency), beriberi (thiamin deficiency), and pellagra (niacin deficiency). Such conditions leave the body vulnerable to infections, depress immunity, slow down healing, disrupt normal growth and development, and promote tissue and organ degeneration. If left untreated all are lethal.

According to the World Health Organization, 70–80% of people in developed nations die from lifestyle- or diet-caused diseases. The majority of cancers are caused by what we put into our bodies. Heart disease, stroke, and atherosclerosis, the biggest killers in industrialized nations, are dietary diseases. Diabetes is a diet related disease. Numerous studies have shown that vitamins, minerals, and other nutrients in foods protect us from these diseases of modern civilization.

When we think of malnutrition, we usually think of emaciated drought victims in Africa or starving people in India. In more affluent countries, the problem is more insidious. Symptoms of malnutrition are not as evident. Overweight people don't look malnourished and methods of diagnosing deficiency diseases require malnutrition to be in an advanced stage before they can be detected.

When a variety of foods is available, few people develop *obvious* symptoms of malnutrition, even when their diets are nutritionally poor. Instead, they suffer from *subclinical malnutrition*. Subclinical malnutrition is a condition where a person consumes just enough essential nutrients to prevent full-blown symptoms of severe malnutrition, but the body is still nutrient deficient and prone to slow, premature degeneration. This condition can go on unnoticed indefinitely. In Western countries the problem of subclinical malnutrition is epidemic. Our foods are sadly depleted of nutrients. We eat, and even overeat, but may still be malnourished because our foods do not contain all the essential nutrients our bodies need to function optimally. As a result, the immune system is chronically depressed, the body cannot fight off infections well, and tissues and cells starving for nutrients slowly degenerate. Disease of modern civilization is the result.

When the body is starved for nutrients, the stage is also set for weight gain. To be successful in losing excess weight and keeping it off, you must address this issue. The following section will explain why.

FOOD CRAVINGS

If you were a cowboy, you would most likely encounter at sometime a horse that had the habit of biting and slobbering on fence posts. Why do you suppose horses chew fence posts? They do it for the same reason cows lick salt, kids eat dirt, and pregnant women eat pickles and ice cream. They do it to satisfy *cravings*. Both animals and humans have food cravings.

Have you ever craved a candy bar, an ice cream cone, or a soda? You may not have been hungry and had no real need for the item, but you just had to have it? Most of us have had feelings such as this at one time or another. Sometimes cravings become so overpowering that we lose all self-control and eat foods we know aren't good for us, but we just couldn't resist. In such cases cravings are as controlling as any narcotic.

Cravings can occur for any type of food or combination of foods. People even crave nonfood items such as dirt, coal, chalk, and wood. Small children often peal off and chew paint or eat clay. One woman troubled with this problem wrote to advice columnist, Dr. Donohue, and said, "I am 29 years old. I suffer from extreme obesity. At the age of 17, I started eating laundry starch. I consumed about a 1 pound box once a week. What makes me do this? Does it add to my weight problem?" There is a term for those who crave nonfood items: it's called *pica*. Why would anyone want to eat laundry starch, paint, or clay? What is it that would drive someone to eat such unsavory items? It certainly isn't the taste.

Food cravings are a direct response to a nutrient deficiency. The body lacking some vitamin or mineral triggers an urge to eat. Hunger may not even be involved. But the urge may be so strong as to be virtually uncontrollable.

Most cravings are caused by a lack of trace minerals in the diet. Minerals perform important functions in the body mostly as components in enzymes and hormones. Some 60 different minerals are needed by the body in order to maintain good health. Most of these are needed in only tiny or trace amounts, but if we don't have them our health suffers. If we cannot get the minerals our bodies need, we begin to get cravings. Some people will eat dirt, paint, or chalk in order to satisfy their need for minerals. Even though these items may taste terrible, cravings can be so powerful they override our natural repulsion to such items and alter our sense of reason. If cravings can be so overpowering as to cause people to eat dirt, what effect do you think it has on those who eat real food? I'll tell you. It causes them to eat and eat and eat without finding lasting satisfaction.

Throughout the history of mankind our water supplies have provided us a source of trace minerals. Rain and spring water leach minerals from rocks and soil. While only 5–8% of the suspended minerals in these waters are actually absorbed and utilized by our bodies, they have provided people an important source of trace minerals throughout history. Modern water filtration and processing methods remove most of these minerals. Hard water, which is particularly rich in calcium and magnesium, is specifically treated to remove these and other minerals. The result is that our drinking water nowadays is minerally depleted and is no longer a good source of trace minerals.

Another traditional source of trace minerals is from salt. All sources of salt come from seawater. Rivers and streams on the crest of mountain peaks dissolve mineral salts out of the rocks in which they traverse as they make their way toward the ocean. The ocean collects these minerals making the water salty. When seawater evaporates it leaves behind these mineral salts. The most abundant of these is sodium chloride, better known as table salt.

Natural, unadulterated sea salt contains all the trace minerals found in nature. Both humans and animals need these trace minerals. For generations ranchers have given their cattle salt blocks to curb salt cravings and provide them with trace minerals. Grass and feed often lack trace minerals and, as a consequence, animals develop a wide assortment of health problems. Ranchers have found that their cattle are healthier when they are given salt. The ranchers don't have to tell the cows to eat it or mix it into their food. A block of salt is left out for them to lick as they please. When the cattle need minerals, cravings develop and they lick the salt block. In this way the animals satisfy their cravings and get the minerals their bodies need.

We, like cattle, crave salt for the trace minerals it naturally contains. Unfortunately, the salt sold in grocery stores and used in almost all prepared foods is highly refined. Processing has removed *all* minerals, leaving only sodium chloride. Table salt provides no trace minerals.

When we have a mineral deficiency our body reacts by producing a craving for salt. We respond by eating salty foods. Most packaged, convenience foods are highly salted to enhance flavor. Most any type of processed food will satisfy salt cravings—*temporarily*. Cravings may be satisfied briefly just after eating because the body anticipates receiving the minerals. When they don't arrive, salt cravings are reinitiated. In this way cravings are never completely satisfied and we end up eating more and more.

Another source of trace minerals is food. Grains and starchy root vegetables are among the richest natural food sources for trace minerals. However, when whole grains are transformed into white flour or white rice these minerals are stripped away, leaving just starch. Our bodies, craving trace minerals, seek grains or other natural starches (like potatoes) to satisfy these cravings, but what we end up eating is white bread, polished white rice, and all manner of sugary foods and drinks. As with salt, we eat high carbohydrate foods to satisfy mineral cravings, yet don't get the nutrients our bodies need. Cravings are never satisfied, so we continue to eat.

Sugar is a carbohydrate. *Craving for sweets is a sign of a mineral deficiency.* Eating a Snickers candy bar isn't going to supply your body with the minerals it needs nor is it going to satisfy your cravings for sweets. Eventually you're going to crave another candy bar, a Coke, or some other sweet. You're going to continue to crave sweets until you solve the underlying problem.

What are the foods we most often crave and overeat? The vast majority are either salty or sweet. Pregnant women have a greater demand placed on them for available nutrients. Eating a nutritionally poor diet leads to food cravings. These cravings often include bizarre food combinations such as pickles (salty) and ice cream (sweet). Our bodies crying for trace minerals signal cravings for salt and carbohydrate—the types of foods which in nature normally provides us with trace minerals. Instead of eating natural salt or complex carbohydrates (grains and starchy vegetables), we give in to donuts, soda, potato chips, cookies, nachos, and candy.

If the foods you ate supplied the missing nutrients, food cravings would disappear. But most of the foods we eat are processed and refined and, sadly, mineral deficient. We eat them until we are stuffed to the gills, which temporarily satisfies the cravings. But since these foods don't supply the needed minerals, cravings return and uncontrolled eating continues. We overeat in a vain attempt to acquire the nutrients our bodies are missing. As a consequence, we pack on more and more weight. When we try to diet, it is shear agony because we still have cravings, but now we refrain from eating and we suffer terribly. A great deal of the pain and suffering we go through when we diet is due to suppressing the cravings of a mineral deficiency. If you could only satisfy those cravings without adding additional calories, dieting would be much more tolerable. That's one thing my eating plan accomplishes.

The best way to satisfy nutrient deficiencies is to avoid all nutritionally depleted foods—processed refined foods like white flour, sugar, vegetable oils, and such. In their place eat foods rich in vitamins and minerals such as whole grains, fruits, vegetables, and natural oils. Whole grains, nuts and seeds are some of the best food sources for minerals. Since our water supply is also mineral depleted it would be wise to supplement the diet with other natural sources of minerals. Mineral supplements are helpful but not enough. Mineral supplements only supply about half dozen of the major minerals. We need about 60 in all. One way to help supply the body's needs for trace minerals is by replacing the processed table salt you may be using now with unrefined sea salt or other natural salt. Use sea salt on your foods and for all of your cooking and baking needs.

Another source of trace minerals is to use one of the many brands of liquid minerals available. While there may be some minor differences between the different brands, most of them seem to offer a wide variety of trace minerals. Some come from sea water; others from humic shale deposits. Liquid mineral supplements provide the most concentrated source of trace minerals.

FAT AND FOOD CRAVINGS

You can use fat to help stamp out food cravings. If you don't get enough fat in your diet you can become malnourished. Fat is essential for good nutrition. Many of the protective antioxidants that shield us from diseases such as cancer and heart disease are fat soluble and are found only in the fatty portion of foods. An adequate amount of fat must be present in our diet in order to properly digest and absorb these vital nutrients.

Besides being necessary for the digestion of fat-soluble vitamins and antioxidants, fat is also necessary for the absorption of minerals. Low-fat diets limit our ability to absorb minerals, thus promoting nutritional deficiencies and food cravings.

Fat slows down the rate at which the stomach empties. When gastric emptying is slowed down the foods are bathed in stomach acids and digestive enzymes for a longer period of time, thus improving digestion and releasing more nutrients. Calcium, for example, needs the action of strong stomach acids in order to make it available to the body. Without enough stomach acid or adequate time in the stomach, calcium is not released or available for assimilation in the intestines and passes on through the digestive tract. Low-fat diets, therefore, promote calcium deficiency and associated complications such as osteoporosis.

Many other essential minerals also need time in the stomach for proper digestion. Magnesium, iron, zinc, and numerous trace minerals require an adequate amount of time in stomach acid to make them bioavailable. Therefore, fat helps us get maximum nutritional benefit from the rest of our foods. As you can see, nutritional deficiencies, particularly with trace minerals, can squash good intentions and foster uncontrollable food cravings that can kill any weight-loss diet. Eating fat helps your body digest and absorb minerals and other nutrients, which prevent food cravings and overeating.

FOOD QUALITY

In order to avoid malnutrition or, more likely, subclinical malnutrition and accompanying food cravings, you need to eat the best quality foods you can get. The highest quality foods are those that contain the highest nutritive value and the least harmful additives or byproducts. The lowest quality foods contain the most calories, the greatest amount of chemical additives, and supply the lowest nutritive value. Generally speaking foods that have had the least amount of processing are of the highest quality. The more processing or refining a food undergoes the lower in quality it becomes.

The way food is grown also affects its quality. Fruits and vegetables grown in artificially fertilized soils or mineral depleted soils are less nutritious than those grown in rich, organic soils. Organically grown foods are produced in naturally fertilized soils and are not contaminated by pesticides, so they are of a higher quality than non-organic foods.

Meat from a grass-fed, organically raised steer is of higher quality than from an animal that came from a stockyard, fed on corn and soy and pumped up with antibiotics and artificial hormones. Meat from either one of these sources is better than that found in processed meats such as hot dogs, which are loaded with preservatives and other additives and incidental contaminants.

Excessive or improper cooking and preparation can lower quality. Cooking not only destroys nutrients, but high heat, such as used in frying, changes the molecular structure of some foods, transforming them into substances unusable by the body and often making them very difficult to digest. This is true for both produce and meats. To retain the quality of foods, they should be eaten raw or only moderately cooked. Oils, and particularly vegetable oils, when heated to high temperatures, as in deep frying, become carcinogenic. The only heat tolerant oil is one that is high in saturated fat, such as coconut. Raw and moderately cooked, organically grown vegetables, fruits, nuts, and seeds are the highest quality foods we can eat. The highest quality meats, eggs, and dairy are those from animals that have been allowed to roam and eat outside (referred to as free-range or grass-fed) and are free of drugs and hormones.

DIETARY SUPPLEMENTS

The best source of all nutrients is from whole foods from good sources. Many foods, even whole foods, are lacking in nutrients. This is because they were grown or raised on nutrient-poor soils. Most farmland, although enriched with chemical fertilizers which supply phosphorous, nitrogen, and potassium, are sadly depleted of trace minerals. After many decades of farming these trace minerals are no longer present in the soils.

Alarmed about the lack of nutrients in most farmland the US Senate issued an official warning, which, in part, states:

"Do you know that most of us today are suffering from certain dangerous diet deficiencies which cannot be remedied until the depleted soils from which our foods come are brought into proper mineral balance?

"The alarming fact is that foods—fruits and vegetables and grains, now being raised on millions of acres of land that no longer contains enough of certain needed minerals, are starving us—no matter how much of them we eat!

"You'd think, wouldn't you, that a carrot is a carrot—that one is about as good as another as far as nourishment is concerned? But it isn't; one carrot may look and taste like another and yet be lacking in the particular mineral element which our system requires and which carrots are supposed to contain.

"Laboratory tests prove that the fruits, the vegetables, the grains, the eggs, and even the milk and the meats of today are not what they were a few generations ago.

"No man of today can eat enough fruits and vegetables to supply his stomach with the mineral salts he requires for perfect health, because his stomach isn't big enough to hold them!

"It is bad news to learn from our leading authorities that 99% of the American people are deficient in these minerals, and that a marked deficiency in any one of the more important minerals actually results in disease. Any upset of the balance, any considerable lack of one or another element, however microscopic the body requirement might be, and we sicken, suffer, and shorten our lives.

"Lacking vitamins, the system can make some use of minerals, but lacking minerals, vitamins are useless."[1]

The fact that our soils are mineral depleted is bad enough, what is even more alarming is that this document was issued in 1936! Our soils are much worse now.

In order to get the same amount of nutrition our ancestors received we must not only eat the best (least processed) foods we can find, but should also consider adding dietary supplements. A source of trace minerals is the most important because foods nowadays are sadly depleted of these important nutrients. Major minerals and vitamins are also valuable because people who have been eating highly processed foods are nutritionally bankrupt and need to rebuild their nutritional savings account. A good daily multiple vitamin and mineral supplement would be beneficial for most people.

You need not worry about getting too much nutrition by taking dietary supplements. The RDA is a *minimum* requirement, not a maximum. Your body can safely handle vitamins and minerals three or four times the RDA, and generally even much more than that. The excess is usually just flushed out of the body in the urine. Taking a dietary supplement is like having insurance, you are protected from nutritional deficiency. For a few pennies a day, vitamin and mineral supplements are the cheapest health insurance you can buy.

GOOD DIGESTION
Good Food May Not Be Enough
You might think that eating wholesome foods would eliminate the risk of subclinical malnutrition and food cravings. For most people this is true, but for some it is not. Eating a healthy diet is one thing, but digesting it is another. Consuming nutritious foods may not be enough to overcome nutrient deficiencies if your body cannot properly digest and absorb the nutrients in these foods. Even vitamin and mineral supplements may be of little help in this situation. Often, a body abused by many years of poor dietary choices may not be able to properly digest and assimilate the nutrients it is given.

In order to eliminate food cravings and urges to overeat, you must satisfy your nutrient needs. No weight-loss diet will ever work unless you address this problem. Most of those who have digestive problems have no idea who they are. Clues would be symptoms such as frequent indigestion, heart burn, nausea, stomach cramps, bloating, constipation, or diarrhea. These symptoms suggest that food isn't being completely digested.

A more direct test would be to look into the toilet after a bowel movement. If you see droplets of oil on the surface of the water or if your stool floats, it suggests that you are not properly digesting fats. A foul smell indicates incomplete protein digestion. If you see undigested food particles, you are not completely digesting carbohydrate or plant foods. If you have any of the conditions listed above, you probably have some level of digestive insufficiency.

If you're not properly digesting foods, you are in real danger of suffering from subclinical malnutrition. Taking dietary supplements may not help. If you have problems digesting foods, you will probably be unable to digest and absorb vitamin supplements as well. In addition to eating wholesome foods and taking vitamin and mineral supplements, you may need some digestive aids, which are discussed below.

The Digestive Process

Digestion begins in the mouth. We chew our food to break it down as much as possible before sending it to the stomach. This mechanical breakdown is very important because a small chunk of food can pass completely through the digestive tract intact. Food particles must be physically broken apart so that digestive enzymes can work on them. Food that is incompletely broken down by chewing can pass all the way through the digestive tract without releasing the nutrients it contains. The body gains no benefit.

To get the most nutrition you should thoroughly chew all your food. Eat slowly and enjoy it. If you don't enjoy what you're eating, don't eat it. Why eat something you don't enjoy? Don't gulp it down because you're in a hurry. In a busy world many of us eat on the run. If you don't have time to sit down and eat, then you don't have time to eat. All foods should be eaten slowly and enjoyed for maximum nutritional benefit. Also, when you eat slowly you end up eating less, thus helping reduce calorie consumption.

As you chew your food it is mixed with saliva. The saliva contains enzymes that begin the chemical process of digestion. The purpose of digestive enzymes is to reduce fat, protein, and carbohydrate into molecules small enough to be transported across the intestinal wall and into the bloodstream. Fat is broken down into fatty acids, protein into amino acids, and carbohydrate into sugars. Our bodies produce many different types of enzymes, all of which have a specific purpose. One group of enzymes called *lipase* digests fat, another called *protease* breaks down protein, and another called *amylase* dismantles carbohydrate. The reason we cannot digest fiber is that we do not produce the enzymes that can do the job. Many animals do have these enzymes and can thrive on very high-fiber foods like grass, leaves, and tree bark.

When food is swallowed it travels down the esophagus and into the stomach. In the stomach, food is mixed with water, hydrochloric acid, and digestive enzymes. This is where protein digesting enzymes are most active. Stomach muscles work to mix and blend digestive juices with the food producing a liquidy mass. This partially digested mass is slowly released

119

from the stomach into the small intestine where the acid is neutralized and digestive enzymes produced by the pancreas complete the job of breaking fats, proteins, and carbohydrates down into absorbable units.

It takes only a couple of hours for the stomach to empty food into the small intestine. Food may remain in the intestine ten times that long as it slowly travels toward the colon. It is in the intestines where most of the digestion and assimilation of nutrients takes place.

When this process works the way it is supposed to, everything moves along fine, nutrients are absorbed and the leftover waste is removed. In some people, however, the digestive process breaks down. They are unable to produce enough digestive juices or enzymes to gain full benefit from the nutrients in the foods they eat.

Low Stomach Acid

When food enters the stomach it is bathed in a solution of hydrochloric acid and protein digestive enzymes. It is in the stomach where the majority of protein digestion takes place. Very little fat and carbohydrate digestion takes place in the stomach. The high concentration of acid also acts as a means to kill potentially harmful microorganisms that enter the body with the food. In some people the acid production goes haywire, resulting in either too much or too little. Either one can cause digestive disorders that affect health.

The stomach enzymes work most efficiently in a fluid with a pH of 2 or lower. This is a level of acidity between lemon juice and battery acid, or one million times more acidic than the blood. The walls of the stomach would be burned by the acid and digested by the protein digesting enzymes if it were not for a thick protective layer of mucus which shields the lining of the stomach from harm. If acidic stomach juices back up and enter the esophagus, they irritate the unprotected tissues, creating a burning sensation referred to as heartburn. If the stomach has difficulty properly digesting food, it may lead to heartburn as well as indigestion and bloating.

Judging from advertising on television and in magazines we are led to believe that too much acid is a common problem. You've seen the ads: "For faster relief from heartburn and acid indigestion try Rolaids" or "TUMS knocks out heartburn fast." Although ads like this promise to bring relief from excess stomach acid, a much more common problem is too *little* acid. In fact, if you experience heartburn, bloating, or indigestion, you are more likely to be suffering from not having enough than from having too much. Taking antacids will only make the situation worse. You may get relief from symptoms, but as stomach acid decreases, digestion also decreases. Food particles pass through the stomach only partially digested.

120

Protein enters the intestine in relatively large chunks, much of it passing through the body. Mineral absorption is severely affected by low stomach acidity. Both trace minerals like zinc and selenium and major minerals like calcium and magnesium need the action of strong stomach acids to make them absorbable. This means that some nutrients don't get assimilated, which may lower your nutrient status and initiate food cravings.

Many people who think they have excess stomach acid are really acid deficient. Based on my experience, I would estimate that about 25% of the adult population have under-acid stomachs. Some physicians have reported 25-50% of their patients have hypochlorhydria (low stomach acidity).[2] I've seen far more people who have too little acid than those who have too much. Most people who have an under-acid stomach aren't even aware they have a problem. Those who know they have a problem assume it to be caused by excess acid and treat it by downing antacids. According to Jonathan Wright, M.D., an expert on digestive disorders, "When we actually measure stomach acid in people who've been taking antacids regularly, better than half have subnormally *low* levels of acidity."[3]

If your food happens to contain harmful bacteria, normal stomach acids will usually kill them. In people with low stomach acid, bacteria can manage to survive and cause illness. At one time it was believed that too much stomach acid was the primary cause of gastric ulcers. We now know that about 93% of all gastric ulcers are caused by a bacteria called *Helicobacter pylori*. This bacteria is only able to survive and infect the stomach lining when acid production is depressed. So ulcers are really a result of too little acid rather than too much. When our bodies are under stress, the digestive process, including the production of stomach acid, slows down. For this reason, people who live stressful lives are prone to digestive and nutritional problems.

Symptoms frequently associated with low stomach acidity include: bloating, belching, heartburn, indigestion, and ulcers. Affected people won't necessarily have each of these symptoms, usually only one or two. Some don't have any. Since low acidity affects nutrient absorption, other signs may include: fingernails which easily peel or break, hair loss in women, and unusual dilation of the capillaries in the cheeks and on the nose.

Health problems that may also be associated with low acidity are: diabetes, underactive and overactive thyroid, frequent yeast infections, childhood asthma, eczema, gallbladder disease, weak adrenals, osteoporosis, rheumatoid arthritis, chronic hives, lupus, chronic hepatitis, vitiligo, and rosacea. Perhaps the most common conditions associated with an under-acid stomach are food allergies and sensitivities. Dr. Wright says, "Food allergy and sensitivity is so frequently associated with low stomach acidity that the finding of one should automatically lead to a consideration of the other." Food that is incompletely digested may find its way into the bloodstream. The immune system identifies these food particles as foreign invaders and attacks them, bringing on symptoms typically associated with allergic reactions.

Age is also associated with low acidity. Acidity normally declines with age. Research has reported that more than 50% of those over age 60 are affected. The more of the conditions listed above that fit you, the more likely you are to have an under-acid stomach.

Your doctor can run tests to make a more precise diagnosis. Stomach acid can be measured directly using a Heidelberg capsule. In this test a radio transmitter inserted into a tiny capsule is swallowed. The capsule sends a signal indicating acidity. A less direct test is a hair analysis. Hair can indicate the mineral status of the body. If several minerals are low it indicates poor mineral absorption which suggests low stomach acidity. A third test is to examine stool specimens, looking for the presence of incompletely digested foods.

Low stomach acidity can be treated by lowering the pH (increase acidity) of the digestive juices. This can be done with dietary supplements. Two types of hydrochloric acid (HCL) are used in over-the-counter dietary supplements—betaine HCL and glutamic acid HCL. These are sold in tablet or capsule form and usually include a mixture of digestive enzymes. If stomach acidity is seriously low, however, supplementation should be done under the supervision of a physician.

Coconut Oil for Digestion

Most digestion-related problems involve incomplete protein digestion. Next in line is fat. Many people have trouble digesting fats. One of the benefits of using coconut oil is that it is easy to digest. The molecules that make up coconut oil are smaller than most other fats and require fewer digestive enzymes to be broken down into individual fatty acids. The medium-chain fatty acids (MCFA) in coconut oil digest so rapidly, in fact, that they don't even need pancreatic enzymes and are absorbed almost immediately as they pass through the stomach into the intestines. The benefit in this is that people who have trouble digesting fats can easily digest coconut oil. They are able to absorb fat-soluble vitamins and minerals and do not suffer from digestive discomfort caused by other fats.

A study conducted in France and published in the *American Journal of Clinical Nutrition* reported that obesity is associated with a defect in fat digestion. A group of obese subjects were given oils containing either long-chain fatty acids (LCFA) which are the ones typically found in most foods and vegetable oils or MCFA derived from coconut oil. The subjects had difficulty completely digesting the LCFA. There was no difficulty seen in those who were given MCFA. The authors of the study recommended foods containing MCFA in place of LCFA as a treatment for obesity.[4]

Because coconut oil is easy to digest, it has been a lifesaver for many people. It is used in special food preparations for those who suffer from malabsorption syndrome such as cystic fibrosis. It is added to hospital and commercial baby formulas because infants, particularly premature infants, have difficulty digesting other fats. It is also beneficial for the treatment of malnutrition. Since it is rapidly absorbed, it can deliver quick nourishment without putting excessive strain on the digestive and enzyme systems, and helps conserve the body's energy that would normally be expended in digesting other fats.

Not only is it easy to digest, but it also enhances the absorption of many other nutrients. When added to the diet, it improves the absorption of minerals (particularly calcium and magnesium), B vitamins, fat-soluble vitamins (A, D, E, K, and beta-carotene), and amino acids from protein.[5] Coconut oil improves the utilization of essential fatty acids. A diet rich in coconut oil can enhance the efficiency of essential fatty acids by as much as 100%.[6] In Third World countries where the poor are often malnourished, simply adding coconut products to their diets has brought recovery from nutritional deficiencies.

Coconut oil doesn't necessarily supply these missing nutrients. What it does is make what nutrients that are already present in the diet more bioavailable so that the body is better able to absorb them. Whether you have digestive problems or not, adding coconut oil to your diet will enhance nutrient absorption.

Gallbladder

If you have had surgery and had your gallbladder removed, you are at high risk of suffering with subclinical malnutrition. The purpose of the gallbladder is to store and regulate the use of bile. The function of bile in the digestive process is often given little notice, but is essential. The liver produces bile at a relatively constant rate. As the bile is secreted, it drains into and is collected by the gallbladder. The gallbladder, being hollow, functions as a container to hold bile. When fats and oils leave the stomach and enter the intestinal tract they stimulate the gallbladder to pump bile into the intestine. An adequate amount of bile is essential for the digestion of fats because it emulsifies the fat, allowing it to freely mix with digestive enzymes. Without bile, fat in the intestine would clump together and pass through the digestive tract unabsorbed.

Having dietary fat pass though the digestive tract without being absorbed may sound like a good thing if you're trying to lose weight, but it can cause serious health problems, one of which is abdominal discomfort. Another is nutritional deficiency. You must have fat in your diet in order to absorb the fat-soluble vitamins, some of which function as important antioxidants that protect you from free-radical destruction.

When the gallbladder is surgically removed, fat digestion is greatly hindered. Without the gallbladder, the bile, which is continually being secreted by the liver, slowly drains into the small intestine. The tiny amount of bile that drains directly from the liver into the intestine is not enough to function adequately in fat digestion when even moderate amounts of fat are consumed. This leads to malabsorption of fat-soluble vitamins and to digestive problems. Bile must be present in the intestine to properly absorb fat-soluble vitamins.

Since coconut oil doesn't require pancreatic enzymes for digestion and absorption, it also doesn't need bile. So if you have had your gallbladder removed, you can get all the nutritional benefits of fat by using coconut oil in place of other fats.

I know people who have had their gallbladders removed who would suffer from indigestion or cramping if they ate too much fat or oil. When they switch to using coconut oil the problem disappears. I've had people report to me that they can take as much as four tablespoons of coconut oil at one time without experiencing any discomfort, when just a small amount of any other oil would cause gastric distress.

Digestive Aids

Poor digestion means poor nutrient absorption. If you have any of the problems listed above, you should consider using foods and supplements that aid digestion. The first thing you should do is begin using coconut oil for all cooking and baking purposes.

The second thing you can do is to improve the natural secretion of gastric juices and enzymes. The best food for this purpose is cayenne pepper. Adding cayenne pepper or any fresh hot pepper or horseradish to meals will stimulate digestive fluids. The more you use, the more effective it is. If you're not accustomed to eating hot foods, go slowly at first. As you become used to it your tolerance for hot foods will increase and you can add a little more as time goes by. Other foods that stimulate digestive juices are lemon and vinegar. Use these to flavor vegetables, salads, meats, etc. A glass of water with a couple of fresh lemon wedges makes an excellent drink.

The easiest way to improve digestion is to take digestive supplements. You can obtain them at drug and health food stores. Take the recommended amount suggested on the container *after* each meal. If you forget to take them immediately after eating, you can still benefit if you can get them down even a half hour or so after a meal. The reason you take them after eating is to allow time for the body to produce all the enzymes it can naturally. Taking the supplement before eating will encourage the body to slow down enzyme production, because the supplement does the job for you. The body, sensing the presence of these enzymes, refrains from producing more.

There are many different brands of digestive supplements that use a variety of different ingredients. Look for one with a combination of protein, carbohydrate, and fat-digesting enzymes in combination with either betaine HCL or glutamic acid HCL. Sometimes vitamins and minerals that support digestive function such as niacin, vitamin B-6, and magnesium chloride, will be added as well. The most important thing is to get the enzymes.

For protein-digesting enzymes, look for terms such as protease, pepsin, papain, bromelain, or trypsin. For carbohydrate-digesting enzymes, look for amylase. For fat-digesting enzymes, look for lipase. Pancreatic enzymes or pancreatin contains all three groups of enzymes.

The most common protein digesting enzymes come from tropical fruits: bromelain from pineapple and papain from papayas. Pancreatic enzymes in supplements come from animal sources and are most like those produced by our own bodies.

Eating tropical fruits after meals can aid in protein digestion. Enzymes in fresh pineapple, papaya, and kiwi can help relieve indigestion and heartburn. In the past I've had heartburn so bad I couldn't sleep at night. Getting up and eating a couple of pieces of freshly cut pineapple settled my stomach in minutes and allowed me to sleep peacefully for the rest of the night. To be effective these fruits must be *raw*. Canned pineapple, for example, has no effect because the enzymes are destroyed in processing.

In time, as you eat a whole foods, natural diet, your health will improve. As your health improves, so will your digestion. Many people happily report to me that as they get away from processed foods and begin eating the foods I recommend their digestive problems disappear. Some of these people have gained relief even after years of suffering with digestive problems.

Chapter 9

HOW TO SUPERCHARGE YOUR METABOLISM ▃

Don't you hate them—those people who are as skinny as rails and eat like horses? They're full of pep and vitality, gorge themselves on all types of fattening foods and never gain an ounce. You, on the other hand, eat a celery stick and immediately gain five pounds. Why is that? The answer—metabolism. Your basal metabolic rate (BMR) is slower than theirs. They burn up more calories with the same amount of physical activity as you. They can eat more than you, but weigh less.

Wouldn't it be nice if you could jump-start your metabolism and kick it into high gear? In this chapter you will learn what causes metabolic problems, but more importantly, you will learn how to revitalize your metabolism and get it humming along at a more normal rate.

We face a serious problem nowadays. A new plague of gigantic proportions is sweeping across the civilized world. With the adoption of modern lifestyles and processed foods a new disease has spread throughout the world claiming millions of victims. You could be one of them. It is estimated that 1 in 4 or about 23% of the population is already affected by it to some degree. Many more are in danger. Unlike the plagues of the past which strike quickly, this new plague is more deceptive. It creeps up on its victims very slowly and often goes undetected for years. By the time you begin to suspect something is wrong, symptoms are far advanced. What is this insidious new plague? It's not an infectious disease, like those in the past. It's a metabolic disorder called thyroid system dysfunction. Thyroid system dysfunction can be divided into two major categories or conditions—hypothyroidism and Wilson's thyroid syndrome.

HYPOTHYROIDISM

When people say they have low metabolism or have a thyroid problem, what they are generally referring to is hypothyroidism. Hypothyroidism is a condition characterized by the underproduction of thyroid hormones. The thyroid is a butterfly shaped gland located in the neck just below the Adam's apple. Thyroid hormones influence every single cell in your body. They regulate body temperature, metabolic rate, reproduction, growth, the making of blood cells, nerve and muscle function, the use of calcium in the body, and more. They affect your cells' ability to utilize blood sugar and insulin and determine the rate at which calories are metabolized, thus having a dramatic effect on body weight.

How can you tell if you have an underactive thyroid? Symptoms of hypothyroidism include overweight, sensitivity to cold, lack of energy, muscle weakness, slow heart rate, dry and flaky skin, hair loss, constipation, irritability, mental depression, slowness or slurring of speech, drooping and swollen eyes, swollen face, recurrent infections, allergies, headaches, calcium metabolism problems, and female problems such as heavy menstrual flow and cramping.

If hypothyroidism occurs in childhood and remains untreated, it may retard growth, delay sexual maturation, and inhibit normal development of the brain.

Severity of the symptoms depends on the degree of thyroid hormone deficiency. Mild deficiency may cause no observable symptoms; severe deficiency may produce many of the above conditions.

Thyroid hormones regulate metabolism. Metabolism controls the rate at which the body uses energy to power the processes within living cells. As energy is consumed by the cells, heat is produced. The heat produced from metabolic processes is fairly constant, normally fluctuating less than a degree or so throughout the day. It is lowest when we are at rest when energy needs are low and increases with physical activity when energy needs are greater. Vigorous physical activity can raise body temperature by as much as two or three degrees.

Normal body temperature is 98.6° F.* During the day body temperature can vary up or down by a full degree. A temperature of 97.6° F could be considered normal depending on the conditions in which the reading was taken. If metabolism is low due to insufficient secretion of thyroid hormone, body temperature would be chronically lower than normal. Obvious symptoms would be sensitivity to cold. Being easily chilled and frequently experiencing cold hands and feet are typical signs of hypothyroidism.

---

*This is oral body temperature, internal body temperature is actually higher.

Another consequence of low metabolism is being overweight. When metabolism is slowed down, less energy is used. If your body doesn't use all the energy supplied in the foods you eat, it converts it into fat. So the lower your metabolism, the more likely you will store fat and gain weight. For this reason, calorie consumption alone is not the cause of overweight. A person with a thyroid problem could eat a normal amount of food and still gain weight.

IODINE DEFICIENCY

What causes hypothyroidism? Many environmental and dietary factors can influence the function of the thyroid gland. Malnutrition is a significant factor. The absence of trace minerals, particularly iodine, can cause hypothyroidism. In severe cases the thyroid will swell up so large that the gland protrudes from the neck. In extreme cases the gland can grow as large as a grapefruit. This condition is called goiter.

Iodine is essential in the production of thyroid hormones. When the iodine level in the blood is low, the cells of the thyroid gland begin to enlarge so as to trap as many atoms of iodine as possible. If the gland enlarges due to an iodine deficiency, until it is visible, the condition is called *simple goiter*. Goiter afflicts about 200 million people throughout the world, most of them in Africa. In 96% of these cases the cause is iodine deficiency.

Simple goiter occurs most commonly in areas of the world where the soil and water are deficient in iodine. Iodine in soil is taken up by plants. We get iodine from the meat and milk of animals that graze on these plants or from crops grown in these soils.

Fahrenheit	Celsius
32.0	0.0
90.0	32.2
96.0	35.6
97.6	36.4
97.8	36.6
98.3	36.8
98.4	36.9
98.6	37.0
98.9	37.2
100.0	37.8
104.0	40.0
107.0	41.7

Temperatures given in this chapter are expressed in degrees Fahrenheit. For those readers who are more familiar with Celsius, please refer to the table at left.

128

Iodine is plentiful in ocean water, so seafood is a good source. Land masses that have at one time been under the ocean are overlain by sedimentary rocks and soils rich in iodine. Some areas are iodine deficient, because they are covered by volcanic rock and soil such as in the inland valleys of Oregon and Idaho or have been stripped of sedimentary rock by glaciers during the ice ages, like in the Great Lakes area of the United States and Canada.

For many years farmers living in iodine poor areas routinely gave their livestock salt blocks. The salt, which was mined from ancient seabeds, supplied iodine to the cattle. Iodine from salt blocks and from what little was in the plants the animals ate was concentrated in their milk fat. Butter made from the milk fat of these cows provided people with just enough iodine to prevent goiter. As long as people ate an adequate amount of butter, goiter wasn't a problem. When the 1930s came along, margarine became popular as a butter substitute. During the Great Depression money was scarce so people began using the cheaper margarine in place of butter. For many people butter was their primary source of iodine. When they switched to margarine, goiter suddenly became a serious health problem. In an effort to prevent goiter, iodine was added to table salt. Even today you see this in the store as iodized salt. In Canada all table salt is iodized.

While simple goiter is not a serious problem for most of us, mild forms of iodine deficiency are still possible, particularly if you eat a low-sodium diet and nutritionally poor foods.

There is a simple test you can do to see if you are deficient in iodine. To do this you need a jar of 2% iodine solution, obtainable from most any drug store. It is sold as a disinfectant. Coat an area on the skin about one-inch in diameter with the iodine. Let it dry (about 5 minutes). It will leave a red stain. You may want to do this on a spot that will be covered by your clothes so you don't draw attention to yourself when you are out in public. If you are getting an adequate amount of iodine in your diet, the stain should remain on your skin for about 24 hours before it completely fades away. If you are deficient, your body will quickly absorb the iodine and the stain will fade before that time. The quicker it disappears the more deficient you are.

Getting your required amount of iodine is easy. You only need a tiny amount. You can increase your iodine intake by using sea salt (which naturally contains iodine) and by eating sea vegetables (such as kelp) and ocean fish. Freshwater fish are not a good source. Dietary supplements are also available. Most natural supplements get their iodine from dried kelp.

DIETARY GOITROGENS

Some of the foods we eat each day depress thyroid activity and promote hypothyroidism. These foods contain antithyroid substances called goitrogens. Goitrogens interfere with the production and function of thyroid hormones and can even induce goiter formation. Goiter caused by toxins in foods is called *toxic goiter*.

Ironically, what some people consider to be health foods contain the most goitrogens. All cruciferous vegetables (the cabbage family) contain goitrogens. This would include cabbage, cauliflower, brussels sprouts, mustard greens, broccoli, turnips, and kale. Legumes also contain goitrogens. This includes soybeans, peas, lentils, bean sprouts, etc. Eight million people worldwide, mostly in Africa, have toxic goiter because of the overconsumption of cruciferous vegetables.

Does this mean that you should avoid all these vegetables? Fortunately, most goitrogens are heat sensitive and are neutralized when cooked. Light cooking destroys the toxins without significantly affecting nutritional content. So if these foods are cooked you can eat all you want without fear.

For most people eating small amounts of these vegetables raw is not harmful. If you suspect you have a thyroid problem, however, it is best that you stay away from them unless they are cooked.

Of all the goitrogenous foods, soybeans pose the greatest threat. The antithyroid substances in soy are not destroyed by cooking. Soy products such as tofu and texturized vegetable protein have gained a great deal of popularity particularly as meat extenders or replacements. But you say you don't eat soy? Think again. If you eat like most people, you're consuming soy in one form or another every single day, whether you know it or not. Since soy is used in a wide assortment of foods, exposure can come from many sources. Soy byproducts have found their way into an incredible number of everyday foods. Soy is often used as a replacement for meat and dairy. It is disguised as everything from cheese, milk, burgers, and hot dogs to ice cream, yogurt, and protein drinks. It's even in baby formula. At least 60% of the foods on America's grocery shelves contain soy derivatives—soy flour, texturized vegetable protein, vegetable oil, partially hydrogenated oil, soy protein isolate, etc. Most every packaged, prepared food you pick up now contains soy in one form or another. It makes me wonder if part of the reason why we are experiencing a growing problem with hypothyroidism and overweight is due to the increasing amount of soy in our food supply.

Many soy containing foods are marketed as low-fat, dairy-free, or high-protein meat substitutes which are eaten by people conscious about their weight. Little do they know that by eating these "low-fat" diet foods they are destroying their thyroid gland, lowering their metabolism, and setting the stage for obesity.

We have been bombarded with the supposed benefits of soy for so long that many people find it hard to believe that soy promotes weight gain by interfering with thyroid function. However, there exists a significant body of research that demonstrates goitrogenic and even carcinogenic effects of soy products.[1] There are many reports of goitrogenic effects on children resulting from the use of soy based infant formula.[2, 3] Even healthy adults can develop thyroid problems when they begin eating soy.[4] Researchers have clearly shown that soy protein (isoflavones) inhibits the thyroid's ability to produce hormones.[5] Soy protein has even been linked to autoimmune thyroid disease—another mechanism that causes hypothyroidism.[6]

Soy protein isn't the only villain. Soybean oil also attacks the thyroid. The oil doesn't necessarily cause goiter but is equally as toxic, because it interferes with the production and utilization of thyroid hormones. Approximately 80% of the oils in our diet come from soy: soybean oil, partially hydrogenated soybean oil, margarine, and shortening. Look at ingredients labels for soybean oil of one type or another.

If you see anything that contains soy, don't touch it. The only exception would be soy products that have undergone a long period of fermentation. The microbial action in fermentation neutralizes most of the toxins. Fermented soy include miso, soy sauce, and tempeh. Small amounts of these items may be okay on occasion. All other soy products should be avoided.

Don't be taken in by the argument that soy products must be safe because the Asians have been eating them for centuries. Contrary to what the soy industry would like you to believe, soy has never been a staple in Asia. A study of the history of soy use in Asia shows that the poor used it during times of extreme food shortage, and only then the soybeans were carefully prepared by fermentation to destroy the toxins. They understood the dangers of soy. Even now most Asians eat very little soy, less than 1–2% of total calories. They use it primarily as a condiment to their meals, unlike in the West where it is eaten in relatively large quantities as a replacement for meat and dairy and as a source of protein.[7]

WILSON'S THYROID SYNDROME
A Treatable Thyroid Problem

Linda started gaining weight after quitting smoking. Her weight swelled to the point that she knew she had to do something. She tried losing weight on her own without success. It was frustrating. Realizing she needed help, she went to a weight-loss clinic and started their program. It didn't help. They even accused her of cheating on the diet because she wasn't losing any weight. She tried another weight-loss clinic with a more strict dietary program. After 6 months limited to just 800 calories a day she lost only 4 pounds.

Discouraged and very depressed, she went to an endocrinologist for help. He determined that her thyroid was underactive and prescribed Synthroid, a synthetic thyroid medicine. It wasn't much help. A year later she was even more depressed, constantly tired, had headaches every day, and was still overweight. Her doctor finally told her she would have to live with herself as she was, overweight and tired. She told her doctor that she refused to live the rest of her life this way. He advised her to see a psychiatrist to help her accept the way she was. This caused her to feel even more hopeless, depressed, and discouraged.

Eventually she learned about a condition known as Wilson's thyroid syndrome (WTS) which could be causing her metabolism to be so sluggish. She began treatment and within a few weeks began to feel more energy and less depressed. In just a couple of months she lost 40 pounds and her fatigue was completely gone. Depression, fatigue, and headaches were no longer a part of Linda's daily life.

Five years ago Debbie was under an extreme amount of stress. During this time she began experiencing headaches, dry and flaky skin, loss of energy, depression, and weight gain. She had put on weight even though her food intake had *decreased*. She began to retain fluid and her feet and ankles became so swollen and painful that, at times, it became uncomfortable for her to stand or walk. She knew something was wrong.

At this point she decided to seek medical help. She went to two different doctors and got the same answers. They could find nothing wrong. Her blood tests were normal. They said there was nothing wrong with her thyroid or her metabolism. They couldn't do anything to help her.

She then learned about the Wilson's Thyroid Syndrome Treatment Center and made an appointment. As she filled out the patient information sheet and checked off all the symptoms, she became embarrassed at the large number of symptoms she had that corresponded with those on the list. Her temperature was taken and registered below normal. She told the nurse, "That's okay It's always low." Her low temperature, however, was a key to her failing health and weight problem.

Although her blood tests showed her thyroid to be "normal," she *did* have a thyroid problem. Those with Wilson's thyroid syndrome often display normal blood test readings, yet they don't have normal thyroid system function.

132

Debbie began treatment and within a week her symptoms began to disappear. Her family and friends could not believe the immediate changes. She said she had almost forgotten what feeling good was all about.

In Linda's case she was diagnosed with low thyroid, but thyroid medication did little to help alleviate her symptoms. Debbie had no measurable thyroid deficiencies, yet she too suffered from a thyroid system problem. Both were victims of Wilson's thyroid syndrome (WTS). Wilson's thyroid syndrome is a cluster of reversible symptoms caused by dysfunction of the thyroid system. WTS is not easily recognized by doctors because it does not show up on standard blood tests for thyroid gland problems. Many thousands of overweight people are affected with WTS without realizing it. Aches, pains, and weight gain associated with Wilson's thyroid syndrome are often attributed to aging or some other cause. People can suffer for years with these symptoms without realizing there is a treatment.

Treatment is very simple and in most cases permanent. With hypothyroidism patients must take thyroid medication for life. But Wilson's thyroid syndrome is a reversible condition that can generally be corrected in a few weeks to a few months time. After treatment is over, no further medication is usually necessary. People who have suffered with overweight and other symptoms for 10, 20, 30 years or more have been able to overcome the problem in a few months and get on the road to recovery and permanent weight loss.

Thyroid System Dysfunction

Many overweight people suspect they have a thyroid problem which causes, or at least contributes to, their weight problem. When someone says they have a thyroid problem what they are generally referring to is the function of the thyroid *gland*. The thyroid gland, however, is only one part of the thyroid *system*. A person can have a thyroid gland that is working normally yet still have a thyroid *system* problem.

Low metabolism can be the result of either an underactive thyroid gland (hypothyroidism) or a dysfunction of the thyroid system. Blood tests can only determine thyroid *gland* function. According to Denis Wilson, M.D., who was the first to identify WTS, most metabolic or thyroid problems are *not* due to hypothyroidism, but to thyroid *system* dysfunction. This is why so many people who suspect metabolic problems have normal blood test results. Wilson's thyroid syndrome is a thyroid *system* problem.

The thyroid gland secretes hormones that regulate metabolism. These hormones are called T4 (thyroxin) and T3 (triiodothyronine). Eighty to ninety percent of the hormones released by the thyroid gland are T4. Synthroid, a common thyroid medication, is composed entirely of T4.

When someone is hypothyroid, their thyroid gland is not producing adequate amounts of T4 and T3. They are considered to have a thyroid *gland* problem.

Many people with low thyroid gland activity are helped by taking medication that supplies the body with the thyroid hormone T4. By increasing the blood concentration of T4 the body receives the hormone it needs to keep metabolism up to normal. Taking T4, however, isn't a cure it's a crutch to assist a thyroid gland that isn't functioning optimally. Thyroid medication must be taken for life.

When T4 is released by the thyroid it circulates in the blood and is absorbed into cells. Here it is converted into T3. The great majority of the T3 in your body comes from conversion of T4 within the cells. T4 has little biological activity. T3, on the other hand, has four times the activity as T4 and, therefore, has far more impact on metabolism. Thyroid system dysfunction occurs when T4 is not adequately converted into T3. The thyroid may make normal amounts of T4, even over produce it, but if it is not converted to T3, metabolism will be depressed. This is what happens in Wilson's thyroid syndrome. T4 may be adequate, but T3 is not. Sometimes people with WTS will be hyperthyroid as well. Treatment with T4 medications does little good because it isn't converted to the more active T3. This is why a person can be given thyroid medications and experience little or no improvement.

Multiple Enzyme Dysfunction

The most characteristic feature of WTS is low or unsteady body temperature. In fact, low body temperature is believed to be the primary cause for the symptoms associated with WTS.

Body temperature is one of those things that is tightly controlled. If your temperature goes too high (107° F), it can cause brain damage. Likewise, a temperature that is too low (below 90° F) can be just as harmful. The ideal temperature, measured orally, is 98.6° F. This is true for all people regardless of genetic background or individuality. Optimal body temperature is a chemical constant, like water freezing at 32° F. Whether you go to the frozen tundra of Alaska or under the hot Hawaii sun, water still freezes at 32° F. Our bodies are structured to function within a very narrow range of temperatures. Normal is considered 98.6°. Any higher or any lower starts to affect body function.

The reason why small variations in temperature are so important is that enzymes function optimally at 98.6°. The farther away from this the temperature gets, the less effective or less active enzymes become. Enzymes are important because they are involved in nearly all the chemical reactions that occur in the body. If enzyme activity slows down, over time health problems can develop. This is called multiple enzyme dysfunction (MED). Low metabolism is caused by multiple enzyme dysfunction. Inappropriate weight gain can be due to MED. Dr. Wilson has identified as many as 60 health problems associated with MED. The most common include:

overweight
cold hands and feet
fatigue
migraines
PMS
irritability
fluid retention/swelling
anxiety and panic attacks
hair loss
depression
decreased memory and
  concentration
low sex drive
dry skin and hair
constipation
irritable bowel syndrome
insomnia
hives
itchiness
asthma
allergies

food intolerances/sensitivities
brittle nails
slow healing from wounds
  and injuries
bruise easily
heat and/or cold intolerance
hypoglycemia
frequent or persistent colds
frequent urinary tract
  infections
frequent yeast infections
depressed immunity
acne
arthritis and joint pain
carpal tunnel syndrome
ulcers
poor coordination
ringing in the ears
acid indigestion
infertility
irregular periods

Chronically low body temperature can be the primary cause or at least a contributing factor for any of these conditions. Those suffering from Wilson's thyroid syndrome won't necessarily have all of these conditions, perhaps only one or two. Some may have many. I've seen people with at least 16 of the above symptoms (all of which, by the way, were significantly reduced or eliminated by the diet and lifestyle changes discussed later in this book).

How can you tell if you have WTS? One way, is to check your symptoms with the list above. Are you experiencing any of these symptoms? Many of these symptoms can also be caused by other conditions, such as hypothyroidism. Some people with mild WTS may have no noticeable symptoms. The best test for WTS is simply taking your temperature. If your body temperature is constantly below normal, enzymes are not working effectively and you probably have a thyroid system problem. If T4 medication is of little or no help, WTS is most likely at fault.

Low body temperature is the most characteristic feature of WTS. Some people may say that their body temperature is "naturally" low, or that it is "normal" for them to have a low temperature. Low body temperature is not normal for anyone. In order for your enzymes to function optimally, your temperature needs to be at or near 98.6°. This temperature does not vary from person to person. When the temperature does vary it indicates a metabolic problem.

Feeling hot all the time is not a good indication of body temperature. Many people, particularly if they are overweight, feel hot, yet their temperatures may be below normal. The reason they "feel" hot is that they have become oversensitive or intolerant to fluctuations in temperature. Often, a person who is always unbearably hot in the summer is also frigidly cold in the winter. If you happen to be married to one of these people, you know the conflict that can take place. During the winter one will be constantly turning up the furnace and stacking on blankets at night, while the other turns it down and sleeps with little covering. During the summer the roles may reverse. It's a constant battle.

What Causes Chronic Low Body Temperature?

Lisa never had much of a weight problem in her youth, but after the birth of her third child the pounds began to stack up. It was almost like someone turned on a switch for increased fat production. Within just a few years after delivery she had gained 30 extra pounds. She didn't eat any differently than she used to, but the weight kept piling on. Headaches, irritability, hypoglycemia, and other health problems began to emerge as well. Like most, she attributed the excess body fat as simply a consequence of gaining weight during pregnancy and as part of the natural process of getting older. Her real problem, however, was that during her last pregnancy she had developed WTS.

Our body's metabolism has basically three settings—fast, medium, and slow. Metabolism shifts between all three during the day depending on different circumstances. At times our body functions best at high speed, at other times it prefers to go slow. Most of the time it runs in neutral or medium, not too fast and not too slow.

Metabolism will shift into high gear in response to certain circumstances. For instance, when we are involved in a physically demanding activity our lungs breathe deeper and faster, our heart rate increases, and a greater amount of oxygen is delivered to our muscles, which is necessary

136

for energy production. If we get an infection and become sick, metabolism increases to accelerate production of antibodies and speed healing and repair.

Metabolism shifts into low gear when we sleep or rest or when food consumption decreases. When we fast or even diet, the body interprets it as a period of starvation. In response, metabolism slows down to conserve energy to ensure survival during the time when food is less plentiful.

A normal, healthy body constantly shifts in and out of all three levels of metabolism. When conditions that cause the body to gear up or gear down are over, metabolism rebounds back to normal. This is the way it's suppose to work. However, in Wilson's thyroid syndrome when conditions that cause the body to slow down are passed, the body doesn't recover, it becomes stuck in low gear. It can stay stuck for a few weeks, months, or years. Subsequent events that shift the metabolism into low gear can crank metabolism down even lower. If metabolism doesn't recover before a new episode hits, it can go lower and lower. As metabolism slows down, body temperature decreases. This is why some people may have a temperature only slightly below normal while others may be off by two or three degrees.

What causes metabolism to get stuck in low gear? It is a combination of both stress and malnutrition. When we are under stress the body responds by increasing its metabolism. If you have to take an important test, run a race, or meet a deadline at work, the body responds by pumping up metabolism. As metabolism increases, cellular processes are all shifted into high gear. The demand for energy to fuel these activities is increased. The need for vitamins and minerals is increased because the enzymes that run all chemical activities in the body depend on these nutrients. So vitamins and minerals are used up at an accelerated rate. If there are enough nutrients in storage, and if the stress is removed after a brief period of time, the body is perfectly able to cope with this shift in metabolism.

A problem arises, however, when stress becomes chronic or severe *and* the body is undernourished. When stress is frequent or very severe, there is a great demand for vitamins and minerals for the utilization of enzymes. If the needed nutrients are not present, the body senses a situation similar to that of starvation and shifts into low gear. When nutrients become depleted the body goes into a state of exhaustion and becomes locked in low gear. It does this as a means of self-preservation to conserve energy and nutrients that are vital to maintaining life. Vitamins and minerals are absolutely necessary for the brain, heart, lungs, and other vital organs to function. If these nutrients become too depleted, permanent damage and even death can result.

If enough nutrients are not supplied to adequately replenish the body's storehouse, metabolism remains stuck in low gear. Repeated episodes of stress drive metabolism even lower, making it harder to recover. What types of stress can bring about this situation? Any type of chronic or severe physical, mental, or emotional stress, such as pregnancy and childbirth, divorce, death of a loved one, job demands, family troubles, surgery, accidents, illness, or lack of sleep. Eighty percent of those who are affected by WTS are women. This is understandable since the number one cause is pregnancy and childbirth.

As you learned from the last chapter, malnutrition, or rather subclinical malnutrition, is very common in our society. Eating sweets, refined grains and oils, and other processed foods, which have been stripped of much of their natural vitamins and minerals, has created a society of people who are on the edge nutritionally. Pregnant women have an increased demand for good nutrition. The unborn child demands ample nutrients for proper growth and development and will steal them from the mother's body if they are not supplied in her diet. If she doesn't eat properly her own nutrient reserves can become dangerously depleted. Add on to that the fact that pregnancy can be a very stressful time. Nine months of stress culminate in several hours of arduous labor and childbirth. It is no wonder why pregnancy and childbirth is the number one cause of WTS.

Certain drugs such as cortisone or steroids can also promote WTS. Cortisone blocks the conversion of T4 to T3. The absence of adequate T3 in the body lowers metabolism and body temperature.

Dieting can worsen WTS. Low-calorie diets, especially those that allow poor quality foods, can be interpreted by the body as starvation. A body already suffering from a lack of good nutrition will shift its metabolism even lower. This makes losing weight harder. When "normal" eating is resumed, weight rebounds, dragging with it a few extra pounds because now metabolism is even lower than it was before. Some people's metabolism is so low that they can gain weight on just 800 calories a day.

How Can You Tell If You Have Wilson's Thyroid Syndrome?

Standard blood tests can't detect WTS. Blood tests measure the amount of hormones in the blood, which give an indication of how well the glands are functioning. WTS doesn't have anything to do with how well glands produce thyroid hormones, it has to do with how well the tissues process these hormones. It is more of a thyroid system imbalance than it is a thyroid hormone deficiency. Thyroid blood tests aren't useful because they can't measure what's happening in the tissues and cells of the body.

138

In WTS the production of thyroid hormone is often normal, but the processing of that hormone in the tissues can slow down, leading to an imbalance that can leave patients with low body temperature and the classic symptoms of low thyroid function.

Often those who have low thyroid hormone production (hypothyroidism) are also affected by WTS. According to Dr. Wilson there are "far more people with WTS than all other low thyroid problems combined." So WTS is a very common condition. If you suspect a metabolic problem, it is likely to be WTS.

The way you can tell if you have WTS is to check for the symptoms. Look over the list of symptoms listed above. Do you have any of these? Keep in mind that even one of them is a sign that something is wrong. Illness is not normal and dysfunction is not normal. The body tries to maintain optimal health so long as it is allowed to. When it doesn't have it, something is out of place.

Overweight is one of the most common symptoms associated with WTS. Obviously metabolism is slow and gaining weight is easy. If you are overweight it may not be simply because you eat too much. Most overweight individuals have metabolic problems that exacerbate their weight problems.

Not everyone who is overweight has thyroid system problems. But a great many do. If you eat little and put on weight, gain weight easily, have been on low-calorie diets in the past, eat junk foods, don't exercise, and experience a lot of stress, then you may have WTS. If you are female and have been pregnant or if you were normal sized as a youth and suddenly packed on weight (within a couple of years), you may also suspect WTS.

The strongest indication of WTS is body temperature. If your average daily temperature is consistently below normal, suspect WTS.

Taking Your Temperature

Simply taking your temperature once during the day isn't a very accurate way to evaluate body temperature. Several factors influence temperature readings such as physical activity, climate, bathing, and eating. Our temperature also fluctuates during the day. Temperature is normally lowest in the morning just as you wake up. As the day progresses, temperature rises, maintains a certain level, and at the end of the day begins to decline. This daily cycle can vary by as much as 1 degree in a relatively healthy individual. If you take your temperature in the morning you will get a lower than normal value, no matter what your "real" temperature is.

To avoid the lows in the morning and evening you should take your temperature during the day when your metabolism is at its peak. When you

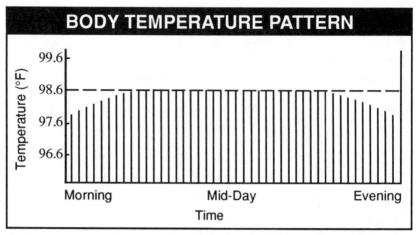

BODY TEMPERATURE PATTERN

Body temperature is normally a little low in the morning and evening. During the day it should be at or near 98.6° F. Those people with WTS usually run about one degree lower throughout the day.

measure your temperature when it is at its highest it should register as normal (98.6° F). For the most accurate evaluation you should take your temperature three times a day and average them together. If your average temperature is normal it should be at or near 98.6° F.

Dr. Wilson advises taking the first temperature 3 hours after arising in the morning, the second 3 hours later, and the third 3 hours after that. For instance, if you wake up at 6:00 a.m., take your first temperature at 9:00 a.m., the second at 12:00 noon, and the third at 3:00 p.m. For each day add the readings together and divide by 3 to get the average. Take readings for at least 5 days. For women body temperature changes during the first few days of the menstrual cycle and the middle day of the cycle, so avoid doing this test at these times.

Temperature should be taken by mouth. Keep the thermometer in your mouth for at least 4 minutes. Foods can affect the temperature of the mouth, so take the reading before or at least 15 minutes after eating or drinking. Also keep in mind that many digital thermometers commonly used have an accuracy of about plus or minus .2 degrees.

When you take your temperature during the day, you are recording you body's normal high temperature. It should be 98.6° plus or minus about .3° F. The farther it is from normal the greater your chances of WTS. If your average temperature is below 98.3° you may have Wilson's thyroid syndrome. Keep in mind, however, that not all low body temperature is caused by WTS. The closer your average temperature is to normal, the less severe your symptoms are likely to be. A person with an average temperature of 98.3° may have no noticeable symptoms, while one who has a temperature of 97.5° may exhibit many. It is not uncommon for people to have mid-day temperatures as low as 96.0° or lower. Dr. Wilson has reported some patients showing signs of WTS with average temperatures as high as 98.4°, but states that most patients with noticeable symptoms have temperatures of 97.8° or less.

If your temperature readings vary significantly, it may also indicate a problem with metabolism. Readings that fluctuate greatly suggest that the body has difficulty maintaining normal temperatures. This can be a sign of possible WTS. It's normal for temperatures to vary 2-3 tenths of a degree under ordinary conditions (not exercising or exposed to extremes in ambient temperatures). If it fluctuates by a degree or more there is clearly a problem. Ideally your temperature should only fluctuate by .6° throughout the day under normal circumstances.

If you have a normal temperature reading, yet you experience many of the symptoms associated with WTS, your thermometer may be wrong. Dr. Wilson advises rechecking your temperature using a different thermometer. He claims that if a person has symptoms of WTS, the chances of having a normal temperature are only about 1 in 200. There's a lot better chance that your thermometer is wrong then there is that your temperature is normal.

Treatment

Treatment for WTS is simple. The conversion of T4 to T3 is depressed because enzymes necessary for this process are sluggish due to low body temperature. If the body temperature can be raised to near normal for a period of time, the enzymes will function properly. Simply raising the temperature of the body will improve T4 to T3 conversion. As more T3 is made, metabolism speeds up in response and body temperature increases. At some point body temperature remains high enough to keep T4 to T3 conversion going at a normal rate. Temperature stays near normal, as it is suppose to, and the body can continue on its own from then on. The entire process can be completed in as little as a few weeks to a few months. In some cases, where thyroid system dysfunction is more severe, it may take longer. Once the correction is made, body temperature remains normal, metabolism remains normal, and enzymes throughout the body function at a normal rate. The result is recovery from conditions caused by multiple enzyme dysfunction, which includes the loss of excess body weight. When metabolism is where it is supposed to be, excess weight is easier to take off with proper dieting.

How is temperature raised to accomplish this? Oral consumption of T3 will raise blood levels of this hormone, which in turn will stimulate metabolism and raise body temperature. T3 must be prescribed by your doctor. Your doctor needs to be familiar with Wilson's thyroid syndrome, not all are. Before giving you any medication, a blood test will probably be required. If your physician isn't familiar with WTS, the tests may only measure T4 and thyroid *gland* function.

Giving the patient T3 to stimulate metabolism and increase temperature brings relief to WTS patients. Dr. Wilson has successfully treated thousands of patients. Many other doctors are also treating WTS patients, but not all have the experience, so choose a physician who is familiar with this condition.

Since T3 is a hormone, it can have a variety of effects on the body, both good and bad. To avoid undesirable side effects, T3 therapy must be administered and monitored by a physician experienced in treating WTS patients.

The hormone must be taken each day following a strict time schedule. If the medicine is skipped only once, or even if taken a few hours late, treatment in most cases must start over. When the medicine is not taken on time, the body shifts back into low gear and the process of jump-starting the metabolism must start from the beginning. The reason T3 works is that it keeps the body's temperature elevated at or near normal for a long enough period of time that it allows the body to adapt and continue the process on its own. This means that the temperature during the day must be constantly maintained near normal for several weeks straight for the process to work.

Another drawback to T3 therapy is that if a patient does not address nutritional needs, she can often relapse next time she encounters a stressful situation. In this case, T3 therapy can be repeated. If a stressful situation can be anticipated, low doses of T3 can help prevent relapse. Unfortunately, stress is a normal part of life. We will never be free from it. Our bodies should be healthy enough to handle stress whenever it hits.

T3 therapy is just one way to treat WTS. For severe cases, T3 therapy may be necessary, however, diet and lifestyle changes can also accomplish the same thing without the need of taking medication. Since the WTS responds to a rise in body temperature, any process that can accomplish that goal has the potential to work.

BOOST YOUR ENERGY

When someone comes to me and says, "I'm always tired, what can I do to get more energy without taking drugs or using caffeine?" My answer is quick and simple, "Use coconut oil."

When I tell people this, at first they're startled, "Won't that make me fat?" I tell them, "No, not so long as you don't overdo it by consuming more calories than your body needs to fuel daily activities." An easy way to do this is to simply replace the oils you are currently using with coconut oil. Coconut oil can give you more energy and help you lose weight.

One of the major differences between coconut oil and other fats is the way in which it is digested and metabolized. Coconut oil is different because it is composed of a special group of fats called medium-chain fatty acids (MCFA). Most all fats in our diet, whether they are saturated or unsaturated, are in the form of large molecules called long-chain fatty acids (LCFA). Both vegetable oils and animal fats are composed almost entirely of long-chain fatty acids (LCFA). The medium-chain fatty acids (MCFA) in coconut are much smaller in size. The size makes a big difference.

When we eat foods containing long-chain fatty acids (LCFA) the fats are slowly broken down by digestive enzymes into units small enough to be absorbed through the intestinal wall. As they pass through the intestinal lining they are gathered together and packaged into little bundles of fat (lipid) and protein called *lipoproteins*. These lipoproteins are sent into the bloodstream, where they circulate throughout the body. As they circulate in the blood, the fats are distributed to all the tissues of the body. These are the fats that end up on artery walls and fill up fat cells. This is how fat builds up in our fat tissues. These lipoproteins continue to circulate in the bloodstream until most all of the fat is distributed. Cholesterol, saturated fat, monounsaturated fat, and polyunsaturated fat are all packaged together into lipoproteins and carried throughout the body in this way. The vast majority of the fats you eat every day are made up of LCFA.

The medium-chain fatty acids (MCFA) in coconut oil, however, are processed differently. Because of their smaller size, MCFA don't require pancreatic enzymes for digestion. By the time these fats reach the intestinal tract they are already broken down into individual molecules and instead of being absorbed through the intestinal wall like LCFA, they are channeled directly into the liver. Here they are converted into energy to fuel metabolism. MCFA are not packaged into lipoproteins like other fats, *so they don't circulate throughout the body adding fat to fat cells.* Coconut oil goes to the liver to produce energy, not body fat. This difference in the way your body processes MCFA is very important in respect to metabolism and body weight.

Eating foods containing MCFA is like putting high-octane fuel into your car. The car runs smoother and gets better gas mileage. Likewise, with MCFA your body performs better. Since MCFA are converted into energy, your energy level increases. This energy boost is not like the kick you get from caffeine, it's more subtle and longer lasting. It is most noticeable as an increase in endurance.

The fact that MCFA are digested immediately to produce energy has led athletes to use them as a means to enhance exercise performance. Some studies indicate this to be the case. In one study, for example, investigators tested the physical endurance of mice that were given MCFA in their daily diet against those that weren't. The study extended over a six-week period. The mice were subjected to a swimming endurance test every other day. They were placed in a pool of water with a constant current. The total swimming time until exhaustion was measured. While at first there was little difference between the groups of mice, those fed MCFA quickly began to out perform the others and continued to improve throughout the testing period.[8] Tests such as this demonstrated that MCFA had the ability to enhance endurance and exercise performance, at least in mice. Another study using human subjects supported the animal studies. In this study conditioned cyclists were used. The cyclists pedaled at 70% of maximum for 2 hours, then immediately embarked on a 40 K time-trial ride (lasting about an additional hour) while drinking one of three beverages: a MCFA solution, a sports drink, or a sports drink/MCFA combination. The cyclists who drank the sports drink/MCFA mixture performed the best.[9]*

Because of these and similar studies many of the powdered sports drinks and energy bars sold at health food stores contain MCFA to provide a quick source of energy.** Athletes and other active people looking for

---

*The authors of the study theorized that the MCFA gave the cyclists an additional source of energy, thus sparing glycogen stores. Glycogen, the energy stored in muscle tissue, would have been used up during the three-hour ride. The more glycogen in the muscles, the greater an athlete's endurance. So any substance that can conserve glycogen while providing energy would be useful to endurance athletes. In a follow-up study to test the glycogen-sparing theory, participants cycled at 60% of their maximum for three hours while drinking one of three beverages as was done in the earlier study. Following the exercise muscle glycogen levels were measured and found to be the same for all three groups. The conclusion was that MCFA did not spare glycogen stores, yet did improve performance. The improvement in performance was not due to glycogen sparing, but must be attributed to some other mechanism.

**The medium-chain fatty acids (MCFA) most often used in sports drinks and energy bars are in the form of medium-chain triglyceride oil. They are usually indicated as "MCT" on food, supplement, and infant formula labels.

nutritional, non-drug methods to enhance exercise performance have begun using them.

Although many studies have shown MCFA to boost energy and endurance, there are other studies which have shown little or no effect, at least when MCFA mixtures are taken in a *single* oral dose. Studies generally show that a single oral dose has little measurable effect. In studies where animals were fed MCFA as a part of their daily diet, however, the results were more significant. From these studies it appears that the best way to increase energy and endurance is to consume MCFA on a daily basis and not a single time just before or during competition.

One of the side effects of being overweight is a lack of energy. Part of this may be due to low thyroid function, or simply because carrying about a lot of excess weight is tiring. This encourages inactivity and further encourages weight gain. Coconut oil can give you a boost of energy that will help keep you more active throughout the day and help you burn off a few extra calories.

A LOW-CALORIE FAT
Not All Fats Are Alike

Replacing the oils you now use with coconut oil may be one of the healthiest dietary decisions you ever make. We often think that the less fat we eat, the better. However, you don't necessarily need to reduce your fat intake, you simply need to choose a fat that is better for you, one that doesn't contribute to weight gain. You can lose unwanted body fat by eating *more* saturated fat (in the form of coconut oil) and *less* polyunsaturated fat (processed vegetable oils).

One of the remarkable things about coconut oil is that it can help you *lose* weight. For this reason coconut oil can quite literally be called a low-calorie fat.

All fats, whether they are saturated or unsaturated, from a cow or from corn, contain the same amount of calories. The MCFA in coconut oil, however, are different. They contain a little less. Because of the small size of the fatty acids that make up coconut oil, they actually yield fewer calories than other fats. Coconut oil has at least 2.56% fewer calories per gram of fat compared with that of long-chain fatty acids (LCFA).[10] This means that by using coconut oil in place of other oils, your calorie intake is less.

This small reduction in calories is only part of the picture. The amount of calories coconut oil contributes is in effect closer to that of carbohydrate or protein because it is digested and processed differently than other fats.

It has been well documented in numerous dietary studies using both animals and humans that replacing LCFA with MCFA results in a decrease in body weight and a reduction in fat deposition.[11-15]

These studies have provided the scientific verification that replacing traditional sources of dietary fat, which are composed primarily of LCFA, with MCFA would yield meals having a lower calorie content. MCFA can be a useful tool in the control of weight or fat deposition. The simplest and best way to replace LCFA with MCFA is to use coconut oil in the preparation of all your food.

A Metabolic Marvel

Wouldn't it be nice to be able to take a pill that would shift our metabolic rate into a higher gear? In a sense that is what happens every time we eat. Food affects our basal metabolic rate. When we eat, many of our body's cells increase their activities to facilitate digestion and assimilation. This stimulation of cellular activity, known as diet-induced *thermogenesis*, equals about 10% of the total food energy taken in. Perhaps you have noticed, particularly on cool days, that you feel warmer after eating a meal. Your body's engines are running at a slightly higher rate so more heat is produced. Different types of foods produce different thermogenic effects. Protein-rich foods, such as meat, increase thermogenesis and have a stimulatory or energizing effect on the body. Protein has a much greater thermogenic effect than either carbohydrate or fat. This is why when people suddenly cut down on meat consumption or become vegetarians they often complain of a lack of energy. This is also one of the reasons high-protein diets promote weight loss, the increase in metabolism burns off more calories.

One food that can rev up your metabolism even more than protein is coconut oil. MCFA shift the body's metabolism into a higher gear, so to speak, so that you burn off more calories. This happens every time you eat MCFA. Because of this effect, coconut oil is a dietary fat that can actually promote weight loss!

MCFA promote weight loss by *increasing* the metabolic rate. A dietary fat that takes off weight rather than putting it on is a strange concept indeed, but that is exactly what happens, so long as calories in excess of the body's needs are not consumed. The reason for this is that MCFA are easily absorbed and are rapidly burned and used as energy for metabolism. This increase in metabolic activity even fuels the burning of the LCFA.[16] So not only are medium-chain fatty acids burned for energy production, but they encourage the consumption of long-chain fatty acids as well.

146

Dr. Julian Whitaker, a best-selling author and well-known authority on nutrition and health, makes an interesting analogy which describes this process. He explains that LCFA are like heavy wet logs that you put on a small campfire. Keep adding the logs, and soon you have more logs than fire. MCFA, on the other hand, are like rolled up newspapers soaked in gasoline. They not only burn brightly, but will burn up the wet logs as well.[17]

Research supports Dr. Whitaker's view. In one study the thermogenic (fat burning) effect of a high-calorie diet containing 40% fat as MCFA was compared to one containing 40% fat as LCFA. The thermogenic effect of the MCFA was almost twice as high as that of the LCFA—120 calories versus 66 calories. The researchers concluded that the excess energy provided by fats in the form of MCFA would not be efficiently stored as fat, but rather would be burned. A follow-up study demonstrated that MCFA given over a six-day period can increase diet-induced thermogenesis by 50%.[18]

In another study, researchers compared single meals of 400 calories composed entirely of MCFA or LCFA.[19] The thermogenic effect of MCFA over 6 hours was 3 times greater than that of LCFA. Researchers concluded that substituting MCFA for LCFA would produce weight loss as long as the calorie level remained the same.

For those who are overweight the news is even better. The thermogenic effects are greater with obese as compared to lean individuals.[20] The thermogenic increase in energy after eating a meal usually lasts only a few hours. The metabolic stimulating effects of MCFA, however, are not only evident a few hours after eating, but for a much longer time.[21]

Studies with both animals and humans consuming MCFA indicate the metabolic effects lower body weight and reduce fat deposits as compared with LCFA consumption.[22-24]

Researchers have shown that replacing LCFA with MCFA for an extended period of time could produce weight loss without decreasing energy intake.[25] So if all you did were to switch from using ordinary cooking oils (which are almost all LCFA) to using coconut oil (which is almost all MCFA), you would lose weight even if you ate the same amount of food. I see this all the time. People report to me that simply switching to coconut oil, without any other dietary change, has resulted in significant weight loss. I discovered the same thing myself when I first started using coconut oil regularly.

A review of all animal and human studies on MCFA and weight management shows that in comparison with LCFA, they have fewer calories, produce a metabolic stimulating effect which increases energy output and calorie consumption, lowers body weight, and reduces body fat. For these reasons many researchers have suggested using MCFA in the treatment or prevention of obesity.[26-31]

Substituting coconut oil for other vegetable oils in your diet will help promote weight loss. The use of refined vegetable oil actually promotes weight gain, not just from its calorie content, but because of its harmful effects on the thyroid and metabolism. Polyunsaturated vegetable oils depress thyroid activity, thus lowering metabolic rate—just the opposite of coconut oil. Eating polyunsaturated oils, like soybean oil, will contribute more to weight gain than any other known fat, even more than beef tallow and lard. According to researcher Ray Peat, Ph.D., unsaturated oils block thyroid hormone secretion, its movement in the circulation, and the response of tissues to the hormone.[32] When thyroid hormones are deficient, metabolism becomes depressed. Polyunsaturated oils are, in essence, high-calorie fats and encourage weight gain more than any other type of fat. If you want to lose weight you would be better off eating lard, because lard doesn't interfere with thyroid function.

Farmers are always looking for ways to fatten their livestock because bigger animals bring bigger profits. Fats and oils have been used as an additive in animal feed as a means of quickly packing on weight in preparing them for market. Saturated fat would seem like a good choice to fatten up livestock and pig farmers tried to feed coconut products to their animals for this purpose, but when it was added to the animal feed, the pigs lost weight![33] Farmers found that the high polyunsaturated oil content of corn and soybeans were able to do what the coconut oil couldn't. Animals fed corn and soybeans packed on pounds quickly and easily. One of the reasons these oils work so well is that the polyunsaturated oils suppress thyroid function, decreasing the animal's metabolic rate. They can eat less food and gain more weight! Many people are in a similar situation. Every time we eat polyunsaturated oils our thyroid function decreases. Weight gain is one of the consequences.

If you want to lose unwanted weight the best thing you could do is to start using coconut oil—the world's only natural, low-calorie fat.

COCONUT OIL AND WTS

I often hear people say how coconut oil has helped them with some health problem. Many report an increase in metabolism and body temperature, better digestion, relief from candida, improved healing from injury or infection, weight loss, and such. I know that using coconut oil has these effects because they are documented in the medical literature. What surprised me was that people would report improvement from many other conditions not described in the medical journals. I knew the oil was good and had many health benefits, but I was hearing things that I had never seen documented by medical research. I'm naturally skeptical about stories, and I was with these as well. You never know how accurate they are or what other events in a person's life may also have contributed to the results they experienced. I made a mental note of them, but paid little attention.

I attributed most of these stories to the placebo effect, it was just wishful thinking on their part, or so I thought. What was interesting to me was that many people reported relief from the same conditions—irritability, insomnia, arthritis, PMS, low sex drive, food cravings, and even hypoglycemia, to mention just a few. I still didn't pay much attention and shrugged it off as just a coincidence.

I then learned about the success some doctors were having treating Wilson's thyroid syndrome. Suddenly, all these testimonials made sense. Standard treatment for WTS involves giving the patient T3 to boost metabolism and raise body temperature. The increase in temperature allows enzymes to function more optimally, thus relieving the symptoms associated with low body temperature and WTS. Coconut oil, used on a regular basis, can also raise metabolism and body temperature and improve enzyme function, thus creating a similar situation. Now I understand why so many people have experienced such a wide variety of health benefits by using coconut oil.

The advantage to coconut oil is that it's a food, rather than a medicine, and can be used safely without fear of side effects. Coconut oil, combined with a good nutritional program, as will be described in Chapter 13, can be a powerful aid to overcoming thyroid system problems and associated symptoms. People who experience severe symptoms of WTS may still need T3 therapy and should check with their doctor.

Since coconut oil is a food it can be eaten every day, which can help prevent relapse if severe stress hits again. Also, eating nutritious foods will supply the body with ample nutrients to protect it from nutritional bankruptcy, so the body is better able to cope with stress as it should.

The following testimonials provide a sampling of what people are experiencing as they use coconut oil:

"I am a celiac and the coconut oil has had very good effects on my intestinal tract. I am the only one left in my immediate family not on thyroid medication right now and the only one not overweight. Something must be right about this. I am 49 and seem to be healthy for my age."
—Tish

"I have tried taking 3 tablespoons of coconut oil per day for a couple of months to help combat chronic fatigue. During this time I have experienced these changes: muscle stamina dramatically better for the first time in 2 years, no herpes outbreaks or mouth sores at all, gum health improved, less stomach/intestinal problems, and more energy."
—Jan (from Sweden)

"I have severe systemic candida overgrowth from decades of poor eating habits, hypothyroidism, and antibiotics. The coconut oil is working miracles for me."
—Audry Mills

"I do like the way my skin feels now. It is much softer, smoother, and less rough. I also never have any constipation since adding coconut oil to my diet. I also seem to have a bit more energy."
—Janet Turner

"I bought some oil for the health benefits, and started it today, as soon as I got it. My temperature (taken as an experiment to see if the oil did raise it) the last few days has been between 97.2° to 97.6° and after taking the oil it rose to 98.8° and was still 98.3° later on in the day. Have to admit this really surprised me, despite having read of it."
—Carole Horsman

"My metabolism is soaring right now!!! My energy is very high and my strength in the gym is increasing. Fantastic product."
—A. Simkins

"Having Hashimoto's Thyroid disease has caused me to experience many severe symptoms for a very long time. Since I added 4 tbsp of my 'heavenly gold' (i.e., coconut oil) to my food, it is the most marvelous change to ALL my body, both inside and out. I wish you could feel my almost 54-year-old skin; my husband says it is now the softest thing he's ever felt, and this newfound skin can be attributed to only one thing because I do not use lotions—it's the precious coconut oil. Thank God I found the coconut-info web site when researching thyroid disease. I cannot praise it highly enough and have told everyone I know about it. And, hey, losing 11 pounds while consuming all the fats is fairly telling about the metabolic effects it has indeed!"
—Linda Passarelli

150

"During the past several months, I have been experiencing severe insomnia. I do not believe in taking drugs to assist in sleeping, but it had gotten so bad that I got a prescription from my doctor. On using the prescription (and I have only tried this a couple of times) I was still only able to increase my night's sleep from about 2 hours to about 4 and after taking the sleeping pills I felt so much worse the next day that I had abandoned that as a solution to my problem. I have noticed that since using the coconut I am now getting a full 8 hours. Also, the pain in my hands and vertebrae and knees from arthritis has almost completely disappeared. I still have the occasional twinge in the knuckle in the little finger on my right hand, but I suspect that is because it has calcified. I almost feel foolish writing this, because I cannot quite believe that I have been the beneficiary of such incredible improvement for all my ails just from consuming coconut milk and oil. I keep expecting the problems to return. Another benefit is that I have lost the chronic irritability that I have had for so long. I can only attribute all of these things to the coconut oil as nothing else about my life has changed."

—Rhea Lust

"Coconut oil seems to be improving my mood too, and I feel like a friendlier person now. I can wave at my neighbor and smile at the same time."

—JDR

"Since I started consuming lots of coconut oil, I've lost weight and even my cellulite seems somewhat diminished although I have *increased*, not decreased my calories!"

—Laura S.

"I have been using coconut oil for about two months. I am sleeping better. I no longer have hypoglycemia symptoms. I use 3½ tablespoons a day most days... My energy level is up. I rarely have fibro pain at night now."

—Beth Percifield

"I've been taking my basal temperature every morning for over three years according to Dr. Broda Barnes instructions. According to Dr. Barnes I have a slightly underactive thyroid. However, in the last few days [after using coconut oil] my temperature is several tenths higher than it has ever been."

—Marilyn J.

ALTERING YOUR METABOLIC RATE

If you are troubled with thyroid system dysfunction (hypothyroidism, WTS, etc.) don't think weight loss is hopeless. There are things you can do to stimulate your metabolism and help you lose excess weight. Your metabolic rate is *not* one of those things in life that is unchangeable. Metabolism can be influenced by lifestyle and diet—factors you have control over. Below are things you can do to revitalize your metabolism.

Diet

One of the most important steps you can take to correct metabolic problems is to make sure you are getting adequate nutrition. Over the past few decades metabolic or thyroid system problems have become commonplace. This rise in incidence suggests that these problems are caused or influenced by dietary or lifestyle choices. The healthier your diet is, the healthier you will be, and the less likely you will have a thyroid system problem. If you have a thyroid system problem, good nutrition is *required* to correct it.

When the body is undernourished it creates an environment where the body is incapable of properly handling stress. We know this situation can push metabolism into low gear and keep it there. Poor nutrition may also affect thyroid gland health. A lack of trace minerals, especially iodine, can adversely affect thyroid gland function. Goitrogens from raw cruciferous vegetables, raw legumes, and especially soy, along with polyunsaturated oils also depress thyroid gland activity.

Your choice of dietary oils is important. Some oils stimulate metabolism while others depress it. Ironically, the oils that are most often recommended in weight-loss diets are the ones that are most likely to lower metabolism and promote weight gain. Polyunsaturated oils promote hypothyroidism. Saturated and monounsaturated oils do not. Coconut oil is a thyroid system builder. It stimulates metabolism and enzyme activity. Judging from the results I've seen, for some people at least, it appears that consistent use of coconut oil can reactivate T4 to T3 conversion. You should make coconut oil a regular part of your diet. Eat it every day, preferably with foods at every meal. Coconut oil and dietary recommendations are outlined in Chapter 13.

Drugs

If possible, you should avoid all drugs that interfere with thyroid system function. Sulfa drugs and antihistamines adversely affect the thyroid gland. Cortisone and other steroids affect the way the body handles thyroid hormones, blocking the conversion of T4 to T3.

The standard medical treatment for hypothyroidism and WTS consists of hormone therapy. Your doctor can prescribe either a synthetic or natural form of thyroid hormone. In the case of hypothyroidism where the thyroid gland is not producing enough hormones, medication must be continued for life. Synthetic hormone medication (e.g., Synthroid), which is by far the most commonly prescribed, is accompanied by some undesirable side effects. One of which is a significant loss of bone calcium. If you take synthetic thyroid hormone medication you should also increase calcium supplementation. In my opinion, natural thyroid (e.g., Armour) is better because the hormone is essentially identical to that produced by your body and there are few, if any, undesirable side effects.

Exercise

Exercise has beneficial effects on metabolism and weight. Regular exercise stimulates metabolism. Metabolism remains at a heightened rate for several hours after exercise has stopped and can remain slightly elevated for up to 2 days afterward. Exercising every day can keep your metabolism purring along at a heightened level of activity, keeping your temperature slightly elevated and helping you burn excess calories. This topic is covered more thoroughly in Chapter 12.

Heat

Saunas or hot baths can elevate your body temperature much like exercise does. If the water or steam is hot enough to raise the body's temperature a few degrees, it can remain elevated for a time afterward. The effects of hot baths are short lived, but can be helpful in raising the body's temperature, at least for an hour or two. During this time sluggish enzymes will be kicked into high gear and bodily processes will run at a heightened level of activity.

Heat therapy has been in use for thousands of years. The effects of stimulating the metabolism have proven useful in cleansing toxins from the body and speeding recovery from illness. Our bodies' own process of fighting infections involves producing a fever to increase circulation and stimulate cellular and glandular activity.

If you have access to a sauna or steam bath at a spa or health club take advantage of it. If you don't, a bathtub filled with hot water will also work. Simply sitting in a tub of hot water or taking a hot shower, however, does not work! You need to be completely submerged, except for your head, and the water must be hot enough to raise your body temperature up to about 100° F.

To do this, start filling the bathtub with hot water, but not hot enough to burn yourself. Sit in the tub as it is filling up, keeping the water as hot as you can tolerate. Filling the tub in this way will help your body adjust to the temperature. After the tub is filled to capacity, turn off the water and submerge your entire body, keeping only your head above water. Relax and rest your head on a towel. While you soak and as the water cools, you can drain some out and add fresh hot water to keep the temperature as hot as necessary. Usually as your body adjusts to the heat, you can withstand a little more hot water. Even though you are covered with water, your body will sweat profusely. Remain in the bath for 20–30 minutes.

A major problem with many bathtubs is that they are too small. In order to make this effective, the entire body, except for the head, needs to be submerged. Many bathtubs are not big enough to do this. One solution to this problem is to buy a plastic sheet, available in various lengths at garden supply stores, and drape it over the tub, water, and yourself like a blanket. You do not wrap it around your body and it is not put in the water with you. It covers the top of the tub to seal in heat. This way if your knees or toes stick out of the water they will still keep warm.

Keep the plastic off your face. The head should be left exposed to cool air. This will allow you to remain in the water longer, gaining full benefit. If you get a headache, the water is too hot. Cool it down with some cold water and apply a cold wet washcloth to your forehead as you soak. You want to heat your body up to about 100° F. This is only 1.4° above normal. A healthy person can easily handle temperatures up to 104°, so there is no need to worry about overheating yourself at 100° F. Use a thermometer to regulate your temperature. If you get too hot, cool down the tub. If you're not hot enough, add more hot water.

Even though you are submerged in water you will do a lot of sweating. The sweat glands can secrete nearly a full pint of water in 15 minutes, so you need to drink plenty of water. Drink a full glass of water before bathing and another glass afterwards. Do not drink cold water because it will cool your body down. Sweating removes salt and minerals from the body so you should make sure to replenish them by eating an adequate amount of salt and taking a mineral supplement afterwards.

To take full advantage of your elevated temperature created by the bath, avoid activities immediately afterwards that will cool you down, such as going out in cold air or consuming cold foods or beverages. Hot baths are relaxing. It is best to do this in the evening so you can relax or go to bed afterwards.

Heat therapy can have a dramatic effect on the body. Those who have multiple sclerosis, hyperthyroidism, hypertension, or serious heart conditions should consult a health professional before trying it.

154

Sunlight

You may wonder why a book on weight loss would include a section on sunlight. Believe it or not, sunlight can help you lose weight! Yes, lying on the beach, under the sun is one way your body can shed excess body fat. What a marvelous way to lose weight! Perhaps that's why sunbathers are so thin? It certainly isn't the only reason, but sunbathing does help.

Sunlight has more influence on health than most of us realize. Getting an adequate amount of exposure to full sunlight is critical for the activation of enzymes and the production of certain hormones necessary for many chemical processes that occur in your body. A lack of sun exposure can cause multiple enzyme dysfunction and the undersecretion of hormones that influence metabolism and body temperature. Too little sun can actually cause you to gain weight and prevent you from losing excess body fat.

Sunlight influences our health by the chemical and electrical activities it ignites in our skin and our brain. For example, when light enters the eye, millions of light-sensitive cells called photoreceptors convert the light into electrical impulses. These impulses travel along the optic nerve to the brain where they trigger the hypothalamus gland to send chemical messages to regulate the autonomic (involuntary) functions of the body. The hypothalamus releases hormones that control the activity of other glands, including the *thyroid gland*. If the hypothalamus is underactive, due to a lack of sunlight, the thyroid gland will also be underactive. I suspect that many people who are affected by hypothyroidism could benefit greatly by simply getting more exposure to sunlight.

Sunlight also influences chemical reactions in the body by activating enzymes under the surface of the skin. For example, ultraviolet (UV) radiation from the sun activates enzymes that convert cholesterol into vitamin D. Most of the vitamin D in our bodies comes from exposure to sunlight. In addition, many vitamins and minerals in our foods are inactive unless we are exposed to sunlight. So a lack of sunlight can contribute to nutritional deficiencies, which, as you've learned in Chapter 8, can cause food cravings and overeating.

It's not so hard to recognize the importance sunlight has on health. We see and feel the sun's influence every day. Haven't you ever noticed an increase in energy or a positive mood when you go outside on a bright sunny day? In contrast, you may notice a lack of enthusiasm or feel tired or depressed when it is overcast and dark.

These effects are clearly evident in plants. Shine some light on a dormant plant and it will spring to life. Sunlight activates enzymes in plants, stimulating metabolism, growth, and activity. A lack of sunlight causes plants to go dormant and humans and animals to sleep or hibernate. Without sunlight plants shrivel up and die, and so do we.

During the winter when the sun's rays are less intense and often blocked by clouds, people are known to develop a condition called *seasonal affective disorder* (SAD) also known as the "winter blues." The symptoms of SAD are depression, irritability, excess sleeping and eating, weight gain, and lowered sex drive. Exposure to sunlight reverses this condition.

Your body requires *full* sunlight. Artificial lighting is not adequate, and research shows it may even be detrimental. Natural sunlight contains a full spectrum of light wavelengths. Natural light contains all possible wavelengths, from infrared to ultraviolet (UV). Each wavelength carries a different level of energy and has a different effect on body tissues. Artificial lighting, both incandescent and fluorescent, lacks the complete balanced spectrum of sunlight.

An analogy can be made between light and nutrients in foods. Natural foods contain a wide variety or spectrum of vitamins and minerals. When foods are processed, many of these nutrients are removed. Likewise, natural sunlight contains a full spectrum of light wavelengths. Artificial light does not. When any wavelength of light is missing, the light becomes imbalanced and can affect health, just as if a food were missing an important nutrient such as vitamin C. That's why artificial lighting is not an adequate replacement for natural sunlight.

Another reason artificial lighting is inferior is because it is far weaker. Most buildings, even with windows, have a light level of 500 lux (the international unit of illumination). Outdoor light has a level of about 50,000 lux, or approximately 100 times more. At night, or in offices where artificial lighting is the only light source, the level drops to 50 lux.

Our body's optimal absorption of vitamins and minerals requires full spectrum sunlight. Windows, windshields, eyeglasses, smog, clouds, and sunscreen all filter out parts of the light spectrum. Research reveals that if some wavelengths aren't present in light, the body can't fully absorb certain nutrients.[34]

Many of us spend 90% or more of our time inside buildings or cars, shielded from direct sunlight. Without adequate sunlight enzyme activity slows down, hormone production tapers off, and nutrients are not properly utilized. The result is a long list of health problems, many of which are the same as for Wilson's thyroid syndrome listed earlier, including weight gain.

If your metabolism is slow because you don't get enough direct sunlight, taking medications isn't going to help. You need to get out into the sun every day. Sunbathe if you can. Any exposure will be of benefit. I recommend you get 15—30 minutes of direct sun every day.

Some people hesitate to go out into the sun for fear of developing skin cancer. Like saturated fat, sunlight has been unjustly criticized in the past as a health hazard. We are warned to avoid overexposure to sunlight because it may cause cancer. Some fanatics even recommend total avoidance of the sun. Research now shows moderate exposure to sunlight is not only harmless, but necessary for good health and can actually *protect* you from cancer. You don't need to fear sunlight.

We are often told to shield ourselves from the "damaging" rays of the sun, especially UV radiation, because it can cause skin cancer. The most deadly form of skin cancer is melanoma. Because of all the publicity blaming sunlight for skin cancer, many people are paranoid about being out in the sun. I've heard people make all sorts of claims about being exposed to the sun as a child and then later developing skin cancer as an adult. One person said that a bad sunburn he received on his back and arms 30 years ago was the cause of the melanoma that recently developed on his foot. Is he saying the sun's rays hit his upper body and took 30 years

HOW TO REV UP YOUR METABOLISM

- Eat a wholesome diet containing a wide variety of nutrients
- Avoid nutritionally poor foods
- Avoid raw cruciferous vegetables and raw legumes
- Avoid all soy products, with the exception of fermented soy
- Avoid processed polyunsaturated oils
- Avoid sulfa drugs, antihistamines, and steroids
- Consume a source of iodine regularly—sea salt, sea food, or dietary supplements
- Get regular exercise
- Use coconut oil daily
- Occasional sauna/hot baths
- Get daily sun exposure
- Use thyroid medication if necessary*

*There are two major types of thyroid hormone used to treat hypothyroidism— Synthroid and Armour. Synthroid is a synthetic hormone which contains only T4. Armour is a natural hormone medication that contains both T4 and T3. Another thyroid medication, Cytomel, contains only T3 and is used to treat WTS patients. All thyroid medications must be prescribed by a physician.

to travel to his foot? If the sun only got his back and arms why is his foot affected? This is normal for melanoma. It occurs not where sun exposure is the greatest, but where it is the least, suggesting that a *lack* of sunlight may be a bigger problem. Recent research seems to verify this. A study carried out by the US Navy compared the risk of melanoma for different naval occupations. It was discovered that those with indoor jobs had the highest incidence of melanoma, while those who worked at least part of the time outdoors had the lowest rate. In addition, a higher rate of melanoma occurred on the trunk of the body which was covered by clothing, as opposed to the head and arms which are more likely to be exposed to sunlight. The author of the study stated that the location of the melanomas suggest a *protective* role for regular exposure to sunlight.[35]

Studies also show vitamin D suppresses the growth of malignant melanoma cells. A vitamin D deficiency, caused by a lack of adequate exposure to sunlight, therefore, can promote melanoma formation.[36] This is consistent with other studies that have shown that sunlight has a protective effect against many forms of cancer. For example, researchers at Johns Hopkins University Medical School in Baltimore, Maryland, showed that exposure to full-spectrum light, including UV light, is *positively* related to the prevention of breast, colon, and rectal cancers.[37]

Chapter 10

SATISFY YOUR HUNGER LONGER ____ ∎

WEIGHT LOSS WITHOUT PAIN

If you lived in Europe during the middle ages and were brought before authorites and charged with a misdeed, you might have ended up in the torture chamber. Here you would be shackled to a rack and stretched until your limbs nearly pop out of their sockets or your flesh might be seared with a red hot iron. Nowadays we're more civilized. We don't send people to the torture chamber for mistakes in judgment, we put them on low-fat diets. The suffering can be just as intense.

Most weight-loss diets are basically the same. To reduce calorie consumption you are limited to tiny portions of food that have had all traces of fat removed. Fat gives food flavor and improves taste. When it is removed, you end up with a small portion of some tasteless gruel. Perhaps the reason for this is that if it tastes bad enough, you won't even want to eat it and you will consume fewer calories. My vision of a satisfying meal is not a grilled tofu patty resting on a bed of raw bean sprouts. If I have to eat this way, I'd rather be fat.

Most weight-loss diets ultimately fail because they make you hungry. The low-calorie foods you are allowed to eat cause you to be hungry because they are not satisfying. Honestly, how long is a bowl of shredded lettuce and a slice of cucumber going to satisfy you? Low-fat diets are inherently doomed to failure because of the mistaken assumption that in order to reduce calories, you must cut out as much fat as possible.

But you say you've lost 50 pounds on one of these low-fat diets or know someone who has. Let me ask you this: are those pounds still gone?

159

If you gained them back, then the diet didn't do you a bit of good. It didn't work. If a weight-loss diet cannot keep the lost weight off permanently, it is useless. In fact, it may be worse than useless because yo-yo dieting encourages weight gain. Statistics show that 95% of those people who go on weight-loss diets eventually regain all their weight back. That's an incredible 95% failure rate!

Why do these low-fat diets fail? Because they are torture! Following such diets is nothing more than slow starvation—literally. You feel hungry and miserable all the time. You rarely feel satisfied. You think about food constantly. When you're trying to stop from eating, continually being reminded of food by a groaning stomach is agony.

An ideal diet is one which lets you eat until you're satisfied and keeps you from being hungry until the next meal. In addition, the food you're allowed to eat is flavorful and delicious. Impossible you say? Yes, if you follow the mistaken idea that eating a low-fat diet is the only way to lose weight. But if you add fat into your diet, while avoiding a few trouble-makers, you can eat to your heart's content, be satisfied, and still lose weight. Since you can eat as much as you please (without gorging yourself, of course) and aren't constantly hungry all the time, or in other words miserable, you can easily maintain this diet indefinitely and, consequently, keep the excess pounds off permanently.

HOW TO SATISFY HUNGER

The problem with most low-fat diets is that they lack satiety. What is satiety? It's the feeling of fullness or satisfaction at the end of a meal, the feeling that you are no longer hungry. The longer you can maintain this feeling, the longer you can go without eating and without overeating at the next meal. Some foods provide greater and longer lasting satiety than others. A T-bone steak provides greater satiety than an apple. A baked potato with butter and cheese offers more satiety than a cucumber, and a bowl of chili with beef more than a bowl of lettuce and tomatoes. Satiety is one of the ingredients for successful weight reduction.

When the volume of food we eat is not adequate enough to achieve satiety, or if the food digests rapidly, we become hungry again long before the next meal. This encourages snacking and feelings of hunger that make dieting a challenge.

It is true that in order to lose weight you must take into account total calorie consumption. Unfortunately, that is all most weight-loss diets focus on. High-calorie foods (i.e., those that contain the most fat) are restricted so you can eat more low-calorie foods. In theory if you cut out high-calorie foods you will be able to eat a larger volume of low-calorie foods and feel satisfied on fewer calories. While this idea may sound logical, in real life it doesn't work. The problem with this approach is that most low-calorie foods aren't very satisfying. For instance, after eating a lettuce and tomato salad, how long can you go without feeling hungry again? If you are like most people, hunger returns after only an hour or two. These low-calorie foods digest very quickly, leaving your stomach empty and complaining. You have to eat again to satisfy your hunger or you must suffer until the next meal. Most of us can only take so much suffering before we call it quits and go back to eating the way we used to.

A diet that allows you to eat until you are satisfied and keeps you from getting hungry until the next meal is a much better way to control total calorie intake. When your stomach is full you don't think about eating, you don't spend time dreaming about foods, you don't suffer, and you don't feel the need to cheat in order to satisfy hunger pangs.

You can control calorie intake easier if the food you eat gives you a feeling of lasting fullness. What you need is a diet that allows you to eat a satisfying volume of food while balancing calorie consumption with energy needs. However, the foods that are the most satisfying are generally the highest in calories.

Fortunately, we don't eat foods based on calories, we eat based on satiety, which is determined by volume, not calorie content. When the stomach is full, hunger is satisfied. It's that simple. And the longer food remains in the stomach, the longer we can go between meals without feeling hungry and without eating. So even though the foods you eat may contain more calories, if they satisfy your hunger and keep you from overeating, your total calorie intake will be less and you will lose weight.

There are certain foods that satisfy hunger and keep us feeling full for several hours. There are other foods that digest quickly and cause us to be hungry sooner. Each of these are discussed in the following sections.

FIBER

If you had your choice between two nearly identical pieces of cake with one having half as many calories as the other, which one would you choose? If you are concerned about your weight you would choose the one with fewer calories.

If the foods you ate had fewer calories, you could eat just as much as you normally do and still lose weight without going hungry. One way to lower the calorie content of your food, without lowering the volume, is to eat foods which are high in fiber. Fiber contains no calories, but does provide bulk and can help with feelings of satiety. High-fiber foods are also good sources of nutrients.

Foods that are high in fiber are generally low in calories and provide bulk, so they are more likely to fill you up, not out. A slice of whole wheat bread, for example, is five times more filling than a slice of white bread. Whole wheat bread also contains fewer calories than white. The same volume of whole wheat bread provides less starch (calorie producing carbohydrate) and more fiber (non-calorie carbohydrate) than white bread. Ounce for ounce the whole wheat bread supplies fewer calories because it contains more fiber (as well as vitamins and minerals).

Fiber not only provides bulk with fewer calories, but it also delays hunger. Fiber tends to linger in the stomach, delaying gastric emptying. Fiber also delays the absorption of carbohydrates and fats in the small intestine. This provides a feeling of fullness and satiety. Increasing your fiber intake will help make your stomach and brain think you are full, even when you are taking in fewer calories.

During a meal it takes about 20 minutes to get the feeling of fullness that prompts us to stop. Whether you eat fast or slow it still takes the same amount of time. In today's fast-paced world many people don't take the time to eat. They quickly gulp down a meal and off they go. Studies show that when people eat meals at a rapid rate, they became hungry again more quickly than when they eat exactly the same volume of food at a slower rate.[1] So the rate at which you eat not only influences how much you eat at a meal, but also influences the length of time a person can go without eating between meals. Fast eaters, therefore, tend to eat more than slow eaters. Several studies have shown that overweight people usually eat more rapidly than slim people. Fiber is helpful here, too. Since fiber is chewy, it takes more time to eat high-fiber foods. Eating is slowed down so we end up eating less.

Eating high fiber foods and adding fiber to your meals is an important step in any permanent weight-loss program. High-fiber meals provide low-calorie bulk, keep your stomach full longer, slow down digestion of other carbohydrates, and slow down eating time so you take in less food. Even a small increase in fiber can make a difference. A study in England discovered that lean adults averaged 19 grams of fiber a day while obese ones consumed only 13. This is a difference of only 6 grams a day.

PROTEIN

An adequate amount of protein in the diet can help you lose weight. The reason is because protein satisfies hunger and is slow to digest. Protein slows down the rate at which the stomach empties. Food remains in the stomach longer, extending the feeling of satiety. Whether the protein is from meat, grains, or vegetables, it doesn't matter.

If you eat a breakfast of ham and eggs (high-protein foods), it will easily hold you over until lunch. A low-protein breakfast, such as a slice of toast, glass of juice, and a half grapefruit won't last long. By lunch time you will be so hungry that you will overeat (if you didn't snack on donuts or candy). The calories you didn't get at breakfast are added on at lunchtime. You will eat faster and your sense of satiety won't kick in until you've loaded up on more calories than you otherwise would. If you also eat a low-protein lunch, the same thing will happen at dinner. You either end up consuming more total calories on the diet or feel miserable all day long.

Studies have shown that eating a high-protein meal is associated with a decrease in hunger afterwards and ultimately eating fewer total calories. Volunteers in these studies were able to wait longer between meals before eating and ate less during the meals. In a study performed in Canada, men were given either high-protein or moderate-protein meals for 6 days, and could eat as much as they liked: those eating more protein took in fewer calories each day. Observations such as this led to the idea that a very high-protein diet may reduce total calorie consumption even more. As a consequence, high-protein weight-loss diets have become popular in recent years.

FAT

For years now fat has been labeled as the primary cause, or at least a contributor, to obesity and overweight. It is ostracized from all weight-loss diets. Indeed, no self-respecting weight-loss diet would be caught dead recommending fat. That is, until now.

Like protein, fat also slows down the digestion of food, allowing the stomach to feel full longer and quenching the pangs of hunger. Fat stimulates the release of hormones that slow down the rate at which food leaves the stomach, allowing you to feel full longer. The small intestine also has fat receptors that act in much the same way. When you eat fatty foods you feel satisfied longer and don't sense a need to snack or to overeat at the next meal. For this reason, *adding fat to your diet can help you lose weight!*

After years of exclusion, fat can now be welcomed back into the diet with open arms. No longer do you need to buy lean cuts of meat or trim off every speck of fat. No longer are you required to eat tasteless non-fat milk and low-fat cheese. You can now add a pat of butter to your vegetables and cook with oil without fear. Adding fat to your foods and eating full-fat foods will help you to eat less and lose weight.

The fact that adding fat to your diet can help you lose weight is backed by medical research. For example, in one study volunteers were given either a high-fat or a low-fat breakfast containing the same number of calories. Those who ate the high-fat breakfast felt full longer and delayed the time of their next meal, thus avoiding between meal snacks.[2]

Research has shown that when people get hungry soon after a meal they tend to overeat at the next. Thus, a high-fat breakfast helps to prevent both between meal snacking and overeating, both of which cut down on needless calories. The end result is the consumption of fewer total calories. When used properly, fat can be an important aid in helping you lose weight and keep it off.

Fat helps to curb appetite. Without fat, food is less filling and so we tend to overeat to get the same feeling of satiety. Also, low-fat foods are not necessarily low-calorie foods. Fat gives food flavor. If you take the fat out, the taste becomes bland and less desirable, so manufacturers add in more sugar to improve the taste. You end up with a low-fat food that has just as many calories as the full-fat version. However, without the fat the food is less satisfying and digests quicker, making you hungry sooner. For this reason, many so-called low-fat and non-fat foods actually promote weight gain!

In another study, a group of women were given a mid-morning yogurt snack and then later served lunch and dinner. There were two choices of yogurt. One was regular full-fat and the other was low-fat. Each was labeled, but there was no mention of total calorie content. Each, however, contained the same number of calories. The only difference was the fat content. Participants were allowed to choose whichever one they wanted. When the women were later served lunch those who had the high-fat yogurt ate *less* than those who ate the low-fat variety. The extra fat in the yogurt snack satisfied their hunger longer and encouraged them to eat less at lunch.

Researchers also wanted to learn if those who ate less at lunch would eventually make up for it at dinner. But at dinner the ones who ate the high-fat yogurt and less food at lunch didn't eat any more than the others. They weren't any hungrier for eating less at lunch. So at the end of the day those women who ate the high-fat yogurt ended up consuming *fewer* total calories than those who ate the low-fat snack.[3]

Some fats exert a greater degree of satiety than other fats. Coconut oil is at the top of the list on the satiety scale. This has been demonstrated in both human and animal studies. For example, in a study conducted in

Japan, rats were given diets containing either coconut oil or vegetable oil.* The amount of food eaten was determined every hour. As early as one hour after feeding, total food intake significantly decreased in the coconut oil-fed animals. Rats were then given a choice between the two foods to confirm if palatability of the diets had any influence. There was no difference in food intake between the two diets.[4] This study showed that coconut oil was more satisfying than other oils, at least in rats.

In a study with human subjects, women were given a drink which contained either coconut oil or vegetable oil. Thirty minutes later they were offered lunch in which they could choose and eat as much as they wanted. The women who had the coconut oil before the meal ate less food, and as the authors of the study stated, "significantly decreased caloric intake in the lunch."[5]

Another study was divided into three phases. In each phase the subjects had free access to high-fat foods for 14 days. The phases differed in the amount of both MCFA (from coconut oil) and LCFA in the foods. The first phase contained 20% MCFA and 40% LCFA of total energy. The second contained equal amounts of MCFA and LCFA. The third had 40% MCFA and 20% LCFA. The total amount of food each subject consumed was recorded. It was found that as MCFA content increased, total food consumption decreased.[6]

In another study normal-weight men were given breakfasts differing only in the type of fat used. Food intakes at lunch and dinner were measured. Those eating breakfasts containing MCFA ate less at lunch time. At dinner there was no difference. This study showed that when MCFA were eaten at one meal, hunger is forestalled for longer and less food is eaten at the next. Also important was that even though subjects ate less at lunch, they did not make up for it by eating more at dinner. Total daily food intake decreased.[7]

These and many other studies suggest that eating coconut oil in place of other oils can provide longer satisfaction and hold off hunger longer, resulting in lower total-calorie consumption.

HIGH WATER CONTENT FOODS

If used wisely, water can also help curb appetite. Like fiber, water provides bulk without adding any calories. Drinking water or eating foods with a high water content can help you feel full on fewer calories. The only drawback with water is that it moves through the digestive system very quickly. It fills you up fast, but leaves you feeling hungry soon afterwards.

---

*The study actually used an oil composed of MCFA derived from coconut oil.

Wisely used, water can help you control your total calorie intake. Water is so vital to weight control that I've included an entire chapter on the subject. Here, however, I will focus only on the role water plays in providing volume and its effects on satiety.

When we sit down to a meal where food is plentiful we normally continue to eat until we feel full or satisfied. When the stomach becomes full it sends a message to the brain that hunger is satisfied and eating should stop. Unfortunately, there is a space of time between the moment the stomach becomes full and reception of the sensation of fullness. It takes several minutes for the brain to receive, recognize, and act. During this time we continue to eat and we consume excess calories that the body doesn't need or want.

It would be desirable to speed the signal from your stomach to your brain and allow you to stop eating sooner. Water can help this happen. In many Asian countries liquids are consumed prior to meals. One of the purposes of this is to stimulate digestive juices to improve digestion. Another reason is to fill the stomach to reduce hunger and prevent over-eating. For the same reason it is a good idea to drink a *full* glass of water about 10 or 15 minutes before eating your meals. The water fills the stomach taking the edge off your hunger and starting the process that signals satiety. The sooner you feel full, the sooner you'll stop eating.

Appetizers work in the same way. When you eat something before the meal it cuts the edge off your hunger, allowing you to eat less. Restaurant owners are well aware of this and that is why appetizers are so common. In order for the appetizer to help you cut calories it must be low in calories, such as a low-calorie drink (like water, tea, or vegetable juice), a salad, or soup—all of which are primarily water. Although salad may look like solid food, salad greens are 90% water. Bread, chips, fried foods, and such aren't good appetizers because they contain too many calories. Water has no calories, so it is a much better choice as are high water content foods such as salad, soup, and vegetable juice. In one study, for example, men who drank a 14-ounce, 88-calorie glass of vegetable juice before lunch took in an average of 136 fewer calories at the meal than did men who weren't given the drink.[8]

When consumed *before* a meal, water and high water content foods help to jump-start feelings of satiety which help prevent you from over-eating. Water by itself, however, does not provide lasting satisfaction. Water is quickly absorbed in the digestive tract. Drinking a lot of water *with* your meals fills your stomach and reduces calories consumed, but feelings of hunger will soon return. This encourages snacking between meals or overeating at the next.

166

Eating a lot of high water content foods such as fruits and vegetables has the same effect. For example, a large slice of watermelon may fill you up, but within an hour you'll be hungry again. The reason is that watermelon is mostly water (92%). When you eat it the bulk fills your stomach and gives you a sense of fullness, but the water is rapidly digested, and before you know it, you're hungry again. Most all fruits and vegetables are predominately water and, therefore, digest very quickly.

Even the fiber content of most fruits and vegetables is rather low compared to whole grains and beans. An apple, for instance, consists of 83% water, 15% carbohydrate, and only 2% fiber. Cauliflower is 92% water, 2% protein, 4% carbohydrate, and only 2% fiber. When fruits and vegetables are eaten, they digest so quickly that they're in and out of the stomach and halfway down the digestive tract within an hour. Consequently, you feel hungry again in a short time. Most low-fat and low-calorie diets focus on eating fruits and vegetables. You can eat them until your eyes bulge out, but within an hour or two you will be hungry again. This is another reason why eating a rabbit-food diet is ineffective for weight loss.

Protein, fat, and fiber slow down digestion. When combined with water, as in a soup, digestion of the soup is slowed down. Vegetable soup with little or no fat or protein is no more filling than a glass of water. Soup with adequate amounts of fat, protein, and fiber takes longer to digest and is more satisfying. For this reason, you should eat fruits and vegetables with foods that supply adequate amounts of fat, protein, and fiber.

A great way to add fiber and volume to soup, without adding any more calories, is to throw in some wheat bran. The bran has no taste and acts as a mild thickener. Add a half or a full cup of bran to your soup and let it cook with the vegetables. If you simmer the soup for an hour or longer the bran dissolves and is undetectable, but still provides bulk and additional nutrients.

Vegetables become more filling and satisfying if combined with a source of fat and/or protein. With a typical low-fat diet vegetables are consumed without much added flavoring. But if you want them to satisfy your hunger until your next meal, you'll eat them with butter, cream, gravy, or sauces and you will enjoy them more, too. Adding coconut oil to your food is one way to make a low-fat or low-protein meal last longer.

Chapter 11

DRINK MORE, WEIGH LESS ▪

Of all the food and beverages we consume, water is by far the most important. Although it contains no calories and provides no energy, it is considered our most vital nutrient. Our bodies require a constant source of water throughout the day in order to maintain bodily functions and to sustain life. We can live for several weeks and even months without other nutrients, but if completely deprived of water we would die of dehydration in a matter of days. A lack of adequate water is, in essence, a death sentence.

Approximately 60% of our body weight is from water. Every function inside the body is regulated by, and depends on, water. Water must be available in sufficient quantities to adequately transport nutrients, oxygen, hormones, and other chemicals to all parts of the body. Water lubricates our joints, protects our brain, facilitates digestion and elimination, and provides the medium in which all chemical reactions in the body occur. Water is so important to the proper function of the body that even a small reduction from normal can have a dramatic effect on your health.

Drinking the proper amount of water every day is vital to good health. If we don't drink enough, our bodies become dehydrated. Severe dehydration can lead to death. Chronic low-grade dehydration creates a state of stress that interferes with many normal bodily functions leading to tissue deterioration, pain, and disease.

Water has another very important purpose. It is necessary in the right amount in order to regulate and manage weight. *Many people are overweight because they don't drink enough water*. Yes, part of the reason you may be overweight is because you don't drink enough pure, clean water.

Diets that ignore fluid intake or that cause the loss of water are dangerously unhealthy! Dieting should improve health, not destroy it. A proper diet that recognizes the importance of water can help you lose weight and improve your health. That's what my plan can do for you. In this chapter we will explore the necessity and purpose of drinking adequate amounts of water and the advantages of dieting without water loss.

DRINK YOUR WATER

"Drink plenty of water." You've probably heard that advice a hundred times, but do you follow it? How much water do you drink each day? I mean real water. Pure water without flavorings, sweeteners, and other chemicals added. Three glasses? One glass perhaps? Maybe none at all? That's fairly typical.

A key element in my weight-loss plan is to drink plenty of water—pure water. In other diets water isn't given much attention. In fact, most fad diets don't want you to drink water because it slows down the rate at which you lose weight. Most of the weight you lose on these diets comes from the loss of water and not fat. You are, therefore, not losing any real weight, just water which the body needs. Quick weight loss is encouraging and compels us to stick with a diet even though it may be unpleasant. You are led to believe that a diet is working to remove fat when in reality you are mostly only eliminating water. This makes it look like your diet is working. This is good for marketing purposes because you tell others about it and praise the program as a success. However, after the body has given up all the water it is going to give without causing serious dehydration and sickness, weight loss slows down, and you hit a plateau. You go on for weeks without losing another pound. This is the time many people give up. Even though you may have lost 30 pounds in 6 weeks' time, you probably only lost 6—12 pounds of fat, the rest was water and lean tissue. The body being severely dehydrated will eventually want to reabsorb some water and you may notice a weight gain, even though you continue to faithfully follow the diet. If you remain on the diet for long and never replenish the water you lost, you could suffer serious health problems due to chronic dehydration. Chronic dehydration is a condition in which the body is continually in need of more water. You don't notice anything at first. But as time goes on cells and tissues thirsty for water become damaged, setting the stage for disease and pain.

The ideal diet is one that doesn't produce quick weight loss due to loss of water, but reduces body fat. It is a diet that can be maintained for life and promotes better health, not dehydration.

Nutritionists have known for years that fad diets promote water loss giving the perception of fat reduction and that such diets are not healthy. It wasn't until the past couple of decades that the importance of water in weight control and health were clearly understood. As incredible as it may sound, one of the reasons you may be overweight is because you don't drink enough water.

THE ELIXIR OF LIFE
The Discovery Made in Prison

Surprisingly, the importance of water in weight management and health in general was discovered by Dr. Fereydoon Batmanghelidj while he was serving time at Evin Prison in Iran. After graduating from medical school in London and working for a time in England, Dr. Batmanghelidj returned to Iran, where he was born, to help the people of his country. In 1979 a violent revolution swept a new government into power. Almost all professional and creative people who had stayed in the country were rounded up and jailed as political prisoners. Dr. Batmanghelidj was among them.

The prison in which he was placed was built to hold only 600, but quickly overflowed with 9,000 inmates. Trained medical personnel were scarce so Dr. Batmanghelidj was given the responsibility of caring for the sick. The prisoner's health was not a high priority with the new government, and consequently, medical supplies were woefully inadequate.

Dr. Batmanghelidj wasn't there long when one night an inmate racked with excruciating stomach pain was brought to him. The man was suffering from peptic ulcer disease and pleaded for something to stop the pain. Dr. Batmanghelidj had nothing at his disposal that would help. The cries of agony from the man were so disturbing that in desperation Batmanghelidj gave him two glasses of water. He simply didn't know what else to do. To his surprise within minutes the man's pain disappeared. He told the patient to drink two glasses of water every few hours. The man did and remained free from pain and disease for the rest of his time in prison.

This was Dr. Batmanghelidj's introduction to the role water can play in health and healing. Had medications been available they would have been used and Dr. Batmanghelidj would probably have never discovered the dangers of chronic dehydration and the importance of water.

Some time later, after a few medications became available, a similar experience occurred with another inmate. Walking past a jail cell Batmanghelidj spotted a man curled up on the floor of his cell semiconscious crying in pain. He had an ulcer that was nearly killing him. He

170

asked the inmate if he had done anything to relieve the pain. He said he had taken three Tagamets and a full bottle of antacid, but the pain only got worse. Remembering his previous experience, Dr. Batmanghelidj gave the man two glasses of water. Within 10 minutes the pain subsided. He had him drink another glass and within four minutes the pain stopped completely. This patient had taken a huge amount of ulcer medication without results, but after drinking only three glasses of water the pain was gone and he was up socializing with his friends.

These instances prompted Dr. Batmanghelidj to start researching the effects water has on health. For nearly 3 years he treated countless numbers of patients for a variety of illnesses using ordinary tap water and nothing else. The government, impressed with his work, released him from prison. He immediately immigrated to the United States where he continued his research and wrote a book titled *Your Body's Many Cries for Water*. Dr. Batmanghelidj claims that many of the degenerative illnesses we suffer from today are to a large extent caused by chronic dehydration. He has treated many thousands of patients with water and has witnessed complete recovery of those suffering from an assortment of conditions such as high blood pressure, migraine headaches, arthritis, asthma, back pain, chronic constipation, colitis, heartburn, chronic fatigue syndrome, and even obesity. Yes, overweight problems can be treated with water.

Dr. Batmanghelidj claims that every single one of these conditions can be caused by dehydration. Severe dehydration is so destructive it causes quick death. But chronic low-grade dehydration causes disease which can lead to a slow death. Health deteriorates so slowly we don't realize what's happening. We attribute it to age. He maintains that most of us are chronically dehydrated because we don't drink enough water. Dehydration causes damage to cells which leads to inflammation, swelling, and pain. Each individual's response to dehydration differs depending on his or her own chemical and physical makeup. For some it manifests itself first as arthritis, and in others migraine headaches. Arthritis occurs when joints become dehydrated and tissue damage occurs. Back pain occurs when discs between vertebrae become dehydrated, as a result, bones and muscles twist out of alignment, causing stress.

A recent study published in the British Medical Association journal *Annals of the Rheumatic Diseases* (July, 2000) found that people who drank more than 3 cups of coffee a day had twice the chance of getting arthritis as those who drank less. This study confirms Dr. Batmanghelidj's observations. Rheumatoid arthritis is more prevalent in coffee drinkers because coffee has a dehydrating effect. Arthritis is considered incurable by conventional medical standards, yet Dr. Batmanghelidj has done what seems to be the impossible. He's cured many people of arthritis by simply having them drink more water and less coffee, tea, and other beverages.

Other researchers have noted that drinking too little water increases the risk of kidney stones, breast cancer, colon cancer, bladder cancer, obesity, mitral valve prolapse (a heart condition), and physical and mental health.[1]

I highly recommend you read Dr. Batmanghelidj's book (see Appendix). He explains the scientific rationale for his claims and provides numerous testimonials from doctors and laymen. He has successfully treated thousands of people simply by having them drink more water. Some of these people suffered from health problems for years despite the use of drugs and medical treatments. The reason these treatments didn't work was because, as he puts it, the problem was not due to a drug deficiency, but a chronic lack of water.

Chronic Dehydration

Because of the work of Dr. Batmanghelidj and others, most health care professionals routinely recommend that their patients drink plenty of water—at least 2–3 quarts a day. This is the amount the body loses from perspiration, respiration, and elimination every day. This is the minimum amount you should consume each day. If you are chronically dehydrated then you need to increase this amount to replenish your reserves.

So why are we dehydrated? We have water and beverages readily available to us almost all the time. One reason is that as we get older our bodies function less efficiently. Our sense of thirst is one of the functions that declines with age. This doesn't mean we don't need as much water when we're older, it means we don't have the urge to drink as much as we should. Ironically, as we cut down on our water consumption our sense of thirst becomes even less active, compounding the problem.

Another reason for chronic dehydration is that most people mistakenly believe that beverages such as coffee, tea, soda, and juice are just as good as water. They're not. Keep in mind that it's water that the cells of your body need and want, not soda pop. Every item of food you eat or beverage you drink must be diluted and processed by the body. Beverages contain a myriad of chemicals that must be processed just like any other food and, therefore, can actually *dehydrate the body*; some more than others. Coffee, tea, alcohol, and soda are some of the worst, but even a sugary fruit juice can have a dehydrating effect. Sugar requires additional water to digest. This is why you get thirsty after eating sweets. Our bodies need about three quarts of pure water every day. If you drink beverages, they don't count as fulfilling this requirement. In fact, for every beverage you drink, you

172

need to add an equal amount of water to your three quart requirement just to stay equal; if you don't, you will become dehydrated. Only water hydrates the body and cures dehydration.

How much water do you need? We often hear the recommendation of six to eight glasses a day. But how big is a glass? Is it 4 ounces, 8 ounces, or 12 ounces? The amount of water you need depends on your size. A large person needs more water than a smaller person. A general rule of thumb is to drink one quart of water for every 50 pounds of bodyweight. A 100-pound person, therefore, needs to drink *at least* two quarts of water a day. A 200-pound person needs four quarts. This is the minimum recommended amount you need just to maintain your current level. If you are chronically dehydrated you may need to drink more to make up for a lack of water. Also, if you are physically active, if you live in a dry or hot climate, if it is summer, or if you eat foods or beverages that have a diuretic effect then you need to drink more than this. Do not count coffee, soda, or other beverages as fulfilling this water requirement.

Chronic dehydration isn't something that happens in a day. It is a slow process that occurs over weeks, months, and years. Consequently, rehydrating the body isn't a one-time event. You can't drink a gallon of water and cure chronic dehydration. The body isn't a sponge that immediately soaks up water. The body must adapt and adjust to an increase in water consumption. Injured cells and tissues must have time to repair themselves.

Salt and Trace Minerals

Increasing water consumption is the first and most important step in reversing chronic dehydration. Another very important part of Dr. Batmanghelidj's water cure is that as you increase your water intake you must also increase the amount of salt you consume. The reason is that as you drink more water you will also eliminate more water; as the water passes through your body it washes out salts and minerals. You need to replace these minerals. I recommend that you use sea salt because it contains many trace minerals, ordinary processed salts do not. These trace mineral salts are washed out of the body so they, too, must be replenished. Dr. Batmanghelidj recommends taking a half teaspoon of salt for every 10 cups (80 ounces) of water.

You can add the salt to your meals during food preparation as you normally would. Don't be afraid of eating salt. A summary of all studies on high blood pressure and salt has shown that in people with normal blood pressure salt has no effect. In people who have high blood pressure only about 3% are affected by salt. Of these 3%, it is believed that they have high blood pressure because they are chronically dehydrated. Dr.

Batmanghelidj's research has shown that drinking more water can lower high blood pressure, and he has been very successful in this area.

Dietary trace mineral supplements made from sea water or other sources could also be of value in replenishing trace minerals. These supplements are usually sold in liquid form and are available in most health food stores.

With people concerned about water safety, home purification systems have become popular. While this may solve one problem, it may cause another. If you drink distilled or filtered water you enhance the loss of tissue salts. Purified water has been stripped of much of its mineral content and will absorb minerals in the body and pull them out. Drinking this type of water could even create a mineral deficiency. So if you drink distilled or filtered water you need to make a special effort to consume more sea salt and take trace mineral supplements.

CHRONIC DEHYDRATION—A SILENT KILLER

Dehydration is serious. Every summer people fall victim to dehydration caused by heatstroke. In August of 2001, newspaper headlines described the death of Korey Stringer, a 27-year-old Pro Bowl offensive tackle with the Minnesota Vikings. Stringer died of dehydration and heatstroke after practicing in 90-degree weather. His death came 6 days after University of Florida freshman, Eraste Autin, died from the same condition. Athletes aren't the only ones who suffer from dehydration. Three residents died in a Detroit nursing home in June. At least 19 deaths were reported in the Chicago area during a heat wave that hit the Midwest. Many more occurred in other cities across the country. News stories similar to these repeat themselves every year during the hot summer months.

Early signs of dehydration include flushed skin, headache, fatigue, dry mouth and eyes, dizziness, and burning sensation in the stomach. If allowed to continue, symptoms progress to difficulty in swallowing, clumsiness, shriveled skin, sunken eyes and dim vision, painful urination, muscle spasms, delirium, coma, and ultimately death. Severe dehydration can kill within a matter of days and even hours.

Dehydration kills, we know that. What is less well known is that subclinical or chronic mild dehydration also kills, but at a much slower pace. In a way it is worse than severe dehydration because it strikes without warning. Chronic mild dehydration is a silent killer. It quietly sneaks up on victims and slowly but steadily drains the life blood out of them. Symptoms don't suddenly appear or cause extreme discomfort; they are subtle and, therefore, usually ignored. Symptoms, such as arthritis, consti-

174

pation, or back pain, come on so gradually that they are ignored and mistaken for signs of aging or stress. Victims continue on with their lives, often masking the symptoms with drugs, never suspecting they are slowly dying of thirst.

Without adequate water the body cannot function properly, waste cannot be effectively removed, chemical processes are slowed down, organ function deteriorates, and the whole body suffers. If the condition becomes chronic, degeneration overtakes the body, accelerating the aging process and bringing on disease, sickness, pain, and premature death.

But you may say, "I'm not dehydrated, I drink lots of fluids during the day and don't feel particularly thirsty." That's just the problem! You don't have to feel thirsty in order to be dehydrated. As a consequence, most of us don't drink enough, and what we do drink is usually coffee, soda, or some other beverage rather than water.

The sensation of thirst, like many other physiological processes, becomes less active as we age.[2] As a result, many older people are dehydrated without even knowing it. Dehydration is so common among the elderly, it has been identified as one of the most frequent causes for hospitalization for people over 65. In one study, half of those hospitalized for dehydration died within a year of admission. Even though these patients knew dehydration was a problem for them, they still weren't drinking enough. Without the thirst sensation we tend not to drink.

While the elderly are most at risk, they aren't the only ones who suffer from chronic dehydration. Often we become so busy at work and in our everyday lives that we don't take the time to satisfy thirst. We put it off until it's more convenient. Ignoring the thirst reflex dulls this sensation. We become so accustomed to ignoring the body's subtle signals of thirst that we don't realize we are becoming dehydrated. So even relatively young people can and do become chronically dehydrated.

Another problem is that we often satisfy thirst with beverages rather than water. Beverages can bring immediate satisfaction, but in the long run, may promote dehydration. If you drink caffeinated beverages to quench your thirst you are not satisfying the body's need for water. Caffeine and sugar will cause the body to become more dehydrated later on. If the beverage is again consumed to quench thirst the problem can escalate.

A study by the National Research Council revealed that on average women (ages 15–49) drink a mere 2.6 cups of water a day.[3] Most of their fluids come from beverages. This finding suggests that a large portion of women may be chronically dehydrated. Another study performed by researchers at Johns Hopkins Hospital in Baltimore discovered that 32–41% of the subjects they tested (both men and women ages 23–44) were chronically dehydrated to one degree or another.[4] Some food consumption surveys indicate that as much as 75% of the population (all ages) is chronically mildly dehydrated.

Dehydration of as little as a 1% decrease in body weight results in impaired physiological function, including cardiovascular performance and temperature regulation.[5-7] Normally, a sensation of thirst manifests after the body has reached a level of dehydration of 0.8% to 2% loss of body weight.[8, 9] At this point the body is in a mild state of dehydration. If this situation persists it can become chronic. Even chronic mild dehydration is dangerous and has many adverse effects on body function and performance. Studies have shown that a 2% loss of water results in significant reductions of arithmetic ability and short-term memory.[10] If a 150-pound person loses 2% of his or her body weight (3 lb), mental as well as physical performance will decrease by 20%.[11, 12]

Usually drinking a glass or two of water can relieve mild dehydration. If the level of dehydration is greater than 3% of body weight, complete rehydration requires more than just drinking a glass of water. Complete rehydration in this case would require many glasses of water over an 18—24 hour period.[13]

Because it only takes a small decrease in water to become dehydrated and we often don't respond to thirst by drinking water, many of us become chronically dehydrated without even realizing it. In the meantime, our bodies laboring under extreme stress caused by dehydration, begin to break down and show signs of malfunction and disease.

Dr. Batmanghelidj discovered many of the health problems associated with chronic mild dehydration. Other researchers have also correlated a lack of water to several common health problems.

The role of water in maintaining good health has been recognized since ancient times. Hippocrates, the father of medicine, recommended increasing the consumption of water to treat and prevent kidney stones. Doctors today also recommend drinking more water for the same purpose. Approximately 12–15% of the population will develop kidney stones at some time in their lives.[14, 15] The prevalence of kidney stones is higher in those who are chronically dehydrated. While several factors, such as age and climate, may influence stone formation, adjusting water consumption is a simple preventative measure that has proven successful since the days of Hippocrates.

One of the most common problems associated with chronic dehydration is constipation. A healthy, well-hydrated individual should have a full bowel movement at least once, if not twice, a day. If you eat three meals a day, then you need to eliminate a *minimum* of once a day. The process should be quick and easy. If it is a strain to eliminate or takes more than a minute or two then you are constipated.

In the colon (the endmost segment of the intestinal tract) a certain amount of water is normally extracted from the feces to facilitate excretion. When the body becomes dehydrated the amount of moisture removed is increased in order to slow down water loss. A greater amount of water than normal is removed from the feces traveling through the colon. As a consequence, fecal matter becomes excessively dry and hard, slowing down elimination. The result is constipation. The solution is simple: drink more water.

It also appears that if you want to avoid cancer, or at least some forms of cancer, you should be drinking plenty of water every day. As simple as it sounds, just drinking five glasses of water can reduce the risk of colon cancer by 45%, urinary tract cancer (bladder, prostate, kidney, testicle) by 50%, and breast cancer by 79%.

Numerous studies have shown a direct correlation between the amount of water consumed and the incidence of cancer.[16-19] For example, Dr. W.A. Bitterman and colleagues found that patients with urinary tract cancer consumed significantly smaller quantities of water compared with healthy controls.[20] Dr. L.R. Wilkens and others showed that total fluid intake, and intake of water in particular, had a strong inverse relationship with lower urinary tract cancer among women.[21] Similar findings have been made regarding colon and breast cancer. In a study carried out in Seattle, Washington, researchers showed that women who drink more than five glasses of water a day had a 45% decreased risk of colon cancer compared to those who consumed two or fewer glasses per day.[22] A study by Dr. J.D. Stookey and colleagues revealed that water consumption had a huge influence on breast cancer, reducing risk by a remarkable 79%.[23]

Wow! Just think of it: water as an anti-cancer treatment! Of course, the opposite is also true; not drinking enough water increases the risk of getting cancer.

One of the most common symptoms of chronic dehydration Dr. Batmanghelidj has observed is pain and cramping. Muscle fatigue, spasms, and cramping occur more frequently when the body is dehydrated.[24] Most of us have had the painful experience of a leg cramp during heavy physical activity. Exercise causes a high rate of perspiration which can easily lead to dehydration which, in turn, promotes muscle cramps. When you get a cramp during exercise the best thing to do is to get a drink of water; if water isn't readily available at least rest in a shady location to allow the body to cool down. Heat increases perspiration and dehydration, and taking a break will allow the body to cool down. Sometimes we experience what's called "swimmer's cramp" while in a pool. We don't feel hot or dehydrated while swimming, but this is a deception. We can become very dehydrated because being in the water desensitizes the thirst mechanism so we don't feel thirsty and, consequently, don't get the water that's needed.

Many people experience chronic neck and back pain. They go to the doctor to get pain killers or the chiropractor to fix subluxations (misalignments in the spine caused by muscle spasms and cramps). The chiropractor will relax the muscles and realign the bones, but if the cause was due to chronic dehydration the muscles will eventually cramp up again and the person is soon back in the chiropractor's office getting another adjustment. Drugs and spinal adjustments cannot cure dehydration.

Since the heart and blood vessels form the plumbing system of the body, it is logical to assume that a decrease in water would affect cardiovascular health. This is true. A drop of only 2.2% in body fluid negatively influences the heart rate. Mild dehydration is known to induce leaky valve syndrome (mitral valve prolapse) where the mitral valve of the heart doesn't close completely, thus decreasing the heart's pumping efficiency.

Fatigue, headaches, fuzzy thinking, and loss of mental ability, strength, coordination, and endurance are all consequences of dehydration. It's interesting how often when we get a headache it is simply due to a lack of water. Most people instead of drinking water to relieve their headaches will take pain pills like aspirin or Tylenol. These pain killers haven't solved the problem; the body is still dehydrated. All they did was deaden the nerves carrying the pain sensation, masking the symptom of dehydration which was brought about by your body to get your attention and tell you it needs more water. It is amazing how many people can relieve their headaches within 15 minutes or so by simply drinking a large glass of water, rather than relying on pain pills. The water solves the problem rather than cover it up by deadening the nerves.

FAD DIET DECEPTION

If a loss of only 1–3% of body water can cause all the symptoms mentioned above, what might happen if 4, 5, or 6% were lost? Or what if a mild state of dehydration of only 1 or 2% were always present? It is easy to see that many health problems can arise. It is for this reason that many quick weight-loss diets are dangerously unhealthy!

I recently saw an ad in the newspaper touting the charms of an herbal weight-loss supplement. Herbs are supposed to be harmless and healthy aren't they? That's what marketers hope you will believe. The title across the page read I LOST 54 POUNDS WITHOUT DIETING OR MEDICA-TION IN LESS THAN 6 WEEKS! Wow, that's a catchy title that would grab any overweight person's attention. The problem is that it's grossly misleading.

As we learned in Chapter 7 it's practically impossible for someone to lose 54 pounds of *fat* in just 6 weeks (9 pounds a week) unless they are grossly obese and calories are severely restricted. But the person pictured in the ad (before she went on the diet) wasn't especially large, and the ad claimed you could eat anything you wanted. No calorie restriction whatsoever!

So what was the secret to this program? If this weight-loss program did not involve any dietary restraints, what made it work? The person may very well have lost 54 pounds, but the weight wasn't from the removal of fat. If it wasn't the removal of fat that produced the weight loss, what was it? Much of it had to be water. The ad boasted that the supplement it was promoting consisted of special herbs that promoted weight loss. It boasted that "some people have lost 13 pounds the first week." While the ad didn't reveal the names of all the herbs, it had no reservations in stating that many of them were diuretics. In other words, the "secret" to the success of this weight-loss gimmick was the removal of water from the body. What a dangerous program!

Some of the herbs also were supposed to rev up the metabolism; they probably used herbs that contained caffeine, which is also a diuretic. Even if these herbs stimulated the metabolism it is only a temporary stimulus at best. Another side effect of dehydration is a decrease in metabolic activity. That's right, dehydration can promote fat deposition. Studies show that even mild dehydration will slow down metabolism as much as 3%. If dehydration is chronic, low metabolism would be also. In this case, taking an herb or drug containing caffeine would have no beneficial effect on the metabolism.

Many fad, reducing diets rely on water loss to give the impression that fat is being taken off. You should avoid all diets that rely on diuretics for weight loss. A sound weight-loss program will encourage drinking plenty of water and the removal of body fat rather than body water.

In recent years low-carbohydrate or high-protein diets have become popular. These, too, can be dangerous if they don't address the water issue. Protein has a strong diuretic effect and pulls water out of the body. People who get on high-protein diets and don't drink adequate amounts of water lose lots of weight quickly, but at first it's almost all water. The result is that they become chronically dehydrated.

Many people don't realize that the arthritis, back pain, or chronic headaches they are suffering from right now may be a result of the weight-loss diets they've been on in the past.

So in order to avoid health problems caused by dehydration you need a diet that provides plenty of water. Drinking plenty of water is an important part of my plan. Since you do not lose water, weight loss is slower. The weight you lose is from the removal of fat rather than water. While weight loss is slower, it is more permanent and far healthier.

DRINK MORE WATER, LOSE MORE WEIGHT

Water is the ultimate diet drink because it contains zero calories, suppresses appetite, and helps remove fat. Yes, drinking water can help you take off fat. Studies have shown that decreasing water consumption causes an increase in fat deposition and an increase in water intake has the opposite effect.

This is the reason. The kidney's job is to filter waste from the blood and maintain electrolyte and pH balance. The kidneys need plenty of water to perform their function properly. If water isn't available, the blood becomes too congested and the kidneys can't do their job effectively. Since maintaining a chemical balance is vital to health the liver jumps in and takes on the task performed by the overworked kidneys. This, in turn, puts undue stress on the liver, which must continue to perform all of its regular jobs as well. One of the jobs of the liver is to convert fat into energy for the body. But if the liver is struggling under excessive stress from helping the kidneys, it too can't function at optimal levels. Less fat is converted into energy and more fat remains stored as fat. So when you drink more water, the kidneys and liver are able to function more efficiently, and more fat is metabolized and removed.

We all need a certain amount of water every day. If you don't normally drink water, you must be getting your fluids from some other source. No other fluid can adequately replace water and most of the beverages we drink actively contribute to our weight problems.

A major key to losing weight is to replace all the beverages you ordinarily drink with plain water. Most beverages contain empty calories. That is, they provide little nutritive value but lots of calories. The more beverages you drink, the more calories you consume. A 16-ounce glass of orange juice contains 220 calories. A 12-ounce can of soda has about 150 calories. Water, on the other hand, has zero calories. By drinking water in place of these other beverages you consume fewer calories.

180

We tend to eat about the same amount of food and get the same amount of calories each day. The calories in drinks, however, are all added calories. Regardless of how much or how little you drink between meals, you will eat about the same. Studies have shown that drinking sugar-laden drinks has little effect on how much people eat at a meal. No matter how many beverages we drink we will still eat the same amount. Drinking water instead of beverages can significantly reduce the number of calories you consume each day.

You may think to yourself "I drink low-calorie beverages so it's okay." It's not. Eating and drinking foods containing artificial sweeteners is not a good idea. They stimulate the sweet tooth keeping addictions alive and thriving. A person who becomes accustomed to drinking and eating artificially sweetened foods establishes a bad habit that leads to overeating, particularly of nutritionally poor foods and drinks.

Another problem with sweet or appetizing beverages is that they stimulate the salivary glands and trick the body into thinking it's going to receive food. The body gears up to handle a hearty meal, but all it gets is a liquid which is digested almost immediately. The body now is primed to receive solid food and you begin to feel "hungry." Consequently, you end up snacking and consuming needless calories.

Beverages, whether they are low-calorie or not, can also make you thirsty and cause you to drink more. For example, caffeinated drinks like coffee and soda have a diuretic effect. You may drink a soda to quench your thirst and gain immediate temporary satisfaction, but the caffeine will draw water out of the body causing you to urinate more frequently and become thirsty again. If you satisfy this thirst with another soda the cycle repeats itself. You gradually become more and more dehydrated while consuming more and more soda and more calories. If you satisfied your initial thirst with water instead of soda, you would not become thirsty as quickly and you would not consume any calories or artificial flavors, caffeine, and other chemicals that stimulate the taste buds and encourage addiction.

An interesting study on coffee was carried out by 12 healthy men and women. They were all coffee drinkers, but abstained from drinking or eating anything containing caffeine for 5 days before the study. They were then allowed to drink 6 cups of coffee per day. The researchers found that when the subjects drank coffee they excreted more water in their urine than they consumed in their foods, so that they had a net loss in water. Total body water decreased by 2.7%. Despite this level of dehydration, only two of the subjects experienced thirst.

Water should replace all alcohol, coffee, black tea, herbal tea, soda, juice (which is often packed with additional sugar), and flavored drinks. The ones you should avoid the most are those that contain sugar, caffeine, or alcohol. These are the ones highest in calories and producing the strongest diuretic or dehydrating effects.

This doesn't mean you can never drink these beverages. If you must drink a beverage now and then, make sure you follow it with an equal amount of water. For instance, if you drink a cup of coffee and a soda, you need to drink an additional two glasses of water to compensate for these beverages. Alcohol poses the biggest problem because it requires 8 times its volume in water for metabolization. So if you drink 1 ounce of alcohol you need to follow it with 8 ounces of water. Don't count this water as part of your daily water requirement. You still need to drink another 6–8 glasses of water a day. If you drink all the water you're supposed to each day you will have little desire to drink additional beverages.

If your goal is to lose weight and keep it off you should try to get into the habit of drinking only water (except perhaps for special occasions). Once you develop this habit you will begin to prefer water over other drinks because it satisfies thirst better. Often people will say they don't like to drink water. What they are really saying is that they are addicted to the chemicals in drinks and they need to satisfy those cravings. Even one soft drink a day can have a significant impact on weight. See the article on next page. While this article focuses on children it is just as applicable to adults who drink "liquid candy."

CALORIE CONTENT IN COMMON BEVERAGES	
Beverage (12 oz)	**Calories**
Beer	146
Cola	121
Ginger ale	124
Root beer	152
Dr. Pepper	151
Kool-Aid with sugar	150
Lemonade	150
Apple juice	174
Grape juice	233
Orange juice	167
Carrot juice	147
Water	0

Childhood Obesity Linked to "Liquid Candy"

An extra soft drink a day gives a child a 60% greater chance of becoming obese, new research suggests. The study, published in *The Lancet* medical journal, says the soft drink-obesity link is independent of the food children eat, how much television or videos they watch, and the amount they exercise. These data suggest that people aren't compensating for the extra calories by cutting back on eating, said the study's lead investigator, Dr. David Ludwig, director of the obesity program at Boston Children's Hospital. The prevalence of obesity among children in the United States increased by 100% over the last 14 years.

The soft drink study involved tracking 548 children ages 11 and 12 from public schools across Massachusetts for two school years. It found that if they increased their daily soft drink intake, each extra soda made them 60% more likely to become obese, regardless of how many sodas they were drinking before. All the children were already drinking some soft drinks at the beginning of the study.

Only 7% of the children did not change their soft drink intake over the two years. Fifty-seven percent increased their intake, with a quarter of them drinking two or more extra cans a day, the study said. Soft drinks tracked in the study included regular sodas, Hawaiian Punch, lemonade, Kool-Aid, sweetened iced tea, or other sugared fruit drinks. "The odds of becoming obese increased significantly for each additional daily serving of sugar-sweetened drink," the study concluded.

Dr. Philip James, chairman of the International Obesity Task Force, an independent worldwide scientific organization which was not connected with the study, said the evidence so far indicates that sugar is only slightly less fattening than fat, but sugar in drinks can be deceptive because the beverages are less filling than food.

He said one explanation might be that while people tend to eat less at a meal if they have overeaten at a previous sitting, evening out the calories, they don't tend to do that if the extra calories come from drinks. They tend to eat a normal-sized meal despite having loaded up on sugar from soft drinks and sugary fruit juices.

In the past 10 years, soft drink consumption has almost doubled among children in the United States, Ludwig said, adding that the average American teenager consumes 15 to 20 extra teaspoons of sugar a day just from soda and other sugared drinks.

Half of all Americans and most adolescents consume soft drinks daily. Childhood obesity has been linked to later development of diabetes, heart disease, cancer, and arthritis.

Source: Associated Press

Simply substituting water for other drinks can have a remarkable impact on your health and weight. For example, Donna Gutkowski replaced the 6 to 8 cans of Mountain Dew she was drinking a day with water. As a result, she lost 35 pounds of excess weight. "I'm able to wear clothes that I thought would never touch my body again." Speaking of her upcoming wedding she says, "I can walk down the aisle looking better than I have looked in 15 years."

Bob Butts says, "I easily took off 15 pound without trying. I eat whatever I want... I can honestly say that you have made losing weight an easy thing to do. I know of two brothers, one lost over 100 pounds and the other lost 30."

Drinking water not only helps prevent consumption of liquid calories but also satisfies hunger, thus reducing the amount of food and calories you eat. This is discussed in the following section.

YOU'RE NOT HUNGRY, YOU'RE THIRSTY

Most of us don't recognize the body's signals for thirst. It is often misinterpreted as hunger and we end up eating when our body is really crying for water. Oh sure, when you get cotton mouth you know you are thirsty, but by the time the body starts exhibiting this symptom you have become seriously dehydrated. Dry mouth is a sign of severe thirst. This stage of dehydration ordinarily could have been prevented if you paid attention to your body's earlier cries for water.

The first sign of thirst is a subtle desire to drink. If we ignore this sensation we become more dehydrated. The body is forced to resort to other means to motivate us to drink. The next sign to appear is an empty feeling in the stomach. When the body becomes desperate for water prompting feelings of hunger may motivate eating foods that would supply enough liquids to prevent dehydration. The body isn't really hungry, it's thirsty. If you continue to ignore the body's signal or if you eat foods that don't supply the needed water, you will develop a dry mouth. A dry mouth is unmistakably a signal that the body needs water. It can be accompanied by fatigue, light-headedness, or headache. By this time you are very dehydrated and symptoms are severe.

A very important concept you need to understand is that if you become hungry between meals it most likely is a sign you are thirsty, not hungry. You have ignored earlier signals of thirst and now the body is crying out for water. The only way to satisfy thirst is with water. Often we make do with something less such as coffee, soda, or a snack of some sort which may bring immediate satisfaction but in the long run will make matters worse.

Let me explain why feelings of hunger between meals are a sign of thirst rather than a need for food. On average we need around 2400 calories a day. Any more than this is excess that is turned into fat. Three meals a day can easily supply 2400 calories. For example, take a typical meal at Burger King: Whopper 640, regular french fries 227, a 12-ounce Coke 151, and cherry pie 240, for a grand total of 1258 calories. Even without the dessert it comes to 1018 calories. A three-piece fish dinner at Long John Silver's contains 1180 calories. A chicken dinner at KFC would contain about the same. So a typical lunch or dinner can easily supply over 1000 calories. If you eat three meals a day you can see that a total of 2400 calories is easy to come by. For most of us, it is far too easy.

Now think about it. Your body gets all of the food and energy it needs for the day from the three meals you eat. Ordinarily you don't need any additional food or calories. Snacking between meals just adds extra calories which are turned into fat. Therefore, when you feel "hungry" between meals it's not true hunger, it's a sign of thirst. You need water between meals, not food and not calorie-loaded beverages. A very important key to losing excess weight is to stop eating between meals and to drink water instead. The only exception to this guideline is if you are hypoglycemic or have some diagnosed medical condition that requires you to eat between meals.

Part of the diet described in this book is to recognize the fact that feelings of hunger between meals are almost always signals that our bodies need water, not food and not beverages. Limit your eating to your regular mealtime. Between meals when you feel "hungry" drink a glass of water. The water will surprisingly satisfy your hunger. The liquid in the stomach will fill it up producing a feeling of satiety. The feeling may only last an hour or two, but that's okay because by then your body needs another drink of water anyway. So give it another drink. Do this throughout the day. When you feel hungry drink water.

This way you will get your required amount of water each day without trying or forcing yourself to drink. As you begin drinking more water your sensation of thirst will become stronger or actually become reactivated and you will be more aware of your need for water. This will help you satisfy thirst before the body has to resort to a sensation of hunger or dry mouth.

Simply drinking water between meals can be very effective in cutting unwanted pounds without discomfort often associated with dieting. Dr. Batmanghelidj says, "I know a man who weighed 480 pounds. He lost 290 pounds in 1 year by drinking water whenever he felt hungry. He had to have two operations to remove the loose skin. Another man lost 156 pounds in a year and a half. He reduced 14 pants sizes. A 15- to 45-pound weight loss with water is possible with minimal effort." Wow! What phenomenal results by simply drinking water.

YOU NEED A SYSTEM

Everybody knows they need to drink adequate amounts of water, usually about 3 quarts a day. But few people actually do it. You can't rely on guesswork. Just knowing that you need to drink plenty of water a day doesn't accomplish it. We tend to forget or overestimate the amount we do drink, especially when we consume beverages. People go all day without a single drink of pure water yet feel they've gotten all the liquids their bodies need. They could not be farther from the truth.

If you kept a record of how much water you drink you would find that more than likely you do not get enough. You may think you are drinking plenty of water, and may drink more than you ordinarily would, but for most people it would still be short of the recommended 1 quart for every 50 pounds of body weight.

To help you get your minimum recommended daily allowance you should use a system where you can keep an accurate record of the amount you consume. One idea is to keep a small notebook and record every glass of water you drink during the day and make sure before the day is over that you get your full amount. Don't wait until just before bedtime and try to down 2 quarts of water or you will be up all night. Make sure you drink throughout the day.

I think the best method is to fill one or more containers in the morning with the amount of water you're going to drink during the day. Drink the water throughout the day with the goal of emptying the container before retiring at night. You may have to use 2 or more containers so you can carry one with you when you go to work.

Although I don't recommend that you drink other beverages, especially coffee, tea, or soda, if you do, then add an equal amount of water to your daily ration. If you keep strictly to this regime you won't drink many additional beverages because you will be downing so much water you won't want anything else to drink.

Keep in mind that the recommended daily allowance is a *minimum*. This is equilavent to the amount of water we lose in urine, feces, perspiration, and respiration each day. So you are just replacing what's lost. You can drink more than this if you need to and in certain circumstances you will want to. If you exercise or if the climate where you live is dry or hot, you may need more water. How much should you add? It all depends on the amount of water you lose. A way in which you can determine that is to observe the color of your urine. If it is a dark yellow or amber color you're dehydrated and need to drink more. You want your urine to be a *very* pale yellow, almost clear in color.

In summary, the important concepts you need to remember from this chapter are:

- Drink water instead of beverages.
- Drink whenever you feel thirsty.
- Drink when you feel "hungry" between meals rather than eating snacks.
- Drink a minimum of 1 quart of water per day for every 50 pounds of body weight.
- If you drink anything other than water, add an equal amount of water to your daily water requirement.
- Set up a system to assure that you get your full recommended daily water requirement.
- If the climate is hot or dry or if you exercise heavily, increase your water intake.

I ask people if they are drinking enough water and they say "Sure, I drink three quarts of water a day." But they are still dehydrated. Why? Because it's 98° F (36.7° C) outside and they're losing more water than usual. People often neglect to account for the environment, and although they drink three quarts of water a day, they still aren't getting enough.

In the summer, especially if you live in a hot, dry climate, you need to increase your total daily water intake by about a quart. If you exercise

	Daily Loss of Water (in milliliters)		
	Normal Temperature (68°F/20°C)	Hot Weather	Prolonged Heavy Exercise
Skin	350	350	350
Respiration	350	250	650
Urine	1400	1200	500
Sweat	100	1400	5000
Feces	100	100	100
Total	2300	3300	6600

Source: *Textbook of Medical Physiology, 8th Ed*, Arthur C. Guyton. 1991, W.B. Saunders Company.

heavily or drink other beverages, add more. This may sound like a lot of water, but your body needs it. Keep in mind, especially if you drink distilled or filtered water, to add a little more salt to your diet.

At a temperature of 68° F (20° C), a sedentary adult loses about 2300 ml (2.4 quarts) of water a day. In hot weather, the loss is about 3300 ml (3.5 quarts), and with prolonged heavy exercise, the loss is 6600 ml (7 quarts) of water. You can see that in warm weather or if you are physically active, you have to significantly increase your water intake to compensate for water loss. If you exercise and perspire heavily, you may need to double the recommended daily allowance of water.

Other factors that increase water loss are a diet high in protein, alcohol, caffeine, sugar, and diuretic drugs and herbs; or eating a lot of dry, dense foods such as crackers, pretzels, chips, dried fruit, jerky, granola, etc. Dry, dense foods demand additional water for metabolization. Living in a high-altitude environment also increases water loss, because it is dryer at higher elevations.

Chapter 12

STEP TOWARD A NEW YOU ▄

If you look at popular magazines you're bound to run across "before" and "after" photos of people who lost weight using some diet, pill, or other weight-loss system. The "before" picture shows a typical couch potato with flabby thighs, a bulging waistline, and a body that looks akin to the Pillsbury Doughboy. The "after" picture shows a trim, he-man, bulging with lean muscle or a slender, well-toned woman with all the appearances of a professional model.

Wow! Can a diet pill do all this? Not hardly. Neither can a diet. To lose fat, as well as tone and build muscle you must get physical—that is exercise. No magic pill will give you a muscular or well-defined body as depicted in these photos. The only way you can do that is through exercise. Exercise not only tones muscles, but burns off excess fat. For this reason, all successful weight-loss programs include some form of exercise. It's one of the secrets to effective weight loss and an important step toward the new you.

Not only will exercise help you take off fat, it will help you keep it off. Exercise is the strongest predictor of long-term success in weight management. *The Physician and Sportsmedicine* recently reported that 90% of women who have lost weight and kept it off exercise on a regular basis. In another study published in the same journal, weight-regain patterns were reported in 40 women who had lost weight in a 16-week treatment program. Over the year that followed treatment, researchers found that the most active third of the participants lost additional weight. The middle third, who exercised about half as much, maintained their full end-of-treatment weight loss. The least active third, in contrast, steadily gained weight throughout the year after treatment.

Exercise is one of the keys to successful weight loss and weight management. I expect you to exercise. Remember, my program is designed to help you achieve better overall health. As your body becomes healthier you will lose excess weight. Exercise is one of the steps you must take toward gaining better health.

Now after saying that, you might moan, "Ugh! I don't like to exercise." Precisely, that's one of the reasons why you're probably overweight. If you don't like to exercise, you don't do it. Generally, overweight people avoid exercise because it isn't fun for them and they feel self-conscience. The heavier you are, the more difficult it is to move your body. Heavy people have more weight to move around, so they often tire more quickly, further discouraging exercise. As you lose weight you will be able to move more easily, you will have more energy, and you will enjoy moving your body.

You may find some relief in that I'm not going to recommend that you go out and start jogging 10 miles every day or join a high-impact aerobics class. You can do that if you are physically up to it, but you don't need to. Exercise doesn't need to be a grueling, tedious, or exhausting affair. It can be enjoyable even for those who are unathletic. Moderate exercise like walking or swimming can provide you with many of the same health benefits you would get from more intense exercise. The secret is choosing the right type of exercise and setting up a schedule in which to do it.

Don't let physical limitations prevent you from gaining the benefits of physical activity. It doesn't matter what shape you are in, most everyone can do some type of exercise. If you have any concerns check with your doctor first.

WHY EXERCISE?
Health and Happiness

There are many reasons why you should exercise. Exercise improves bodily functions, helps prevent illness, burns off excess calories, improves appearance, increases self-respect, enhances mood, improves your quality of life, and helps you feel better about yourself and about life.

The health-enhancing benefits of exercise have been known for many years. As far back as the 1930s researchers were able to decrease the incidence of tumors in a strain of cancer-prone mice from 88 to 16% by restricting their calories and increasing physical activity. In 1960, scientists

190

discovered that an extract of exercised muscle, when injected into mice with cancer, slowed the growth of tumors and sometimes eliminated them entirely. An extract of nonexercised muscle had no effect.

Exercise has been successfully used to treat depression and is a potent defense against most all forms of degenerative disease. The health benefits of exercise are well established. Studies have shown exercise to have the following effects:

- Decrease risk of degenerative diseases such as heart disease, atherosclerosis, cancer, and diabetes.
- Increase energy.
- Improve joint mobility.
- Reduce joint swelling and pain from arthritis.
- Reduce depression and anxiety.
- Relieve stress.
- Improve blood and lymph circulation.
- Improve flexibility.
- Enhance immune system function.
- Improve brain and nerve function.
- Enhance healing.
- Improve digestion and bowel function.
- Weight loss and management.
- Lower cholesterol and triglyceride levels.
- Prevent insomnia.
- Improve strength and endurance.
- Normalize hormone secretion.
- Prevent osteoporosis.
- Prevent gallstones.
- Prevent diverticular disease.
- Improve memory and cognitive skills.

That's quite an impressive list. Who wouldn't want to enjoy all of these health benefits? Not only will the quality of your life improve as you exercise, but your chances of dying from a number of degenerative conditions will decrease.

There is a large body of evidence that suggests that the more physically active you are, the less likely you are to die prematurely. In a study reported recently in *The Journal of the American Medical Association* researchers from the University of Helsinki reported that taking brisk, 30-minute walks just six times a month cuts the risk of premature death by 44%. This study was unique because it involved only twins and was, therefore, able to separate out mortality due to genetics versus mortality due to fitness. The study tracked almost 16,000 healthy men and women in a national registry of twins in Finland for an average of 19 years. The researchers found that even occasional exercisers—those who did less than the equivalent of 6 brisk, 30-minute walks a month—were 30% less likely to die during the study than their sedentary twins. More vigorous exercisers—those who did at least the equivalent of 6 brisk walks or jogs lasting 30 minutes each month—were 44% less likely to die early.

In another study researchers from the University of Virginia also found that exercise helps prevent illness and prolongs life. During a 12-year period covered by the study, researchers found that people who walked 2 miles a day cut their risk of death almost in half. The risk of death was especially lower from cancer. Those who walked infrequently were about two and a half times more likely to die of cancer than were those who walked at least 2 miles a day. The researchers calculated that for every extra mile walked per day the death rate drops by 19%.

The US Surgeon General recommends that we should each get enough physical activity to burn at least 150 calories a day. This would amount to a half-hour of walking daily or 20 minutes of swimming laps. This is a minimum. Walking 2 or 3 miles at a moderate pace is within the ability of most of us.

How Exercise Helps You Lose Weight

As you recall from Chapter 7, body weight is a function of calorie input versus calorie output. If we put more calories into our bodies than we use, the excess is stored as fat. Increasing our level of physical activity burns off more calories. This is true regardless of other factors, such as metabolic rate. Whether a person has a high or a low metabolic rate, if calories in are greater than calories out, body weight increases and vice versa. Increasing our level of physical activity is one way we can compensate for the calories we eat. When exercise is combined with calorie restriction you have two factors working in your favor.

The fat burning effects of exercise increase with duration of the activity. Our bodies need a constant supply of energy to fuel metabolic processes. Glucose supplies the majority of our energy, but when the body's glucose supply begins to run low, fat is utilized for this purpose. The longer the duration of exercise, the greater the contribution fat makes to the total energy used. For this reason, it is best to exercise on an empty stomach while glucose reserves are low. This way glucose reserves can be quickly used up so the body must rely more on fat for its energy requirements. The more fat that is burned the less that remains. This is one reason why it is

192

recommended that we exercise at least 30 minutes a day. As exercise begins our bodies burn mostly glucose and toward the end it burns more fat. The longer you exercise the more fat you burn.

While engaged in a physical activity your body's need for energy increases. Consequently, metabolism and the rate at which calories are burned, increases. Breathing and heart rate increase, your body becomes warmer, everything is running at an accelerated rate. When sitting down and relaxed, a 150-pound man burns about 82 calories an hour. But, when involved in a physical activity, like walking (3 mph), the rate increases to 225 calories an hour. That's an additional 143 calories that are burned off. Jogging (7.5 mph) increases the rate to 510 calories an hour for an increased loss of 428 calories.

What makes this even better is the fact that once exercise is ended, metabolism remains elevated and fat continues to be burned at an accelerated rate. Evidence suggests that metabolism is stimulated by about 25% for as long as 3 hours after intensive exercise and may still be running 10% faster 2 days later. You will be burning off extra calories even while you're relaxing in front of the television.

Changes occur in your body as it adapts to a more active lifestyle. Just 20 minutes of aerobic activity (walking, jogging, swimming laps, etc.) 3 times each week, stimulates even the untrained body to adapt by packing its cells with more fat-burning enzymes. The better conditioned you become the more fat you burn for energy because you have more of these fat-burning enzymes. People who are less conditioned burn more carbohydrate instead.

Lean, muscular people generally have a higher metabolic rate than out of shape, overweight people. It's not because they were born that way, but because muscle tissue consumes calories at a higher rate than does fatty tissue. The more muscle you have, the more calories your body burns. Each additional pound of muscle uses about 50 extra calories per day. This may not seem like much, but it adds up quickly. In one year that amounts to 18,000 fewer calories worth of fat hanging off your body.*

A very important reason why weight-loss diets *must* include exercise in order to be successful is because dieting causes metabolism to slow down

---

* This is equivalent to a little more than 5 pounds. This is 5 pounds of excess fat that is burned off without any additional effort on your part. One of the best ways to build muscle mass is through weightlifting or resistance training. A typical weightlifting program can add 3 pounds of muscle in about 3 months. In 1 year, 3 additional pounds of lean muscle tissue would burn off an extra 55,000 calories or the equivalent of almost 16 pounds of fat.

to a snail's pace. As metabolism slows down weight loss becomes harder. The dieter must reduce calorie consumption even further to continue losing weight. As weight is lost the metabolism slows even further. You end up eating lettuce and celery just to maintain the progress you've made. The joy of eating is gone. If you do relax your regimen even just a little, your weight quickly bounces back up. However, when exercise is combined with dieting, metabolism is kept elevated and you avoid this problem.

Many people believe that exercise increases appetite and, therefore, you'll tend to eat more if you exercise and negate any weight loss. This is not true. Most people who work out moderately (up to an hour a day) actually eat less than sedentary people. If you have extra fat, you will react differently to exercise than those who are lean. Unless you exercise to excess, your appetite will generally not increase from the exercise, because when the body has excess stores of fat, the appetite is not stimulated by moderate exercise.

With all the advantages of exercise listed here it should be clear to you how important physical activity is in weight loss and weight maintenance.

YOUR EXERCISE PROGRAM

What type of exercise should you do? The type of exercise you choose is very important. It must be convenient, economical, enjoyable, not too strenuous, and yet effective. What works for someone else may not be the best for you. The important thing is that you exercise regularly. However, you should avoid stressful exercise that may cause injury or discouragement. You should choose an activity that you can enjoy. This way you are more likely to make it a regular part of your life. It should be convenient so that you can do it easily, rain or shine. And it should fit your budget.

Many people lack the motivation to exercise or they get discouraged easily. To make your exercise program successful, you need to make it a habit. Even if you've always avoided exercise, once you have made up your mind to do it and make it a habit, many of the psychological barriers vanish and you will actually come to enjoy it. The following are some guidelines to help you set up and maintain a successful exercise program.

Commitment

The first step is to make a commitment to yourself. Set a goal to exercise regularly. The American College of Sports Medicine and the National Institutes of Health recommend 30 minutes or more of moderate-intensity activity per day on all, or most, days of the week in order to obtain significant health benefits. Three days a week would be an absolute minimum, 5 to 6 days a week is better.

Duration

Exercise at least 30 minutes at each session and longer if you can. The more time you can spend, the more benefit you will receive. If you're not accustomed to exercise start off slow. You may only be able to do 10 minutes the first day. That's okay. Keep with it. Gradually add more time as your strength and endurance increase.

Activity

Choose an activity you enjoy. The more you enjoy your workout, the more likely you will stick with it. I recommend walking, rebounding, and swimming. These are activities most people can participate in regardless of their fitness level. You can adjust the intensity of your workout from very mild to very demanding depending on your preferences and progress.

Convenience

An ideal exercise will be one that you can do at most any time. Joining a health spa is fine, although it is not the most convenient, nor is it normally cheap. But if you like that sort of thing and it encourages you to exercise regularly, then do it.

Schedule

You need to set a specific time to exercise and stick strictly to it. This is very important! If you do not set aside a specific time for exercise, you will not keep it up. Other things always have a way of popping up, and before you know it, there is no time to exercise. Scheduling is a most important step in developing a successful exercise program. When you set a time to exercise, you adjust all other activities around your exercise schedule so nothing else interferes. Having a set time will also psychologically prepare you for the workout. Before the habit is formed, you may argue with yourself after a hard day at work: "I'm too tired; I've got to make dinner; I've got to do this or that." But if you have a schedule, it will encourage you to exercise regardless of the excuses. You can choose any time that is most suitable for you. Some people like to do it the first thing in the morning because it gives them a boost of energy for the entire day. Others like to do it in the evening because it is relaxing and separates them from work and other responsibilities. Others who have the time, prefer to exercise on their lunch break. Some people who have a limited time for lunch find they can eat while they are taking a walk. This way they can get in a 20- or 30-minute walk as well as lunch.

Place

Choose a place to exercise and do it in the same place each time, a room in the house, the garage, a health club, or follow a preplanned route outdoors. Your mind associates this place with exercise, mentally you feel more prepared, and your desire to exercise is increased. One reason some people prefer to exercise at health spas is that the atmosphere there helps get them into the mood.

Clothes

Some people can get into the mood of exercising better by changing into an exercise outfit. If this helps encourage you, then do it. Special clothes are also recommended if your exercise is vigorous enough to cause you to perspire, which it should.

Set Goals

Set goals for yourself and focus on accomplishing those goals. You should have at least two goals, one long-range and one short-range. The long-range goal would be to lose excess weight. This is your primary purpose in initiating an exercise program. Short-range goals will be based on performance, such as time or distance. The short-range goals will make your workouts more enjoyable and give you feelings of accomplishment and of progress. Make the goals realistic, not too easy, yet achievable in a matter of months. Once you have achieved one goal, set a new goal and go for it. Continue to set new goals as you accomplish old ones. Setting goals will give your workout more purpose and allow you to see the improvement you are making.

Don't Overdo It

Avoid stressful exercises or overextending yourself. Tiring yourself out may lead to injury and may make you so exhausted that all you want to do afterwards is rest. Exercise should be vigorous enough to give you a good workout, yet not so demanding as to sap all your strength and make you exhausted for the rest of the day. If you injure yourself, then you will need to take time off to recuperate. Also, stressful exercise may make you dread working out. The right amount of exercise will tire you temporarily, but you will shortly gain renewed vigor and alertness. You should be able to carry on a conversation while you are exercising. If you are too out of breath to do that, ease up. Warning signals of pain or excessive fatigue must be heeded, but they're signs to ease up, not to stop entirely.

Bathe

Take a hot soothing shower or bath after you exercise. This is part of your reward for exercising. The bath will soothe tired muscles, wash off perspiration, and refresh you.

Make It a Part of Your Life

Don't limit your physical activity to just your regular exercise program. Take an opportunity to exercise whenever you can. Go bowling, take tennis lessons, play baseball, or get involved in other activities. Since exercise will make you more physically fit, take advantage of it. Instead of driving to a friend's house, walk or ride a bicycle. When you go to work, park your car at the far end of the lot and walk the rest of the way. Instead of taking the elevator, use the stairs. Take spontaneous walks outside. Go to the park and eat your lunch. Avoid sitting for extended periods. Get up, move about, and get your blood circulating.

WALKING

When Diane Carbonell, 33, decided it was time to lose weight, she didn't turn to a magic pill or embark on a special personalized diet plan. She didn't starve herself either, or resort to eating cabbage soup or rice cakes. Instead she started walking.

Years of relative inactivity caused her to tire quickly at first, but with persistence the length of her walks gradually increased. She chose walking rather than going to a gym because she said she was too embarrassed by her size to join one. After a year on her walking program she lost 135 pounds, dropping from a size 26 to a size 8.

When Diane first began walking around her neighborhood, the 5-foot-9 mother of three weighed more than 250 pounds. Despite having children at home at the time she still managed to go on regular walks. "It isn't easy when you have young children, but I was so determined to lose the weight that I went ahead and put my children in a stroller and took them with me on my walks," says Diane.

Friends she hasn't seen for awhile often don't recognize her now. "My husband and I ran into a group of people he used to work with, and they had no idea who I was," Diane said. "One of them later told my husband that they were all wondering who that woman was with him. It feels good when people I've known for years pass right by me in the grocery store."

Frances James, 44, knows the value of exercise. She lost 35 pounds and has maintained her new weight for 6 years. She says she notices women 20 years younger who never seem to have any energy because of their sedentary lifestyles. "I get up in the morning to do my exercises because I am too tired to do it in the evening," says Frances. "I really look forward to it now. It's such a part of my normal routine now, and it gives me so much energy throughout the day."

Jim Hunt lost 30 pounds by exercising. "I like to pick up 30 pounds of weights, see how heavy it feels, and remember that was how much unwanted baggage I used to carry around," says Jim. "No wonder I was tired all the time."

When the word exercise is mentioned most people think of jogging or lifting weights rather than walking. Many don't even consider walking to be exercise, yet it is one of the best forms of exercise you can do, especially if you are overweight or out of shape. You can get just as much benefit from walking as you can from jogging or bicycling or any other aerobic activity.

Walking is the most convenient and economic exercise there is and definitely the easiest. You can do it anywhere, and with the proper attire, anytime. Regardless of age or fitness level, most people can walk. The adage, "no pain, no gain," is a myth. Engaging in even moderate activity can counteract the effects of a sedentary lifestyle. Although walking is a relatively mild form of exercise, it provides enough physical activity to burn up excess calories and jump-start your metabolism. You don't need to run a marathon or indulge in strenuous activities to benefit from exercise.

Walking outside, especially among trees and foliage, adds a dimension to the activity that increases its enjoyment. With the abundance of shopping malls, mall walking has become a popular activity, especially with older people. Malls are relatively safe and weatherproof. The shops and people give the walk an added dimension of interest.

Since most people who are concerned about weight loss are physically inactive, I recommend starting out slowly. Walk at a leisurely pace for 10 minutes the first day you start. Stick to 10 minutes a day, 5 to 6 days a week for the first week. After 1 week, add 5 minutes to your walk. The following week add another 5 minutes. Keep adding 5 minutes each week until your walks last a full 30 minutes. If you follow this schedule you'll be doing 30 minutes after just 4 weeks.

Most fitness experts recommend the walking pace to be brisk. This would be 3 miles per hour or more. Once you're up to 30 minutes a day at a leisurely pace, you can focus on speed. Three miles per hour is not that fast, but it's not leisurely either. Plan out your course by driving it in your car and recording the distance. You can judge your speed by how fast you cover the distance you've plotted. At 3 mph you would walk a quarter of a mile every 5 minutes. You cover 1 mile in 20 minutes, a mile and a half in 30 minutes, 2 miles in 40 minutes, and 3 miles in 60 minutes. If you can't go that fast, do whatever you can.

Set goals for yourself and strive for improvement. Your first short-term goal may be to do 10 minutes a day for a week. Another goal would be to reach 30 minutes a day. One of your primary goals should be to strive for 30 minutes a day, 5 days a week, at 3 mph (abbreviated as 30-5-3). The 30-5-3 is a goal everyone should shoot for and maintain as a *minimum* amount of exercise.

Once you've reached the 30-5-3 goal and feel comfortable with it you may consider lengthening out the time, increasing the number of days, or increasing your speed. The Institute for Aerobics Research recommends the following:

Minimum For Moderate Fitness

Women: Walk 2 miles in 30 minutes or less 3 days a week, or walk 2 miles in 30–40 minutes 5–6 days a week.
Men: Walk 2 miles in 27 minutes or less at least 3 days a week, or walk 2 miles in 30–40 minutes 6–7 days a week.

Minimum For High Fitness

Women: Walk 2 miles in 30 minutes 5–6 days a week.
Men: Walk 2.5 miles in 38 minutes 6–7 days a week.

REBOUND EXERCISE

Rebound exercise or rebounding, as it is sometimes called, consists of jumping on a cushioned surface. Trampolining is a form of rebound exercise. You don't need a trampoline to rebound however. There are smaller versions known as mini-traps or indoor joggers. The portable type used for most rebound exercise nowadays is called a rebounder. The rebounder, rather than a trampoline, is what I would recommend for most people interested in starting an exercising program.

Rebound exercise is almost as convenient as walking. You can do it anywhere at anytime. One advantage it has over walking is that you can do it in the comfort of your home when it is scorching hot or blustery cold outside. However, you do not get the change of scenery that many walkers enjoy.

Rebounders are cheap. You can get an inexpensive model for about $30. Heavy-duty models cost as much as $300, but are worth the price. The better models are built to absorb the shock of impact and have more spring. They also last many times longer than ordinary rebounders. One model can even fold up to the size of a large briefcase and fit into a nylon case that can be carried over the shoulder.

Rebound exercise has been described as the most efficient, most effective form of exercise yet devised by man. Rebound exercise provides all the benefits of ordinary exercise plus many others unique to rebounding. Muscles are exercised and strengthen as they contract and relax, regardless of the type of exercise you do. One of the reasons rebound exercise is so good is because it works the entire body, not just the leg muscles. *All* the muscles in the body contract and relax with each bounce. This means that not only the muscles in your legs, but also the muscles in your arms, your shoulders, your back, and neck. Every single muscle in your entire body gets a workout. Standing with both feet on the mat and jumping with both feet at the same time your muscles will contract and relax about 120 times a minute—once for each bounce. After 20 minutes your muscles have contracted 2,400 times, after 30 minutes 3,600 times. That's a lot of work! If you want to increase the intensity of the exercise you either jump higher or jump while holding on to hand weights, or both.

You may be wondering: isn't jumping highly stressful and would it be safe for me? One of the remarkable advantages of rebounding is that it is one of the safest and least stressful exercises you can do. The springs and mat absorb nearly 90% of the force of impact, cushioning each bounce you make. It is so gentle on the body that it produces less trauma than walking! I've had people who couldn't walk or do any type of exercise, but they could rebound. One lady for example, had broken her foot several years earlier and it never healed properly. She couldn't walk more then 10 minutes at a time before experiencing excruciating pain. Consequently, she never participated in any type of exercise. Walking is about as gentle an exercise as you can do, but she couldn't even do that. I told her about the advantages of rebounding and she came back to me a week later and reported that she could jump on the rebounder for 20 minutes straight without pain. She was overjoyed! I had an MS patient who was so crippled by the disease that she couldn't get around without the assistance of a walker and a wheelchair. She could not walk a single step without assistance. I helped her up onto a rebounder, literally having to lift one of her legs onto the mat because she couldn't do it herself. Holding onto her arms she was able to jump using her own power and without discomfort. While she couldn't walk, she was able to jump on a rebounder. She was so thrilled because this was the only exercise she had been able to do in years. For people who have trouble standing or balancing, a stabilizing bar can be attached to the rebounder. People can hold onto that as they bounce so there is no fear of falling or losing balance.

Rebounding can be done by people of any age and almost any physical condition. With assistance, even wheelchair-bound people can benefit. In fact, rebounding has been used to reverse the effects of severe arthritis where people have lost all mobility of their legs.

The intensity of rebound exercise can vary to fit your level of fitness. It can be gentle enough for those who are physically handicapped or have severe degenerative conditions, or it can be as intense as running a record-breaking mile.

Bounces can be made by both feet at the same time or alternating legs as if you were jogging. The jogging action provides more of an aerobic workout. There are dozens of different types of jumping movements you can do to work the entire body and add variety to your workout. You can even listen to the radio, watch TV, or talk on the phone at the same time.

Another advantage of rebounding is that the effects are cumulative. You don't have to do your full workout all at one time. You can break it up into increments spread throughout the day. In fact, it is actually more beneficial to do it this way. If your total workout time is say 15 minutes, you can split it up into three 5-minute sessions or five 3-minute sessions. For people who don't have a 30-minute block of time to spare this is the exercise for them. They can do a few minutes here and a few minutes there. By the end of the day you could accumulate a full 30 minutes. You could do it while putting a load of laundry in the wash or while you're waiting for a pot of water to boil. Your whole day could be spent with short periods of rebound exercise. Having a regular schedule is best. A good time to exercise is just before breakfast, lunch, and dinner. This would help you to remember to exercise, and if you do it just before eating, it decreases your appetite so you eat less.

Thousands of people have discovered the therapeutic and weight-loss benefits of exercise simply by doing it. Dorothy Ross had arthritis in her right knee and both ankles, bursitis in her right shoulder and both hips; suffered constant back aches and headaches, and was chronically fatigued. "All this had been going on for years on end," she says. "I was constantly under a doctor's care. He told me I was just getting old and had to expect this sort of thing." Her husband Walt had severe problems too. He suffered a heart attack, was diabetic, and had gone through four cancer surgeries.

This all changed when Walt brought home a rebounder. "He was excited, but I was skeptical," she says. "For three days I watched him bounce for 30 seconds at a time. Each day he seemed brighter and had more energy. His disposition turned happy and sunny and he literally began to whistle while he worked, something I hadn't heard for a long time."

Following his example Dorothy decided to give it a try. At first she couldn't keep her balance so Walt held her hands. She began jumping twice a day. "Sure enough," she says, "I began to feel better too! In 2 weeks my blood pressure dropped 30 points! I had more stamina, and I lost 8 pounds. I began to sing while I worked—literally sing! Life took on a whole new outlook. I had hurt and been tired for so long, I had actually forgotten how it felt to feel really good—no, really great! After just two and a half months, my back aches and headaches were gone. No more arthritis or bursitis pain. The leg and foot cramps that woke me up every night disappeared. I went from a size 24 to a size 18!"

Walt lost 18 pounds, dropped his cholesterol down to normal, and lowered his heart rate 8 beats per minute. Even his eyesight improved. "The doctor says that he is now in better physical condition than any time since he has known him!"

Whether you choose rebounding, walking, swimming, or some combination of these, you will experience a change for the better. You will lose excess weight and your health will improve. The benefits of regular exercise are so well documented that no health or weight-loss program would be complete without it. All you need to do to convince yourself is to try it and see the difference it makes. Set a goal for 30 minutes a day and see how much better you look and feel. Once you see the difference you won't want to quit.

THE HEALTHY LIFESTYLE PLAN _____ ∎

NINE STEPS TO BETTER HEALTH

In this chapter I tie everything that was discussed in previous chapters together into a program which I call the Healthy Lifestyle Plan. As stated earlier, the Healthy Lifestyle Plan is designed primarily to help your body achieve its maximum potential for health. The Plan is structured to help correct metabolic problems that contribute to overweight, diabetes, hypoglycemia, and a host of other health problems. Not only will you lose excess weight, but you will also break addictions, stop food cravings, overcome health destroying habits, revitalize your metabolism, resensitize taste receptors, and accustom yourself to a new way of living and eating that will keep your weight down and greatly improve your health.

As your body becomes healthier you will lose excess fat. Health problems will diminish. You will gain more pep and vitality. You will look and feel younger and healthier.

The Healthy Lifestyle Plan is more than just a diet, it is a complete program. The diet is only one aspect of the Plan. In fact, one of the novel aspects about the Plan is that it can work with a number of different diets. You don't have to follow *one* particular dietary plan. If you believe that low-carbohydrate dieting is the way to go, then you can use this type of diet in the Healthy Lifestyle Plan. If you prefer a low-protein or vegetarian approach, that will also work. The Plan is incredibly versatile.

The Healthy Lifestyle Plan has nine steps or requirements which are:

(1) Eat a low-refined-carbohydrate diet.
(2) Eat three meals a day.

(3) Drink an adequate amount of water.

(4) Avoid nutritionally poor foods.

(5) Eat healthy foods.

(6) Use coconut oil daily.

(7) Take dietary supplements.

(8) Get regular exercise.

(9) Get daily sunshine.

It sounds very simple and it is. There is nothing difficult about this Plan. Each of these requirements is explained in detail below.

A LOW-REFINED-CARBOHYDRATE DIET

The primary feature to look for in selecting a diet is one that could be classified as a low-refined-carbohydrate diet—a diet which is low in sweets and processed grains. There are many diets from which you could choose. For your convenience, I've provided two diets that have proven to be successful with this program. One is a low-carbohydrate diet (moderately high in animal protein) and the other is a raw-foods diet (moderately low in animal protein). Each is discussed in detail in the following two chapters. Since coconut plays a central role in the Healthy Lifestyle Plan, I call them the Low-Carbohydrate Coconut Diet and the Raw-Foods Coconut Diet.

Many diets are ineffective because they allow addictions and bad habits to continue even while dieting. It makes dieting torturous and eventually doomed to failure. Sweets are your number one enemy. If you are overweight, you undoubtedly have a sweet tooth. You crave sweets, starches, or refined carbohydrates. Chips, cookies, and ice cream seem to call for you to come eat them. Artificial sweeteners, although low in calories, continue to fuel the fires of addiction to sweets and encourage cravings and overeating.

People frequently tell me they just can't give up their sweets. They can give up other foods but not sweets. They say this because they're addicted. Their sweet tooth controls their actions much like a drug addict. They've become slaves to their appetites and addictions. Giving up sweets for a time is not impossible. You will be amazed that refraining from all sweets will break these addictions. You will lose that uncontrollable urge to stick something sweet into your mouth.

I know what it's like, I used to get urges for something sweet before I changed the way I ate. Back then I often had urges for sweets. If I didn't have anything on hand I would give one of my kids some money and tell them to go buy us a couple of candy bars. I even started buying bags of candy and keeping them in my desk drawer to satisfy my sweet tooth when it would act up during the day. Once I learned how to eat right and how to break my sweet addictions, I no longer had these cravings. I had a bag of candy in my desk drawer where I worked every day and didn't touch it for over a year. I finally just threw it out because I never thought about eating it and had no desire to. This program will break you from addictions to sweets and refined carbohydrates. That is why a low-refined-carbohydrate diet is important.

There are a variety of diets around that are low in refined carbohydrate. Most of the low-carb diets that are popular now fit this description and will work. While these diets have differences, all you need to do is modify them slightly or make adjustments so that they fit the Healthy Lifestyle Plan, as described below. For example, if one recommends canola oil or margarine, use coconut oil instead. If another diet allows bread, make it whole grain bread, not white. If artificial sweeteners are permitted, just don't use them or use stevia or fruit instead. Following the Healthy Lifestyle Plan will make these other diets much more successful.

THREE MEALS A DAY

Often we get into a habit of eating without even realizing it. We eat as a response to signals in our environment rather than from hunger. Like many people, you may be in the habit of eating a mid-morning or mid-day snack whether you're hungry or not simply because the clock says 10:00 am or 3:30 pm. You may have a habit of eating while watching TV. Just the act of watching TV will create a desire to eat. For weight loss to be successful you need to break free from these fat promoting habits. The way to do that is to eat three meals a day and *only* three meals..

Eating three meals a day is important to establish good eating habits. Many people skip breakfast, but breakfast supplies us with needed energy and sets the tone for the rest of the day. Take time to eat breakfast. When you eat three meals a day you aren't famished when mealtime comes. When people skip a meal they often become so hungry that they tend to overeat at the next. In addition, skipping meals encourages snacking, which generally involves sweets or junk foods.

Eat three meals a day and *only* three meals. This is all the nutrition and energy the body needs each day. When you snack between meals you are only consuming unneeded calories and packing fat onto your body. Your body is capable of storing plenty of energy between meals to supply your needs, even if you are very physically active.

If you must snack on something because you are hypoglycemic or have some other medical problem, I recommend you limit it to a glass of vegetable juice or milk, or a piece of fresh coconut. The best choice is the coconut. Coconut meat is high in fiber and oil and low in carbohydrate. It can satisfy hunger without adding too many calories and provides a source of thermogenic, fat-burning oil. If you follow the Healthy Lifestyle Plan, symptoms of hypoglycemia will eventually lessen and in most cases can be completely overcome.

It is important to keep in mind that overeating leads to weight gain no matter what diet you use. It doesn't matter what you eat, if you consume too many calories whether they are from cabbage or from candy, you won't lose weight. During mealtime, eat until you are satisfied, but don't go overboard. Often we get into the habit of eating until we are stuffed. Cut back if you need to and eat just until your hunger is satisfied.

ADEQUATE WATER

When we get "hungry" between meals it usually isn't a signal that our bodies need food. Rather, it is a sign of thirst. We simply misinterpret it as hunger. Between meals when you feel hungry or get the urge to eat, drink a glass of water. The Healthy Lifestyle Plan requires you to drink 1 quart of water for every 50 pounds of body weight. That's a lot more water than most people drink in a day. During the summer you need to increase the amount of water you drink. If you follow this rule you will be drinking so much water that you won't feel hungry between meals.

When I recommend water, I mean *pure* water, not juices or drinks made with water. Most all beverages contain other stuff. This other stuff is usually accompanied by additional calories or some type of sweetener. Both need to be avoided. Unsweetened herbal tea is all right, but does not fulfill your water requirement.

If you do drink any beverage other than water you need to add an equal amount of water to your daily requirement. The only exception is milk or vegetable juice which you can drink along *with your meals*. Milk and vegetable juice are foods so don't drink them between meals. However, at mealtime you are free to drink as much as you like. Fresh vegetable juice contains lots of vitamins and minerals and I recommend you add it to your meals whenever possible.

If water begins to taste stale or unsatisfying to you, add a wedge or two of lemon or a little sea salt. Water often loses its appeal if your body is in need of salt. Adding more salt to your meals will also help. Dr. Batmanghelidj recommends taking a half teaspoon of salt for every 10 cups

(80 ounces) of water consumed. If you drink 3 quarts in a day that would be 12 cups. So you would need just over ¹/₂ teaspoon of salt. Don't eat it all at once, but spread it out over the day. Use it in your foods or put it in your water.

The type of salt you use is also important. I recommend sea salt or minimally processed rock salt that originally came from an ancient sea. Ordinary salt has been stripped of all trace minerals that naturally accompany it and man-made chemicals are added. It is much like the process done with wheat when they convert it to white flour, nutrients are removed and chemicals added. Ordinary table salt usually has an aluminum compound such as silicoaluminate added as an anticaking agent. It's nice for keeping the salt from becoming lumpy, but it is also toxic. The small amount used is *presumed* to be harmless. But I wouldn't want to add poison to my food regardless of the amount.

Water quality is also an issue you should consider. Municipal water supplies contain chlorine, fluorine, and numerous other chemicals, some of which are known to be carcinogenic. Since you drink lots of water on this program you can be exposed to high level of chemicals. To reduce exposure I suggest you use a water filter and drink filtered water whenever possible.

NUTRITIONALLY POOR FOODS

Our modern diet is loaded with nutrition-poor, weight-promoting, health-destroying foods. One of the biggest causes of overweight is refined carbohydrates—sugar and white flour. Foods made from these are devoid of nutrition and packed with calories. Their consumption leads to subclinical malnutrition, food cravings, continued feelings of hunger, and can be overpoweringly addictive. Artificial sweeteners are no different and carry the risk of many additional health problems.

Processed, refined vegetable oils, hydrogenated oils, margarine, and shortening supply little nutrition, rob the body of antioxidant nutrients, depress thyroid function, and cause a great deal of distress on body function. Artificial fats are even worse.

Polyunsaturated oils and oxidized fats create dangerous free radicals that contribute to degenerative disease and premature aging.

Below is a listing of all the foods you should completely avoid:

- Refined grains (white rice and white flour products)
- Refined sugars (sucrose, fructose, corn syrup, etc.)
- Artificial sweeteners
- Artificial fats (olestra, etc.)

- Partially hydrogenated vegetable oil
- Margarine
- Shortening
- Processed, refined vegetable oils (canola, corn, soybean, safflower, cottonseed, etc.)
- Processed lunch meats (hot dogs, baloney, salami, pepperoni, beef sticks, etc.)
- Powdered/dehydrated eggs and dairy (milk, cheese, and butter)
- Pasteurized, homogenized milk

This isn't a complete list of all poor quality foods. These are the biggest troublemakers: Frankenfoods—the ones that contribute the most to poor health and obesity. Get into the habit of reading ingredient labels. If an item lists any of the above, don't eat it. Generally if a food has one of more of these ingredients, it also has other things which are not good as well, such as artificial preservatives, coloring agents, and other chemical additives.

One of the hardest things for most people to do is to stop eating foods made with refined sugar and white flour. Unless you can overcome this addiction you cannot achieve success with *any* weight-loss program. In order to break additions to refined carbohydrates you need to go cold turkey just like a recovering drug addict would have to do. You need to eliminate these foods from your diet completely and let your body heal and recover. Once the addiction is overcome, that doesn't mean you are free to eat these foods with impunity. Once an addict, always an addict. If you start eating refined carbohydrates they will quickly overpower and control you just as they did before. You need to say good-buy to them forever. Once you learn to eat and enjoy natural foods, you won't miss them at all.

HEALTHY FOODS

The best foods are those that have nourished people for generations— *fresh* fruits and vegetables, whole grains, nuts, and seeds, as well as meat, fish, poultry, eggs, and dairy.

You are encouraged to eat a healthy amount of fresh raw vegetables. Most vegetables can be eaten either cooked or raw. Cruciferous family vegetables—cabbage, broccoli, cauliflower—are best cooked if you suspect you have thyroid or metabolism problems, otherwise you can eat them raw. For the same reason, soy products are discouraged. Fermented soy— tempeh, miso, and soy sauce—are okay because the antithyroid substances in them are neutralized during the fermentation process.

As noted above, pasteurized, homogenized milk is not recommended. Raw milk and dairy are preferred (see Appendix for resources). Cultured dairy, even if it has been pasteurized, is okay. Choose whole and full-fat dairy products and avoid the non- and reduced-fat varieties.

The best oils to use for cooking and food preparation are coconut oil and extra virgin olive oil. Other good choices are butter, lard, and tallow. You are encouraged to eat fat, particularly from coconut. Fat is an important part of a healthy diet. Eat the natural fats in your foods. Don't trim it off your meat. Fat gives foods flavor. The best tasting and finest choices of meat are marbled with fat. Fat helps digest your food and increases nutrient absorption, so don't be afraid of it. Enjoy the flavor. Use fat and oil liberally in cooking, frying, baking, and all your food preparation needs.

If you eat grains they should be unrefined—whole wheat and brown rice. Stores nowadays sell a variety of whole grain products such as rolls, tortillas, pasta, etc.

Natural sweeteners such as raw honey, grade B or C maple syrup, molasses, rice syrup, and sucanat (raw sugar from dried sugarcane juice) can be eaten, but *in moderation only.* You can reactivate your sweet tooth very easily with natural sources. Eating sweets should not be an everyday affair, but should be reserved for special occasions. Stevia is still your best choice.

Besides the type of food you eat, you should also be aware of the quality of your food. Our foods are processed and prepared in a variety of ways, some of which lessen their nutritional quality and add harmful contaminants.

The best foods are those that have gone through the least amount of processing. Fresh produce is preferable over frozen, and frozen is superior to canned. Buy fresh produce whenever possible and prepare meals at home. This may take more time, but this way you avoid many of the chemical food additives and incidental contaminants that often accompany prepackaged, prepared foods.

Our foods become contaminated in many different ways. Man-made chemicals of all types are routinely added to our food supply in the form of pesticides, herbicides, fungicides, growth hormones, antibiotics, and the like. While most foods only retain trace amounts of these chemicals, even trace amounts eaten every day over time can have an accumulative effect. If possible, it is best to eat foods grown or raised like they were in our great-grandparents day, without chemicals. Look for produce that are organically grown, eggs from cage-free or free-range hens, meats from animals that were raised without hormones or antibiotics, preferably grass-fed or pasture-raised. Fish should not be farm-raised but caught wild. These foods should be labeled so you can tell them apart from those that are produced conventionally. Game meats are considered organic since they were caught in the wild. Many major supermarkets are now carrying these types of foods. If your local grocery store doesn't, then try a health food store or a farmer's market.

COCONUT DAILY

Because of the satiety and metabolic effects of coconut oil, you are encouraged to eat at least 1 tablespoon of the oil at each meal. You may cook your food in it, mix it in afterwards, or take it by the spoonful like a dietary supplement. Salad dressings made with coconut oil are a good way to add it into your diet. Chapter 16 contains recipes for meals using coconut oil.

As you begin to use coconut oil you will notice one interesting characteristic. Coconut oil solidifies at temperatures below 76° F (25° C). If your kitchen is below this temperature the oil will be solid and white. Above this temperature the oil melts into a clear liquid. In liquid form you can use the oil just as you would any other vegetable oil. If solid all you need to do is warm it up. Putting the oil container in hot water for a few minutes will melt it quickly. If you're using it in cooking you don't need to melt it first, just take a knife and spoon the solidified oil out of the container. Some people keep the oil in the refrigerator, but you don't need to. Coconut oil is very stable chemically and doesn't oxidize easily like polyunsaturated oils do. You can store it in the cupboard for many months without fear of it going rancid.

If you eat a meal that doesn't involve any oil, such as fresh fruit, you need to include the oil either by taking it by the spoonful or in combination with some other food. Taking two spoonfuls at another meal does *not* satisfy the one tablespoon per meal requirement. The reason you use coconut oil is because it satisfies hunger longer and pumps up metabolism. This is particularly important for those who have a slow metabolism because skipping the oil, even for one meal, can slow down your progress.

Virgin coconut oil has a delightful flavor and is pleasant enough to eat by the spoon. Virgin coconut oil has been minimally processed so that it retains its coconut aroma and flavor. Some brands taste so good it's almost like eating coconut cream. Ordinary coconut oil has been refined and deodorized so that it has little or no taste or smell. I'm not against using refined coconut oil because it still offers many health benefits, but I do like the taste of virgin oil better. Both varieties of coconut oil are available at health food stores and by mail order from numerous dealers. You can find mail order dealers on the Internet under "coconut."

If you prefer not to take the oil straight you can mix it with other foods. Combining it with a beverage is one way. One of my favorite methods is to add virgin coconut oil to raw milk. This creates a very tasty coconut cream-like drink.

To make this drink, warm 1 cup of milk to room temperature. Mix in 1 tablespoon of melted coconut oil. Stir vigorously. The oil doesn't mix completely in the milk, so drink it immediately.

If you don't have access to raw milk, you can use $1/2$ cup of cream. Dilute with $1/2$ cup of water and drink it that way. Or you can leave out the water and add a little fruit instead. All ingredients need to be at room temperature so the oil remains liquid.

You can also add the oil to fresh vegetable juice. Stir it in vigorously and drink immediately before the oil separates. It tastes surprisingly good.

Put the oil in a fruit smoothie. Make a smoothie as you normally would and just before turning off the blender dribble in some melted coconut oil. This way the oil mixes fairly well even though the smoothie is cold. Don't add the oil before the smoothie is completely mixed or the oil will solidify forming little lumps in the drink.

Coconut oil mixes well with cottage cheese or yogurt. Combine a half cup of cottage cheese with a tablespoon of coconut oil. Mix thoroughly, pulverizing the curds. The oil will blend into the cottage cheese. Add a little pineapple and you've got a delightful treat.

It is important that you get at least 3 tablespoons of coconut oil a day in order to benefit from its metabolic stimulating and health promoting properties. This is especially important at first because most overweight people have low metabolism. *Regular* consumption coconut oil (a minimum of 3 times daily) will help boost body temperature allowing enzymes to become more active and support thyroid system function.

DIETARY SUPPLEMENTS
Vitamin and Mineral Supplements

A good multivitamin and mineral supplement is also recommended to assure adequate nutrient intake. Most people are subclinically malnourished because they live on overly processed foods that are nutrient deficient. A multivitamin is helpful, especially at first, to make up for this deficiency and overcome addictions and cravings.

VITAMINS AND MINERALS

Vitamin/Mineral	US RDA	Recommended
Vitamin A	1,000 RE	
Vitamin B1(Thiamin)	1.5 mg	
Vitamin B2 (Riboflavin)	1.7 mg	
Vitamin B3 (Niacin)	20 mg	
Vitamin B6	2.0 mg	
Vitamin B12	6 mcg	
Vitamin C	60 mg	500 mg
Vitamin D	400 IU	
Vitamin E	30 IU	400 IU
Folate	0.4 mg	
Calcium	1,200 mg	
Magnesium	400 mg	800-1,200 mg
Selenium	70 mcg	
Pantothenic acid	10 mg*	
Biotin	30 mcg*	
Chromium	50-200 mcg*	200-500 mcg
Copper	2.0 mg*	
Manganese	5.0 mg*	
Molybdenum	250 mcg*	
Zinc	15 mg	
Iodine	150 mcg	
Trace Minerals**	Trace	

*FDA estimated safe and adequate intake.
**The body requires about 60 trace minerals in minuscule quantities.

You should make sure you get at least the Recommended Dietary Allowance of the major vitamins and minerals and an adequate amount of trace minerals each day.

The vitamins and minerals listed above are just some of the basic ones you need. You can benefit with a supplement that contains others that are not listed here. There are many different brands available. Use one that supplies as many on this list as possible. Take at least the Recommended Dietary Allowance (RDA) each day. In addition, I recommend higher amounts of certain vitamins because of their antioxidant or metabolic benefits.

Trace Minerals

In order to get a wide range of trace minerals, you need to also take a liquid trace-mineral supplement. While sea salt contains many trace minerals, most people don't eat enough of it to completely satisfy their needs. The addition of a trace mineral supplement is very important. It supplies a full spectrum of trace minerals which are used to activate thousands of different enzymes in the body. Unlike the major minerals such as calcium and magnesium, you only need a very small amount of most minerals. There are about 60 trace minerals that are important to your health, such as iodine, titanium, cobalt, barium, etc. If we don't get them our health suffers. Our grandparents were able to get all the trace minerals they needed from their water and food. Today our water is processed and our foods grown in mineral depleted soils so that they are deficient in these important trace elements. Furthermore, modern food processing removes many nutrients making the situation even worse.

As with all supplements, there are many brands available. You want a *liquid* supplement because the minerals are more bioavailable in this form. The best place to find a liquid trace mineral supplement is at a health food store.

These mineral solutions by themselves taste very unpleasant. Some combine the minerals with flavors and sweeteners to make them somewhat more palatable. Take the supplement according to directions on the container. Take them once or twice a day immediately after meals. The small amount of sweetener they may contain should not be a problem if you take it at mealtime. You may also combine the minerals with ¼ to ⅓ cup of juice. Vegetable juice is preferred over fruit juice because it contains less sugar.

If you experience leg cramps at night it is a sign of a mineral deficiency. Taking a little sea salt or liquid minerals with a full glass of water will help relieve this condition.

Essential Fatty Acids

Some fats are classified as "essential" nutrients because our bodies cannot manufacture them from other nutrients in our foods. Essential fatty acids are often included in dietary supplements. There are two fatty acids that are considered as being essential, they are linoleic and alpha-linolenic. You often hear the terms omega-6 and omega-3 associated with these fatty acids. Linoleic acid is an omega-6 fatty acid. Alpha-linolenic acid is an omega-3 fatty acid.

Omega-6 fatty acids are abundant in fresh produce, nuts, seeds, grains, vegetable oils, and meats. They are so common in our foods that there is no risk of not getting enough. In fact, we actually get too much. Nearly everything you eat every day contains omega-6 fatty acids. Most processed vegetable oils are almost totally omega-6 fats.

We get omega-3 fatty acids from green leafy vegetables, nuts, grains, and fish. All seafoods contain omega-3s—fish, crab, lobster, clams, and seaweed. Grass-fed beef is also a good source of omega-3 fatty acids. Regular beef is not. Eggs also contain omega-3s. Flaxseed and cod liver oil are common supplementary sources for omega-3 fatty acids.

Our need for essential fatty acids is very small. The World Health Organization recommends that 3% of our total daily calories come from essential fatty acids. You can easily get this amount from the foods you eat. If your main dietary oil is from coconut then you need even less. A diet rich in coconut oil can enhance the efficiency of essential fatty acids by as much as 100% so that you need only half the recommended amount.

If your diet consists predominately of a variety of fresh fruits, vegetables, grains, fish, and grass-fed or free-range meats, eggs, and dairy, you don't need to worry about getting enough essential fatty acids.

REGULAR EXERCISE

Another important aspect of the Healthy Lifestyle Plan is exercise. An element that is found in all traditional societies as well as in the lifestyle of our forefathers is ample physical activity. Our ancestors were, for the most part, farmers who worked hard all their lives. The people in the longest living societies today still do physically demanding work even into old age.

Modern technology has taken away much of the need for physical labor. As a result, we have become inactive for the most part. The lack of adequate exercise contributes to a host of health problems including overweight. Regular exercise can improve or reverse many of these conditions.

Fortunately, you don't need to work as hard as a marathon runner or a bodybuilder in order to benefit from exercise. Moderate exercise can be just as good as heavy exercise in regard to health benefits. Walking is an excellent form of exercise that can be enjoyed by most anybody.

If you haven't done any exercise for years you probably should start off slowly. A 10-minute walk each day would be a good place to start. In order to benefit from exercise you need to do it at least three times a week. I recommend you exercise five to six times a week. Start by walking 10 minutes a day. That's a simple enough task. If you do it regularly it will become a habit. After a week, add 5 minutes so that you walk 15 minutes a day. In another week add another 5 minutes so you walk 20 minutes a day. Continue until you reach a *minimum* of 30 minutes a day. If you can spare the time, 60 minutes a day would be even better.

Walking is simple. You can do it most anywhere at any time. You don't need to buy any special equipment so there is little expense. While not everyone can run or lift weights, most people can walk. If you have trouble walking I highly recommend you rebound instead.

Rebound exercise is extraordinarily versatile. It can be gentle enough for someone who is handicapped, yet can be strenuous enough for a professional athlete. It all depends on the intensity and types of exercises you do.

Beware of cheap rebounders, they don't have the spring nor shock absorbing capacity of the better quality models. I don't recommend the type normally sold at sporting goods stores. They are too cheaply made and will only last a few months with regular use and perhaps only a few weeks. I bought two of these and neither one lasted more than a couple of months. The brand I personally recommend is called a ReboundAir. It is more expensive than the generic brands, but well worth the price. The bounce and feel is far superior and the materials are built to last through many years of hard use. For more information on how to obtain a ReboundAir rebounder see the Appendix.

DAILY SUNSHINE

You need to expose your skin to direct sunlight for at least 15–30 minutes every day to activate enzymes, stimulate hormone production, and improve nutrient absorption. You need to be *outdoors* in the sunlight; standing behind a window is not sufficient. When sunlight passes through glass it filters out some of the wavelengths and decreases its intensity.

Sunbathe, if you can, to expose as much of your skin as possible to the healing rays of the sun. If this is not possible, at least get sun on your arms and face. If this is all you can do, you need to stay in the sun longer to get the same amount of exposure. Sun intensity is greatest at mid-day when the sun is directly overhead. During the summer, this is the best time for sun exposure if you live at a latitude of 40° or more. At lower latitudes the sun can be very intense during this time, so you need less exposure, or you can go out in the late morning or late afternoon when the sun isn't quite as intense. During the winter, sun exposure is best at mid-day for all latitudes above 30°.*

---

*Forty degrees and greater is roughly north of Denver, Indianapolis, Philadelphia, Madrid (Spain), and Naples (Italy); 30° and greater includes most all of the United States except the southern portions of Texas and Florida.

Since you are also encouraged to exercise every day, going for a walk during the day is a good way to get both your exercise and your sunlight at the same time. If you like to jump on a rebounder, place it outdoors. This way you are accomplishing two of The Healthy Lifestyle Plan requirements at once.

Do not use any type of sunscreen or suntan lotion, and do not wear sunglasses. You want the full benefit of the sun's rays. The light needs to enter your eyes and your skin in order to activate chemical reactions that stimulate metabolism, raise body temperature, and promote health.

Some people are paranoid about going out into the sun for fear they will get skin cancer. You don't need to fear being harmed by the sun as long as you don't get sunburned. If you feel like you're starting to burn, then you've had enough. At first, you might want to limit your exposure to just 10 minutes or so and gradually increase your time under the sun as your body adapts.

If you still have some apprehension about going out into the sun, I suggest that you apply a layer of coconut oil to your exposed skin. Coconut oil has been used for ages as a natural sunscreen. The Polynesian Islanders who live in very hot, sunny climates use it every day to protect them from the sun. It is the best natural sun lotion you can use. Unlike sunscreen, which blocks the sun's rays, coconut oil doesn't appear to do that, yet it offers protection against sunburn. In the islands it is used as a medicine to treat burns and speed healing. You can use coconut oil on your skin to help prevent sunburn while still getting the benefits of full sunlight.

Coconut oil is, without question, the best hand and body lotion you could ever use. Its healing properties make skin soft and supple. I've seen it work wonders for numerous skin problems. People who have been troubled by extremely dry, rough skin have found relief within weeks after using coconut oil. Once you start using it on your skin, you won't want to use anything else.

WHAT IF YOU HAVE TROUBLE LOSING WEIGHT?
Watch What You Eat

Although many people lose weight quickly on this program, it is not designed for *quick* weight loss. It is designed for *fat* loss. There is a big difference. This program focuses on removing excess body fat, not simply reducing weight. Most all weight-loss programs lose weight by loss of water and lean muscle mass, as well as fat. I would say most weight-loss diets really lose more muscle tissue and water than fat and that's why

216

results with some weight-loss programs, at first, are so dramatic as well as unhealthy. This program is designed to take off fat while improving your health. Exercise helps keep you from losing lean muscle tissue. Drinking throughout the day prevents water loss. So the weight you lose on this plan is almost all fat. Consequently, weight loss is moderate, but more permanent. It's better to lose 2 pounds a week and keep it off than to lose 10 pounds a week and gain it all back a few months later.

We are all different and the rate at which you lose weight will be different from that of others. Some will lose weight quickly, others less so. Larger people tend to lose weight quicker than smaller people. Strict observance of the guidelines I've outlined in this chapter should work for most all people. This means no cheating. If you cheat now and then, it can keep you from overcoming addictions. Get rid of all temptations you have in your home. Remove all sugar, white flour, beverages, and anything else not allowed on the Plan. Give them to a neighbor or friend or just throw them away. Also, do not neglect getting regular exercise, wishful thinking isn't enough, you need physical activity.

Janice started the Plan using a low-carbohydrate approach and was able to lose a few pounds at first, but hit a plateau and couldn't lose any more. She was still about 40 pounds overweight and couldn't understand why she wasn't losing. I asked her if she was cheating. She said no. I asked her if she was following the Plan. She said she was. I asked her to describe what she ate during the day. For breakfast she would have a four-egg omelet with bacon or sausage. At lunch she would typically eat a cheese, cream, and vegetable casserole or something similar. For dinner she would have a couple of pork chops or a large steak and vegetables sautéed in butter. She often got hungry between meals and snacked on roasted nuts. We estimated she was consuming somewhere around 3,000 calories a day! No wonder she wasn't losing any weight.

You can't eat a ton of food and expect to lose weight. You can gain weight on any food, even broccoli, if you eat too much of it. A good example of this is found on the tiny South Pacific island of Tonga. Tonga has one of the world's highest obesity rates. Sixty-six percent of the island's population is obese. You might not suspect this because coconut in one form or another is one of their traditional foods. As you have learned in this book, coconut can help you lose weight. That's only true as long as you don't consume more calories than your body needs. The people of Tonga eat coconut, but they also eat a lot of imported foods as well. In fact, they eat huge amounts. Their diet consists of 5,500 calories a day! The average person needs around 2,000 to 2,500 a day, less than half of what the Tongans eat.

You need to pay attention to the amount of food as well as the type of food you eat. Eat until you are satisfied, not until you are stuffed. As you eat less your body will adjust and you gradually become satisfied on less food. In time it will be easier for you to eat less.

Normally, we keep eating until our stomach sends a signal to our brain telling us that it is filled and it's time to stop. This signal is slow. It takes about 20 minutes from the time we begin eating until we receive the signal to stop. If you eat fast then you can eat twice as much as a slow eater before you feel full.

One thing you can do to avoid this problem is to eat slowly. Have you ever known someone who is a slow eater? You sit down to eat a meal and when everyone else is finished this person has barely gotten started? What did this person look like? I'll bet you anything he or she was slender. Slow eaters usually don't overeat because they get the signal of fullness before they can finish their meal. In contrast, people who eat fast are often overweight. They eat so fast they can pack in an extra 500 calories before they get the signal to stop. And by all means, when you sense the feelings of fullness *stop eating!* Sometimes we enjoy the food so much we keep on eating even though we know we are full and will probably feel gorged for the next 2 hours.

Another way to help keep you from eating too much is to wait at least five or 10 minutes before taking seconds. When you wait like this it gives the stomach time to signal the brain. Have you ever been interrupted in the middle of a meal to answer the phone or the door and came back several minutes later and decided you weren't hungry any longer? This is because your stomach was already full before the interruption. Taking time out allows the signal to reach your brain. If you had continued to sit and eat you would have consumed more calories than your body needed.

Pay attention to the amount of water you drink during the day. Make sure you are drinking at least 1 quart of water for every 50 pounds of body weight. One of the problems with Janice, described above, was that she wasn't drinking enough water, which caused her to snack between meals. Many people think they can mentally gauge the amount of water they need. Unfortunately, 90% of them are wrong. Most of us underestimate the amount of water we drink. That is why I recommend you to set up a system where you can accurately measure the exact amount of water you consume each day. Between meals if you get hungry it means you are not drinking enough water. So drink more often. This would significantly cut down on the calories Janice consumed. Keep in mind that if your climate is hot or dry or if you exercise heavily you need to increase the amount of water you drink, up to 1.25–1.5 quarts per 50 pounds of body weight.

Another way to help keep you from overeating is to drink a full glass of water, milk, or vegetable juice about 10 to 15 minutes before sitting down to eat a meal. The fluids help to fill the stomach and intestines which begins sending signals of satiety. When you eat you will get the feeling of being full quicker.

The reason we feel full after eating is due to an appetite suppressing hormone that is released by the intestines. As the amount of this hormone increases in our bloodstream, hunger declines. Scientists seeking new ways to curb hunger have reasoned that if they could isolate this hormone it could be used as a weight-loss drug. This idea was recently tested and reported in the journal *Nature*. Researchers at Imperial College in London enlisted the aid of 24 volunteers. Half of the volunteers were injected with the hormone and half with a placebo. Two hours later the volunteers were allowed access to a buffet where they could eat all they wanted. Those who received the appetite suppressing hormone ate 36% less food than those who received the placebo. This study showed the drug had potential.

The drug is still in the developmental stages, however, so it will be years before it is available for general use. One drawback to this drug is that it must be administered by injection. The appetite suppressing hormone is a protein, and as such is completely digested when it enters the stomach. So it cannot be administered orally. In a few years we may see overweight people carrying around syringes so that they can inject themselves with this drug before eating.

A much easier way to reduce your appetite is to let the body do it naturally. You can take advantage of your own appetite suppressing hormones by following the recommendations listed above: eat slower; refrain from eating for 5–10 minutes before taking seconds; consume water, tea, or soup a few minutes before eating a meal; and eat only until you are satisfied, not until you are stuffed.

Keep Your Metabolism Up

The body always seeks a balance. If you consume 2,200 calories in your food and expend 2,200 calories in physical activity, your weight will remain constant. The amount of calories going into your body equals the amount of calories going out. If you drop your calorie consumption to 2,000 but continue to burn off 2,200 calories a day, your body will need to get 200 of those calories from stored fat. Consequently, you lose weight.

Let's look at an example, ignoring metabolic fluctuations for the moment. Suppose your weight is stable at 200 pounds on a diet consisting of 2,200 calories. This means you eat and burn 2,200 a day. You are in balance. If you dropped your calorie consumption down to 2,000 calories, but you continued to burn 2,200 calories, you would gradually lose weight. Let's say you drop down to 140 pounds on a 2,000 calorie diet. You can then resume eating 2,200 like you did before. Since you burn 2,200 calories a day, you will maintain your new weight of 140 pounds.

A conscious effort to reduce calorie consumption will allow you to lose weight. As long as you don't consume more than 2,200 calories a day, you will stay at 140 pounds. You can lose more simply by restricting the amount of calories you eat. This way you can lose weight and keep it off permanently.

Susan was following a low-carbohydrate diet and lost 15 pounds in the first 5 weeks. She was thrilled because it didn't seem like a diet to her. It took her another 2 weeks to lose the next pound and then her progress stalled. She had to make a focused effort to reduce her calorie intake to rid herself of that last pound and to keep off what she had already lost. She was still about 35 pounds overweight.

I asked her if she was following the diet. She said she was. I asked her if she was eating any coconut and using coconut oil. "Sometimes," she said. She mostly used bacon grease or butter in her cooking. That was her first mistake.

I then asked her if she was exercising every day. She said, "no." That was her second mistake.

The problem is that normally, when people reduce the amount of calories they consume, their metabolism slows down. When this happens they don't burn as many calories as they did before they started the diet. This makes losing weight much more difficult. And when you get off the diet and resume eating 2,200 calories, your metabolism has slowed so much that you may only burn 2,000 calories a day. You will gain back the weight you lost.

The Healthy Lifestyle Plan has the answer to that problem. You are encouraged to eat coconut oil every day to stimulate your metabolism, so it does not fall. Protein also has a metabolic stimulating effect. Exercise is very important for the same reason. It has the added benefit of increasing the amount of calories you consume so that you lose weight quicker. This makes exercise an essential part of any weight-loss program.

When you eat adequate protein, add coconut oil wherever possible, and exercise regularly, your metabolism remains stable even when your calorie consumption decreases. This way, when you reduce your calorie intake you lose weight. And when you begin eating more carbohydrate-rich foods you don't gain it all back, plus some. Weight loss is permanent. Getting regular exercise and eating coconut oil are important elements in this Plan, so don't leave them out!

You should be exercising at least 30 minutes a day, preferably 5 to 6 days a week. Keep in mind that 30 minutes is a minimum. Your success at losing body fat can improve if you exercise for longer periods of time. If you have difficulty losing weight I suggest gradually increasing your exercise time to 60 minutes or more a day.

From the evidence I've seen, some people who have an underactive thyroid system problem can reactivate their metabolism by taking coconut oil at least three times a day—without fail. The oil helps to keep metabolism slightly elevated during the day so that enzymes function more normally. This can have a positive effect on all body systems as well as encourage weight loss.

You Will Have Success

You should continue to do the things I recommend in this chapter for the rest of your life. That is why I call this program a Healthy *Lifestyle* Plan. You make it a permanent part of your life. If you do this you will have a trim waistline, a spring in your step, a smile on your face, and a positive outlook on life. You will be free from many of the degenerative health problems that often plague people in our society.

If you follow the Healthy Lifestyle Plan as I've explained it, I know it will improve your life. I would like to invite you to write to me and tell me how the Healthy Lifestyle Plan has helped you. You can write to me at HealthWise Publications, P.O. Box 25203, Colorado Springs, CO 80936. For more information on diet and health write and ask for a free copy of the HealthWise Newsletter.

Chapter 14

LOW-CARBOHYDRATE COCONUT DIET ▬

In many ways the Low-Carbohydrate Coconut Diet described in this chapter is similar to other low-carb diets. The biggest difference is the use of coconut oil and the exclusion of all refined or processesed vegetable oils.

There are three phases in the Low-Carb Coconut Diet. Each phase consists of slightly different foods. The first phase is designed to help you lose excess weight, to help your body overcome addictions to sugar and refined carbohydrates, to restore sensitivity to taste (particularly to sweets), and to begin the process of restoring good health. The second phase is designed to continue what was started in Phase I and to serve as a transition to the final phase. The first two phases are designed to help your body overcome weight and health problems and establish good habits. Both are temporary diets used as stepping-stones to the final or maintenance phase of the Low-Carb Coconut Diet. Phase III is patterned after the diet of our forefathers—the diet that has nourished and protected our ancestors from modern degenerative diseases for thousands of years. It provides complete, balanced nutrition for maintaining optimal health. It's a diet you could maintain for life. Because it includes a wide variety of foods, it is a diet that can be eaten with enjoyment for a lifetime.

PHASE I

The foods in this diet are rich and tasty so you don't miss the sweets as much. Unlike a low-fat, rabbit food diet where all you can eat are salad greens, with this diet you get to eat a variety of delicious food—roast, steak, bacon, sausage, eggs, gravy, cream, and cheese.

One aspect of Phase I, in fact of all three phases of the diet, is that there is no restriction on the amount of fat you can eat. This is not a low-fat diet. You are encouraged to eat fat. Fat is an important part of a healthy diet. Eat the natural fats in your foods. Don't be afraid of them. Enjoy the flavor. Use fat and oil liberally in cooking, frying, baking, and all your food preparation needs.

In the first phase of the Low-Carb Coconut Diet your primary foods are meat, fish, fowl, eggs, butter, cream, vegetables, and select fruits, nuts, and oils. You are encouraged to eat a healthy amount of vegetables, both raw and cooked. Eat plenty of raw green salads. I encourage you to eat one salad a day. For example, a chef's salad for lunch or a small dinner salad with your evening meal. It's important that you don't eat just meat, eggs, and cream. Such foods do not supply all essential vitamins and minerals for optimal health. You need vegetables too.

While grains and flour in general aren't allowed in this phase of the Diet, wheat bran is. Wheat bran is a good source of fiber that's low in effective carbohydrate and helps clean out bowels and keep the intestines working smoothly. Bran can be used as a thickener in sauces, gravies, and casseroles. Because bran provides many benefits to health I recommend adding a bit to your meals wherever you can.

The primary restrictions in Phase I are high-carbohydrate foods such as sugars, grains, and most legumes and fruits. Both simple and complex carbohydrate foods are restricted. That means all sugar and white flour products as well as whole wheat bread, legumes, potatoes, and other starchy vegetables and fruits. Although some of these foods provide lots of good fiber and nutrition, when you are suffering from carbohydrate addiction, even a small amount can slow down progress. While complex carbohydrates are normally good and nutritious foods, you need to keep away from high-carbohydrate foods at this time.

The only grain products you are allowed are wheat bran and gluten. Bran is rich in health promoting fiber and can help to regulate blood sugar by slowing down the absorption of carbohydrate. Gluten is wheat protein and not carbohydrate. It is useful in that it can be used in certain recipes in place of flour. A couple of tablespoons of whole wheat flour is permitted to thicken gravies or casseroles.

Like any treatment or recovery program, Phase I is designed as a temporary measure to correct health problems. It is not meant to be a permanent diet for the rest of your life. Its purpose is to break addictions, revitalize metabolism, resensitize taste receptors, and lose unwanted weight. It is a restorative diet. It limits dietary choices and restricts many good foods rich in vitamins and minerals.

I equate it to a diet you would give someone who is ill. For example, if you had the flu and were nauseous and vomiting, you would not want to eat solid foods, even if the foods were very nutritious and otherwise health promoting. You would need to drink plenty of fluids and eat soups and broths until you felt better and your stomach could keep solids down. Although a liquid diet would help you recover from the flu and keep you from becoming dehydrated, you would not want to eat a liquid diet all your life. Once you regained your health you would resume eating solid foods which would provide you with complete, balanced nutrition. The same holds true with this diet. Phase I is a temporary diet.

Once your body is on its way to recovery you can then move on to the next phase of the Low-Carb Coconut Diet. I recommend that everyone start with Phase I. Remain on this portion of the Diet for at least *3 weeks*. If you have a lot of weight to lose or you still have cravings for sweets, you might remain at this phase for 2 to 4 months.

One of the primary purposes of Phase I is to break addictions to sweets. You can tell when it's time to move to the next phase when you have lost all cravings for sweets and refined carbohydrates (e.g., candy, ice cream, donuts, cookies, chips, soft drinks). This doesn't mean you aren't tempted by them, but you don't dream of eating these foods or have desires to eat them when nobody's looking. When you can resist eating a tempting treat when no one is around then you're on the road to conquering food addictions.

Unless you are obese and need to lose a lot of weight, I recommend you move on to Phase II after about 3 or 4 months, even if you still have cravings. Phase II will continue to help you to lose weight and fight sugar cravings while allowing you a wider selection of foods.

PHASE II

Phase II is designed to continue the progress made in Phase I and to assist the body in cleansing and rebuilding. This diet is a little more lenient than the first phase and accomplishes much of the same. You can maintain this diet indefinitely if you had to. But generally, I recommend you eventually work up to Phase III.

Everything that was allowed in Phase I is included here. You have a slightly wider selection of foods with the addition of fruits, nuts and seeds, and most legumes. The addition of new foods slightly increases the amount of carbohydrate you may eat, but it is still a low-carbohydrate diet. All grains and starchy fruits and vegetables are restricted. Starchy fruits include: banana, mango, and papaya. Starchy vegetables are potatoes, sweet potatoes, and yams. All dried fruits are restricted because drying concentrates the sugars into a smaller volume of food.

Phase II allows two sweeteners—fresh fruit and stevia extract. If you want to sweeten up a dish, add fruit or stevia or both. There is no limit on the amount of stevia you are allowed to use. It has essentially no calories. Fruit is limited to one piece or one cup serving per meal. Some beverages other than water and herbal tea are allowed. Stevia can be used to sweeten these beverages.

If while you are on this phase of the diet you begin to gain weight, back up and resume Phase I or cut down on the amount of food you may be eating. Make sure you aren't cheating and that you are following the plan as it's given. If you start to make a few allowances here and there you are just sabotaging your success.

If your weight has dropped to within your target range, you no longer have urges for sweets, and food cravings have gone, then you are ready to move on to the next phase. If not, stay at this phase until you are ready. It may take several months, a year, or more to accomplish this. Keep in mind that it took you years to get to the state you are presently in, it will take some time to get you out.

PHASE III

Phase III is a maintenance diet. As the name implies, it is meant to maintain the progress you've made with the first two phases of the Low-Carb Coconut Diet. You can eat everything in the first two phases of the Diet as well as all other fruits and vegetables, including the starchy varieties. Whole grains and beans of all types are permitted. In fact, I recommend you cut down on your meat consumption and add some whole grains. The only restrictions that remain are primarily white flour products, white rice, and other processed grains, as well as refined sugars, artificial sweeteners, and processed vegetable oils.

Even though you are allowed more foods, you can still lose excess weight at this level, but it will be slower. This is actually the healthiest phase of the diet because it allows the greatest volume and range of nutrients along with adequate fiber necessary for optimal health. It is basically the diet of our forefathers—the diet that our great-grandparents and their parents ate, when obesity, heart disease, diabetes, and cancer were rare. It is a diet that incorporates the essential elements of the traditional diets around the world where people live to be 100 years old without suffering from obesity or crippling degenerative disease.

Now that you've lost excess body weight and your taste receptors have become resensitized you can eat carbohydrate-rich foods again, so long as you avoid the real troublemakers—refined grains and sugars. Natural sweeteners, such as honey, are allowed. Eat only whole grain products—whole wheat bread, brown rice, oats, etc. Whole grains and beans are the richest sources of health promoting fiber. Most fruits and vegetables are only modest sources of fiber. They are 85-95% water and supply on average only 1–4 grams of fiber per serving. Beans, on the other hand, contain much less water and provide 10–20 grams of fiber per serving.

If you find that you are gaining weight you should cut down on your calorie consumption or your carbohydrates. Are you eating too many sweets? This is most often the cause. You may want to go back to Phase I or II for a while.

The third phase of the Low-Carb Coconut Diet is one you can remain on for life. It allows a wide variety of wholesome meats, vegetables, fruits, dairy, oils, and sweeteners that you can use to make an endless array of delicious, healthy meals. Because the foods are rich in protein, fiber, and fat, they satisfy and fill the stomach helping to ward off pangs of hunger and addictive cravings. You need not eat coconut oil at every meal, but use it as your primary dietary oil.

BASIC FOOD CHOICES

I have tried to make the diets in the Low-Carb Coconut Diet easy to use and follow by not burdening you with weights and measures and needless restrictions. I've included very few limits on portion sizes. For the most part, you are allowed to eat all you want of the foods within your particular phase. But you can't eat like a pig and expect to lose weight. Eat until you are satisfied, not until you are stuffed.

Foods allowed under each phase of the Diet are shown on the following lists. Under each main heading, such as "Meat, Fish, Eggs" or "Vegetables" I have four subheadings "Phase I", "Phase II", "Phase III", and "Restricted." If you are on Phase I, eat only those foods listed under that heading. If you are on Phase II eat only those food under that heading and the Phase I heading. For Phase III you can eat anything under all three programs. The last heading lists restricted foods. These foods should be avoided completely, as much as possible. They are restricted because they promote weight gain, nutrient deficiency, and poor health. While eating restricted foods once in a blue moon won't do much harm, the problem is that if you eat a little here and there, you will gradually eat more and more until you become addicted to them again, become a slave to your food, and slide down the path to obesity and poor health. Even people who have strong willpower have a difficult time restraining themselves if they allow themselves to "cheat" once in awhile. Therefore, it is wise to avoid these foods as much as possible.

MEAT, FISH, EGGS
Phase I

Beef	Chicken	Lamb
Pork	Turkey	Game meats
Fish	Shellfish	Eggs

Phase II
Same

Phase III
Same

Restricted
Lunch and hard meats (with nitrites, sugar, flavorings, preservatives, and other additives)
Dehydrated eggs

Virtually all types of meat, fish, and eggs are allowed. The only restrictions are preserved meats with added sugar, MSG, nitrites, and other chemicals. Fresh or frozen meats are best but canned meats can be used sparingly. Canned fish should be packed in water or olive oil and not soybean or any other vegetable oil. Avoid dehydrated eggs and any product that contains them. Dehydration oxidizes the fat and cholesterol in the eggs making them dangerous for the heart and arteries. Do not overcook meat. It is best if only cooked to medium-rare, never burnt or blackened.

VEGETABLES
Phase I

Artichokes	Asparagus	Bamboo shoots
Beets and beet greens	Bok choy	Broccoli
Brussels sprouts	Chili peppers	Cabbage
Chinese cabbage	Carrots	Cauliflower
Celery	Chard	Collards
Cucumbers	Cauliflower	Eggplant

Endive	Garlic	Jerusalem artichoke
Jicama	Kale	Kohlrabi
Leeks	Lettuce (all types)	Mushrooms
Mustard greens	Okra	Olives
Onions	Parsley	Parsnips
Peppers (sweet and hot)	Pickles	Radishes
Rutabaga	Sauerkraut	Seaweed
Shallots	Spinach	Sprouts (all varieties)
Summer squash	Tomatoes	Turnips/turnip greens
Water chestnuts	Watercress	

Phase II
Same

Phase III
Potatoes
Yams and sweet potatoes
Winter squash

Restricted
None

There are a wide variety of vegetables to choose from. All vegetables are good and nutritious and you should have plenty of them in your diet. With the exception of the starchy vegetables (winter squash and potatoes), a weight-loss diet should include plenty. Starchy vegetables such as winter squash, potatoes, and yams should be eaten in moderation and always with fats, such as butter and cream along with a variety of other foods to slow down and moderate the digestion and absorption of carbohydrate. Vegetable juices are also good and can be eaten along with meals.

LEGUMES
Phase I
Green beans	Wax beans	Bean sprouts
Snow peas	Green peas	Tempeh

Phase II
Dried beans (kidney, garbanzo, pinto, black beans, black-eyed peas, etc.)
Lentils	Lima beans	Split peas

Phase III
Same

Restricted
Soybeans and tofu

Most legumes are high in starch. Fortunately, they are also very high in fiber and fairly good sources of protein as well. Fiber helps to slow down the digestion of the starch. But because they are generally high in starch they are limited in the first phase of the diet.

Soybeans and soybean products, like tofu and soy milk, contain substances that slow down metabolism so they are not desirable foods for those who are interested in weight loss. The antithyroid chemicals in soy are neutralized during fermentation. So fermented soy products are okay. These include tempeh, soy sauce, and miso. All other soy products should be avoided.

FRUIT
Phase I

Avocado	Grapefruit
Lemon	Lime

Phase II
(Limit to one piece or 1 cup serving per meal and eat with other foods.)

Apple	Apricots	Blackberries
Blueberries	Boysenberries	Cantaloupe
Cherries	Cranberries	Elderberries
Figs	Gooseberries	Grapes
Guava	Kiwi	Kumquat
Melons	Nectarine	Orange
Passion fruit	Peach	Pear
Persimmon	Pineapple	Plum
Raspberries	Strawberries	Tangerine

Phase III
(These sweet and starchy fruits should be eaten in moderation. Dried fruits are especially high in sugar.)

Banana	Mango	Papaya
Dates	Dried fruits (raisins, prunes, fruit leather)	

Restricted
None

Fruits are limited to one piece or 1 cup serving per meal because of their high sugar content. One piece means 1 small whole fruit like an apricot or plum. Very small fruits like berries and large fruits like melons should be limited to 1 cup. A limit is placed on fruit because eating too much can keep sugar cravings alive. Eat fruit with other foods to slow down the digestion of sugars.

In Phase III there is no restriction on the amount of fruit you can eat each day, however, dried fruits, which are rich in sugar, should be eaten in moderation.

DAIRY AND DAIRY SUBSTITUTES
Phase I

Butter	Heavy cream	Sour cream
Raw whole milk	Goat milk	Hard cheese
Soft cheese	Cottage cheese	Cream cheese
Coconut milk	Yogurt (unsweetened)	

Phase II
Same

Phase III
Same

Restricted

Ice cream	Eggnog	Frozen yogurt
Chocolate milk	Artificial creamers	Soy milk

Pasteurized/homogenized milk
Dehydrated dairy products (milk, butter, cheese, cream)
Non-fat and low-fat dairy products

Avoid pasteurized and homogenized milk. Use fresh raw milk if it is available in your area. If not, use diluted cream or coconut milk in recipes that call for milk. Avoid all non-fat or low-fat dairy products. Fat is necessary for complete nutrient absorption and satiety.

Low-fat and reduced-fat milks, cream, and other dairy products often have powdered milk added. You don't want to eat anything with powdered milk because it contains oxidized (rancid) cholesterol. Oxidized cholesterol damages the arteries. All powdered milks, even non-fat powdered milk contain some oxidized cholesterol. You should avoid any dehydrated dairy products for the same reason. Many packaged foods contain dried dairy products. Look on the ingredient labels for dehydrated or powdered butter, cream, milk, cheese, etc. Dried, grated cheese such as Parmesan and Romano should be avoided. Use them only if you can get them fresh and ungrated like other cheeses.

GRAINS AND BREAD
Phase I
Wheat bran   Wheat gluten

Phase II
Same

Phase III

Amaranth	Barley	Brown rice
Buckwheat (kashi)	Cereals*	Corn
Millet	Oat	Quinoa
Spelt	Whole wheat	

Restricted
Products made with white flour, polished rice, and other processed grains

Grains are restricted at first because of their high carbohydrate content. Wheat bran is allowed, and encouraged, in all phases of the Low-Carb Coconut Diet. Bran is composed primarily of indigestible fiber and is also relatively high in protein. If you have difficulty with bowel eliminations bran can help move things along. Many people who eat a great deal of meat and dairy and not enough grains and vegetables often become constipated. Bran can help relieve this problem.

The use of bran is recommended in all three phases of the Diet because it provides a good source of fiber for healthy bowel function as well as many other benefits. Bran can be added to soups, casseroles, and eggs without affecting the flavor. It makes a mild thickener for soups and chili. If bran causes abdominal discomfort it means you are not drinking enough water. Water softens the fiber and allows it to move through your digestive system without problem.

---

*Whole grain cereals without added sugar.

Wheat gluten is allowed in all three phases of the Diet. Gluten is protein from grains. It is not a carbohydrate. It is useful for making some of the low-carbohydrate foods described in the recipe chapter.

A small amount of whole wheat flour is permitted to thicken sauces and gravies.

Corn and products made with it are allowed in Phase III. Avoid chips and tortillas cooked in vegetable oil. You can cook tortillas yourself in coconut oil or lard, or bake them without oil. Tortillas cooked in saturated oils or baked without oil make great chips, just add a little salt.

BEVERAGES
Phase I
Water
Lemon water
Herbal teas (no sugar added)

Phase II
Coffee substitutes (ROMA, Postum)
Cocoa (without added sugar)

Phase III
Fresh vegetable juices
Fresh fruit juice (in moderation)

Restricted

Soft drinks	Sweetened fruit juices	Powdered drink mixes
Coffee	Black tea	Alcohol

You need to drink 1 quart of water for every 50 pounds of body weight. Between meals drink as much as you can. This will keep the body hydrated and help prevent hunger. It will also help keep you from eating snack foods which only add calories and pounds.

In Phase I of this eating plan drink only water. You may add a wedge or two of lemon to the water for added flavor. Herbal teas are okay to use occasionally. Many of them have a diuretic effect which promotes dehydration and hunger.

Coffee and tea are not recommended because they are addictive and provide no nutritional benefit. They are a source of added calories especially when sweeteners are used. The caffeine has a dehydrating effect that can stimulate "feelings" of hunger which encourages eating.

NUTS AND SEEDS
Phase I

Almond	Coconut	Macadamia
Pecans	Sesame seed	Peanuts

Phase II

Pumpkin seed	Sunflower seed	Filberts
Cashews	Pine nuts	Pistachios
Walnuts		

Phase III
Same

Restricted
None

Nuts should be dry roasted without added oils or sugar. Limit consumption to about 1/3 cup per day. There is no limit on the amount of coconut you can eat. Fresh coconut makes an excellent snack food. Nut butters such as peanut butter are okay so long as they do not contain sugar or hydrogenated oil.

FATS AND OILS
Phase I
Coconut oil
Palm/palm kernel oil
Olive oil
Butter
Ghee
Animal fat (lard, beef tallow)

Phase II
Same

Phase III
Same

Restricted
Vegetable oils (corn, safflower, sunflower, cottonseed, soybean, canola)
Margarine and shortening

Partially hydrogenated oils (any and all products that contain these oils)

Because of its thermogenic effect and its many health benefits you should use coconut oil whenever possible in your cooking and food preparation. Use olive oil, butter, and animal fat when you want to add their flavors to your foods.

Avoid all margarine, shortening, and partially hydrogenated vegetable oils and foods that contain them. Most packaged, convenience foods nowadays contain partially hydrogenated vegetable oils. Read the labels.

CONDIMENTS
Phase I
Fresh herbs and spices
Salt (sea salt, unrefined)
Herbal seasonings
Salt substitutes (Spike, Mrs. Dash, etc.)
Soy sauce, miso
Worcestershire sauce
Coconut mayonnaise (see recipe in Chapter 16)
Olive oil-based salad dressings (without added sugar, preservatives, or chemical additives)
Vinegar
Mustard
Horseradish
Dill pickle relish
Low sugar ketchup

Phase II
Same

Phase III
Same

Restricted
Mayonnaise (and other vegetable oil-based condiments)
Ketchup, barbecue sauce, and other highly sweetened condiments

This is not a complete listing of all possible condiments. Most condiments are allowed even if they contain restricted ingredients if used in moderation only. There are a couple of exceptions. Ketchup is not

234

allowed because it is loaded with sugar and some people use a lot of it. Use low sugar ketchup or make your own.

Polyunsaturated oil-based dressings are not allowed because of the large amount of oil in these products. Use olive oil-, vinegar-, or cream-based dressings. Vinegar is an excellent food and there are many different types and flavorings. Vinegar alone makes a superb salad dressing.

If you want to add something crispy to your salads or as a topping to casseroles and vegetables try pork rinds. Pork rinds are made by removing the fat from pig skin. What's left is the protein matrix of the skin.

SWEETENERS
Phase I
None

Phase II
Stevia
Fresh fruit

Phase III
Honey (raw)
Rice syrup
Maple syrup (grade C or B only)
Sucanat (raw sugar from sugarcane)
Maple sugar
Molasses
Apple butter (no sugar added)
Fruit spread (100% fruit, no jam or preserves with sugar of any type)

Restricted
Processed sugar (sucrose, fructose, dextrose, corn syrup, brown sugar, etc.)
Artificial sweeteners (Nutrasweet, saccharine, sorbitol, mannitol, etc.)
Highly processed natural sweeteners such as honey and grade A maple syrup

Stevia is the only sweetener that is nonaddicting. It should be your first choice. Limited amounts of natural sweeteners are permitted, but you must be careful. I've seen people go overboard on the natural sweeteners and end up addicted and packing on weight.

SAMPLE MEALS

A typical breakfast in Phase I would be a bacon and cheese omelet. For lunch a hearty chef's salad topped with hard boiled eggs, turkey, and cheese. Dinner would be a pork chop or a steak along with a side dish of steamed broccoli with cheese and asparagus topped with butter.

When you look at the foods you are able to eat in this program you may think dieting never looked so good. With a little ingenuity you can make meals a pleasant experience. Below are a few examples of the types of meals you can make and enjoy even on the most restrictive phase of the Low-Carb Coconut Diet.

Breakfast

Ham and eggs
Cheese omelet
Vegetable omelet
Scrambled eggs with sausage and zucchini
Bran muffins

Lunch

Beef stew
Chunky chicken soup
Minestrone
Beef and vegetable chili
Clam chowder

Dinner

Roast chicken with roasted vegetables
Chicken fried steak with sautéed vegetables
Chicken stir-fry with vegetables
Roast beef and gravy with vegetable medley
Broiled salmon with artichoke and tossed salad
Cheesy zucchini casserole

GENERAL SUGGESTIONS
Meats

Meat, poultry, and fish can be baked, broiled, barbecued, roasted, and fried or used as an ingredient in soups and casseroles. In the first two phases of the Healthy Eating Plan meats generally take center stage. Unless you are trying to maintain a vegetarian diet, meat of one type or another is the star of most of your meals.

236

Eggs

Eggs are traditionally eaten for breakfast, but they can make great meals for lunch and dinner as well. Eggs provide a complete protein and wide variety of nutrients. You can eat them poached, boiled, scrambled, fried, and baked in a variety of ways. They make an excellent base for meat and vegetable soufflés, omelets, and quiches.

A typical breakfast can consist of eggs cooked any way you like accompanied by breakfast meats—bacon, ham, or sausage. Combining vegetables such as mushrooms, onions, zucchini, sour cream, and the like can give omelets variety so that every day brings something different.

Dairy

Cheese and cream add zest and taste to many meals. Cheese and cream liven up any vegetable dish. Cheese adds spark to eggs. Delicious rich, creamy soups and chowders can be made with heavy cream or coconut milk. Examples include clam chowder, oyster stew, and cheesy vegetable chowder.

Vegetables

Most meals should have a couple of hearty servings of vegetables. Vegetables are packed with vital nutrients that help to keep us healthy and protect us from disease. One of the reasons most people are subclinically malnourished is because they don't eat enough of them. Vegetables are necessary to round out the protein-rich foods on the diet and supply the necessary nutrients these foods lack.

Sautéed or stir-fried vegetables make a great complement to meats. Frying them in fat or meat drippings adds a wonderful flavor. Vegetables can be grilled or broiled, steamed, and roasted. When you roast meat in the oven throw in a variety of vegetables along with it and let them cook and absorb the flavor of the meat juices. Any vegetable, especially lightly steamed vegetables, taste great under a layer of melted cheese. Add cheese to broccoli, cauliflower, brussels sprouts, zucchini, etc.

Don't use just salt, pepper, and butter on your vegetables, experiment with cheese sauces, toasted nuts, spices, soy sauce, and other condiments for variety.

The hardest transition most people make in using vegetables is eliminating potatoes. Potatoes aren't allowed except in Phase III. Potatoes are most everyone's favorite vegetable and many recipes call for them. Cauliflower can take on a reasonable resemblance to potatoes in many recipes. You can use most of these recipes by substituting cauliflower for potatoes. Use cauliflower in soups and casseroles instead of potatoes. For example, instead of mashed potatoes, have mashed cauliflower and gravy. Use cauliflower in place of potatoes in recipes for potato salad, au gratin potatoes, and the like.

Hearty meat and vegetable soups and stews make delightful meals which are good for lunch or dinner. A thick beef soup with plenty of chunky vegetables is a meal all in itself.

Grains

Eat only whole grain products. Although grains are restricted in the first two phases, grains provide many important nutrients and are an essential part to any long-term nutritional program. The important thing to remember is to stay completely away from refined flour and all products made with it.

When purchasing whole wheat bread look for the term "whole wheat" and not just "wheat." Commercially made wheat bread is mostly white flour with a little whole wheat added along with molasses to make it brown so it looks like whole wheat. Avoid all bread that contains white flour or, as they often label it, "wheat flour." The terms are confusing to customers and manufacturers do this on purpose to make buyers think they're getting whole wheat when in fact they are not. You can be sure that wheat flour really is "white flour" when it says *enriched* wheat flour. Enriched means that the manufacturer added some vitamins because it is white processed wheat flour. To be sure you're getting 100% whole wheat, look for the words "whole wheat" on the ingredient label.

Bread is not the only bakery item that is made with 100% whole wheat flour. Health food bakeries make a variety of whole grain products including rolls, tortillas, pocket bread, hamburger buns, etc. Just about any style of bread or wheat product you find in the grocery store has a whole grain equivalent. There are also a variety of breads and bakery items made with spelt, rye, oats, and other grains. You can even get whole grain pasta. There is whole wheat, brown rice, corn, and spelt pastas. They all taste remarkably similar to regular white flour pasta we ordinarily see in the grocery store. Not all stores carry whole grain products. The best place to look for them is in a health food store.

Wheat bran can be added to many dishes to increase their fiber content. Bran can be used to thicken stews and casseroles. I recommend that you add bran in your meals wherever you can so that you can enjoy the many health benefits it offers. You are allowed to use a few tablespoons of whole wheat flour along with bran to thicken gravies and sauces on any of the diets. A tablespoon of whole wheat flour in a meal isn't going to have a negative effect.

238

When using bran as a thickener, you don't need to mix it with water before adding it to a hot mixture like you do flour or corn starch. You can add the bran directly to the hot mixture and stir it in. As it cooks it absorbs the liquid, thickening the dish. Bran has little taste so it does not affect the flavor of the food you add it to. It can easily be added to omelets, scrambled eggs, and other egg dishes as well as soups and casseroles. It does not thicken as much as flour and is not the best for gravies, but is good in stews, chili, and things like that. Use bran instead of flour as a coating when making fried chicken or chicken fried steak.

Several recipes in this book use wheat gluten. Gluten is the natural protein in wheat. It is basically wheat flour with the starch removed. It is used by the baking industry to produce lighter, better tasting breads. Because it is primarily a protein it can be freely used in any of the diets. You can make delicious, wheat-free, low-carbohydrate muffins using gluten and bran in place of wheat flour (see the All Bran muffin recipes). You can find wheat gluten at most health food stores and many grocery stores.

Fats and Oils

Use coconut oil in cooking and food preparation as much as possible. Butter, olive oil, and meat fat may also be used and adds a wonderful flavor to vegetables and casseroles. Because coconut oil hardens at temperatures below 76° F (25° C) it doesn't make the best salad oil, although many people do use it for that purpose. Olive oil is best for oil-based dressings. Both olive oil and coconut oil can be used to make mayonnaise. Olive oil can give mayonnaise a rather strong flavor which isn't agreeable to everyone. Coconut oil, however, can produce a more mild flavored mayonnaise that can be used for any recipe that calls for it.

FINAL NOTE

The first two phases of the Low-Carb Coconut Diet are the most difficult because of the restrictions on grains, beans, and potatoes—foods that normally make up most of our diet. Learning to prepare low-carb meals without these items takes a little practice. Because of the popularity of low-carb diets nowadays, there are several cookbooks available that can help. The Internet also offers many low-carb recipes. I've provided a few recipes in Chapter 16 to get you started.

You can use many recipes from standard or low-carb cookbooks by substituting ingredients where necessary. For example, if a recipe calls for margarine or soybean oil, use coconut oil instead. In place of pasteurized milk, use cream (diluted with a little water if necessary) or coconut milk.

Along with the dietary recommendations noted above you should follow the remaining steps of the Healthy Lifestyle Plan. This means you eat only three meals a day, drink an adequate amount of water, make wise food choices, use coconut oil daily, take dietary supplements, get regular exercise, and get sunlight.

Not all diets work for everyone. If after following all the recommendations for the Low-Carb Coconut Diet, or other low-carb diet, you still have difficulty losing weight, I suggest the Raw-Foods Coconut Diet outlined in the following chapter. Many people who have difficulty with low-carb dieting find success with this diet.

Chapter 15

RAW-FOODS COCONUT DIET _____ ∎

A RAW-FOOD DIET

A raw-food diet sounds unappetizing to many people. When most of us think of eating raw foods, we visualize celery sticks and lettuce leaves. Don't fear, there is much more to it than this. In fact, raw meals can be delicious and very satisfying. Although the focus is on raw foods, you are allowed some cooked foods as well. So there is a great deal of variety.

The diet is simple. You are allowed to eat most any type of food so long as it is raw or cultured. Cultured or fermented foods are included because they contain live bacteria and, therefore, are considered a living food. Food choices include raw fruits, vegetables, nuts, seeds and raw milk and cultured foods like yogurt, cottage cheese, and hard cheese. Condiments you can use are apple cider or wine vinegar, herbs, spices, sea salt, coconut mayonnaise, and vinaigrette dressing, etc., (recipes given in Chapter 16). Extra virgin olive oil and coconut oil are the only oils recommended.

In addition to raw and cultured foods you are allowed a limited amount of cooked foods. At least 75% of the foods you eat should be raw. Up to 25% can be cooked. A 100% raw diet would be the most effective for weight loss, but it would make the diet so restrictive that few people would stick with it. Allowing up to 25% cooked foods gives the diet variety and makes it easier to follow.

All foods are permitted on this diet except those outlined in Chapter 13—refined and artificial sweeteners, refined grains, processed and hydrogenated vegetable oils, dehydrated dairy and eggs, homogenized milk, and highly processed meats. Also avoid raw cruciferous vegetables and soy products (except fermented soy—miso, tempeh, and soy sauce). Fruit juices are discouraged, even if they are made with fresh fruit, because they contain a high concentration of sugar. Vegetable juices are okay if you make them fresh with your own juicer.

You are allowed to eat whole grain bread, legumes, potatoes, meat, eggs, poultry, and other foods that require cooking, but only up to 25% of your total daily intake. You can eat a steak if you like, but you will need to eat a salad or some other raw food equivalent to 3 times the size of the meat. You need not weigh or measure your food. To make it easy for you to judge the size of food portions, use visual comparison. A simple way to do this is to mentally divide your dinner plate into 4 equal sections. The meat, or other cooked food, would occupy one section. Raw foods would occupy the other three sections (see illustration on next page).

Beverages such as raw milk or raw vegetable juice count as part of the raw food total. Sometimes you will use a variety of dishes. You might have a salad in a bowl, a fish filet on a plate, and a glass of juice. In cases like this, just estimate portion sizes the best you can. You don't have to be exact, but be honest and as accurate as you can. If you cheat, you're only hurting yourself. If you want good results it's better to eat less than 25% cooked food than it is to eat more.

At times you may want to eat a meal that has more cooked food than 25%. If you do, you must make up for it at the next meal or account for it in the previous meal. For example, if you eat a meal that is 50% cooked and 50% raw, you will need to eat 100% raw foods at the next meal or at the previous meal. Don't eat more than 50% cooked food at any one meal. Limit 50/50 meals. Do not do them every day. The more raw foods you eat the better this diet works.

If you find that you are not losing excess weight or you begin to gain weight, you need to cut down on the amount of cooked foods you are eating. Often, when people "eyeball" food portions they overestimate the raw food and underestimate the cooked food portion. They end up eating far more cooked food than just 25%.

The speed at which you lose weight will depend greatly on the amount of cooked food you allow in your diet. The more raw food you eat, the greater will be your weight loss. Although the guidelines specify that you can eat *up to* 25% of your food cooked, you may need to eat less than the maximum allowed. You might be better off without the cooked food and eat a nearly 100% raw-food diet. It all depends on how well you lose weight. Keep in mind that a reduction of 1 or 2 pounds a week is good progress. You don't need to lose 20 pounds all at once. Be patient. Work at it gradually. If you lost only 1 pound a week, that will add up to nearly 50 pounds by the end of the year. So small losses can add up to big results.

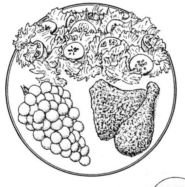

To estimate raw and cooked food portion sizes divide plate into quarters.

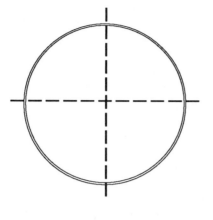

Three of the quarters comprise the raw foods and one quarter the cooked.

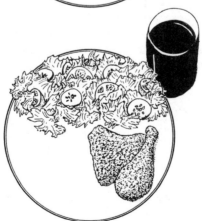

Raw liquids, such as fresh vegetable juice, count as part of the raw food portion.

ADAPT RECIPES

As you can guess, fresh green salads are an important part of this diet, as are whole fruits and vegetables. You should eat as much fresh fruit and vegetables as you can. You are allowed to eat as much as you like during mealtime, but avoid stuffing yourself. Eat only until your hunger is satisfied.

Several salad and salad dressing recipes are included in Chapter 16. Suitable recipes may be found in your own cookbook. Adapt standard recipes, if necessary, to the guidelines of this diet.

Many salad recipes, such as coleslaw, use cruciferous vegetables (e.g. cabbage, cauliflower, broccoli). Because these vegetables contain goitrogens that affect the thyroid, it's best not to eat too much of them, especially if you suspect you have a metabolism problem. One or two individual raw cauliflower or broccoli florets in a salad is a good limit.

You can use other vegetables in their place in many recipes, such as diakon radish, jicama, and Jerusalem artichokes. Each of these can often be found in your local grocery store.

Diakon radish is common to parts of Asia. It grows to the size and shape of a very large carrot. It is white and looks somewhat like a large parsnip. It is not quite as hot as most radishes. It gives salads a little bite similar to what you would expect from cabbage and makes a good replacement for cabbage in salad recipes.

Jicama (pronounced hic-a-maw) is a tuberous root, native of tropical regions in South and Central America. It is about the size of a small cantaloupe and has the coloring of a russet potato. It has a mild, slightly sweet flavor, excellent for salads.

The Jerusalem artichoke belongs to the sunflower family. It has no similarity to the artichoke you typically see in the grocery store. It is a tuber. It grows to about the size of a small potato and looks similar to ginger root. It has a mild potato-like taste and is good eaten raw in salads.

GENERAL GUIDELINES

The same general guidelines given in the Healthy Lifestyle Plan are applicable in the Raw-Foods Coconut Diet—eat three meals a day, drink water between meals, take multiple vitamin and liquid mineral supplements, exercise daily, and get out into the sunlight. One thing that is different with this diet is that you are allowed, and even encouraged, to snack on fresh coconut between meals *if* you are hungry.

According to Dr. Batmanghelidj, if you drink the amount of water recommended, you need to add a half teaspoon of salt a day. Since the majority of the food you eat is fresh fruits and vegetables, salt consumption can be easily neglected. You must make a conscious effort to eat a little salt throughout the day. A good way to do this is to add it to vegetable juices or water. A pinch of salt in a glass of water is essentially undetectable and provides a convenient way to get both your salt and water requirement.

Coconut plays a central role in this diet. You are encouraged to include fresh coconut or coconut oil with *every* meal. The reason for this is to get the metabolic benefits the oil provides. If you eat a salad, use a dressing made with coconut oil. If you eat fresh fruit for a meal you can include a piece of fresh coconut as well. Instead of eating fresh coconut you may also eat a tablespoon of coconut oil. You simply take it like you would a liquid dietary supplement. If you use virgin coconut oil it is actually very tasty.

You are allowed to eat as much raw fruits and vegetables as you like during mealtime. If you get hungry between meals drink plenty of water and eat fresh coconut. I recommend you consume about 3 to 6 tablespoons of coconut oil a day, depending on your size. If you are small, say 120 pounds or less, 3 tablespoons should do. If you weigh 300 pounds or more, 6 tablespoons would be more in order. Don't eat this much oil all at once, spread it out over the day. You can count the oil in fresh coconut as a part of the total. There are about 7 tablespoons of coconut oil in one large coconut. One ounce of fresh coconut contains $1/2$ tablespoon of oil. An ounce of coconut is about $2^1/_2$–3 inches in diameter.

Do not eat dried, sweetened coconut commonly sold in stores, get whole fresh coconuts and remove the meat yourself.

The benefit of the Raw-Foods Coconut Diet is that you can take full advantage of the metabolic effects of coconut. You also get a high concentration of vitamins, minerals, phytonutrients, and fiber. Because fresh raw foods are very high in water, they are also very low in calories. This is a low-calorie, high-water diet. The fresh produce combined with the coconut creates a low-calorie, metabolically energized diet that can help people with even the most difficult weight problems. For some people this diet will melt excess pounds off very quickly.

HOW TO SELECT AND OPEN A COCONUT

Most grocery stores, and even health food stores, sell fresh coconuts. In most areas coconuts must be shipped in, some coming far distances such as Mexico, the Caribbean, or even Fiji. Since coconuts are imported long distances, many of them go bad before they even reach the grocery store. When I first started buying fresh coconuts and bringing them home, I was lucky to get one good one out of three that was edible. Now I can spot the bad ones and my success rate is nine out of 10.

To find a good coconut look for one that is filled with liquid. The liquid inside a coconut is called *coconut water* not *coconut milk*. Coconut milk is made by crushing and squeezing the juice out of coconut meat and has a different color, texture, and flavor than the water that naturally forms in the nut. You want to select a coconut that is full of water. Shake it. If there is little or no water present that means the shell is cracked and the meat will probably be contaminated with mold. When you crack open a coconut the meat should be pure white. If there is any yellow or brown discoloring of the meat it is contaminated with mold. The flavor of the meat should be mild with a fresh coconut flavor. Any strong or strange flavors are caused by mold.

Look at the shell before you buy it. Look for cracks and the presence of mold. Greenish or white mold often forms around the eyes on the outside of the coconut. If the coconut has mold growing on the outside it most likely has mold on the inside as well. If it's moldy don't buy it.

If you've never opened and extracted coconut meat before, it can be a little tricky. To crack open a coconut, first locate the coconut's face— three marks that resemble two eyes and a mouth. The eye marks have a slight ridge over them that resemble eyebrows. The one that is located at the position of the mouth is relatively soft. Puncture it with an ice pick, knife, or screwdriver. Drain the liquid. The liquid will drain faster if you puncture a second hole in one of the eyes. The eyes are a little more difficult to penetrate. Some people use a hammer and nail. I use an ice pick.

After the liquid is drained, place the coconut on a hard surface and hit it sharply with a hammer. It will take a few blows to break up completely. You can do this without draining the coconut first, but it is obviously more messy that way.

Take a knife and pry the coconut meat off the shell. The side of the meat that was against the shell will have a thin brown membrane. You can remove this with a vegetable peeler. Store the meat inside a plastic bag and keep it in the refrigerator. It will stay good in the refrigerator for 5 or 6 days. If you plan to keep the coconut around longer than that you can freeze it. Unopened coconuts can be stored in the refrigerator for a couple of weeks.

SAMPLE MEALS

Below are some examples of the types of meals you can make on this diet.

Breakfast

- Fruit smoothie
- Bowl of fresh fruit
- Pancakes topped with yogurt and fresh fruit
- Hard-boiled egg and fresh fruit
- Oatmeal and raw milk with fresh fruit

Lunch

- Melon or fresh mixed fruit
- Fruit or vegetable salad
- Cheese sandwich and apple
- Avocado sandwich and peach

Dinner

- Dinner salad with hard-boiled eggs
- Shrimp salad and toast
- Fruit or vegetable salad with steamed vegetables
- Fruit or vegetable salad with baked fish
- Fruit or vegetable salad with 3-oz steak and fresh vegetable juice

When preparing your meals keep in mind that you need to get at least 75% percent from raw foods. Raw milk or fresh vegetable juice counts as part of the requirement for the raw foods portion. The best meals would be 100% raw like fresh fruit or a salad. Below, however, are examples of some mixed meals.

Pancakes and Yogurt

This makes a great breakfast. No syrup or sweetening is needed other than the fruit. Make whole wheat pancakes with coconut oil (see whole wheat coconut pancake recipe in Chapter 16). Top with mixture of yogurt, chopped fresh fruit, and pecans. Fruits that work well include: strawberries, raspberries, blueberries, kiwi, and peaches. Since coconut oil is used in this recipe it satisfies the 1 tablespoon per meal requirement.

Oatmeal and Fruit

Combine $1/2$ to $3/4$ cup of hot oatmeal with 1 to $1^1/_2$ cups fresh chopped fruit and $1/2$ cup of raw milk. If raw milk is not available you can substitute yogurt. If needed, you may add a little raw honey or maple syrup. This is delicious with strawberries, but works well with a number of fruits. Add a tablespoon of coconut oil for a pleasant way to get your coconut oil requirement. Serve with a glass of raw milk or fresh vegetable juice.

Cheese Sandwich

Cut two thin slices of whole wheat (or other whole grain) bread. Layer one slice with fresh cheese, thinly sliced onion, sliced tomatoes, lettuce, pickle, and sliced avocado. On the other slice add butter, coconut mayonnaise (see Chapter 16 for recipe), salt and pepper or herbal seasoning. Eat with a glass of raw milk, fresh vegetable juice, or a serving of fresh fruit.

You can add a number of different vegetables to this sandwich for variety. Others you might consider are green pepper, cucumber, sprouts, carrots, and celery. Also, instead of sliced bread, you can use whole wheat pocket bread. Your coconut oil requirement is contained in the coconut mayonnaise.

Avocado Sandwich

Cut two thin slices of whole wheat (or pocket) bread. Layer one slice with sliced avocado, sliced tomato, thinly sliced onion, and lettuce. On the other slice add butter, mayonnaise, salt and pepper or herbal seasoning. Eat with a glass of raw milk or vegetable juice. In place of the mayonnaise you may try the Spicy Coconut Oil Dressing described in Chapter 16. Either one supplies the coconut oil you need.

Vegetable Juice

Fresh vegetable juice is a great way to add raw food to your diet. I recommend that you drink juice with meals and water between meals. Juice is food. It is a concentrated liquid source of vitamins and minerals. It is well worth your time to buy a juicer and use it.

Make just enough juice so that you can drink it all within one day. Fresh juice loses its nutritional value quickly. Don't keep it longer than 24 hours. It's at its nutritional peak just after extraction. This is the best time to consume it. Store leftover juice in an airtight container in the refrigerator.

Most people think of carrots when juicing is mentioned. Carrots, like fruits, are high in sugar. You should avoid sweet juices. That's why I don't recommend straight fruit juice or carrot juice. This doesn't mean you can't ever use carrots or fruits in juicing. They can be used in combination with vegetable juices. Together they can make great tasting drinks.

Good juicy vegetables are celery, cucumbers, bell peppers, and tomatoes. Green leafy vegetables include loose-leaf lettuce, romaine, endive, escarole, spinach, chard, watercress, parsley, cilantro, and beat tops. You can use most any vegetable, even those typically served cooked such as beets, asparagus, zucchini, and okra. Other vegetables to consider are radishes, parsnips, and jicama. Jicama contains a high amount of liquid and is slightly sweet making a good juicing vegetable. Be creative and try different vegetables. Be careful about using cruciferous vegetables, they give juices a strong bite and contain goitrogens. Garlic has many health benefits and a little of it in a juice can spark it up.

Adding a small amount of carrots, grapes, apples, or oranges can sweeten vegetable juice and greatly improve the flavor. Fresh cranberries can also give juices a nice fruity flavor. Lemon and lime give a tangy tartness to juice.

When you open a fresh coconut, you may want to save the water and combine it with your juice. Coconut water is very sweet so I recommend that you dilute it. Once coconut water is removed from the coconut you can keep it in the refrigerator for a couple of days. If you want to keep it around longer than that you need to freeze it to prevent it from spoiling.

Be creative and try different combinations. Rotate the vegetables you use for variety. Adding a tablespoon of coconut oil to vegetable juice makes a great way to get your daily quota. When you combine juice and coconut oil make sure the juice is at or near room temperature so the oil does not solidify.

Some people wonder what they should do with the leftover pulp. The pulp is almost entirely fiber. Fiber has many health benefits. After juicing, you can eat the pulp like a mixed salad. The taste of the pulp can be improved by adding nuts or seeds. Sunflower, pumpkin, and sesame seeds are good, so are chopped almonds, pecans, and macadamia nuts. Shredded coconut can greatly improve the flavor of the pulp. If the pulp is too dry for your liking you can add back a little of the juice to make vegetable porridge.

Fruit Smoothies

The advantage smoothies have over juicing is that you eat both the juice and fiber. Smoothies provide another way to eat fruits and vegetables. There are many ways to make smoothies. What you need is a blender, liquids, and fruit or vegetables. For liquids you can use water, milk, cream, or yogurt. Cottage cheese can be used with water to give the smoothie a tart, creamy flavor.

You might try adding some of the leftover pulp from juicing to your fruit smoothie. This will increase the fiber content and provide bulk that can fill you up without adding much in the way of calories.

AFTER YOU'VE REACHED YOUR GOAL

After you've reached your weight-loss goal, you need to continue to eat so that you maintain the progress you've made. Does that mean you must stay with a 75% raw, 25% cooked diet? Not necessarily. Many people can increase the amount of cooked food in their diets without regaining weight. This is particularly true if you continue to do all the other things outlined in The Healthy Lifestyle Plan.

Many people find that they enjoy the improved health and energy they've gained from eating a 75/25 raw-foods diet and don't want to change. That's fine. Others miss some of the cooked foods they've done without. At this point, you have the option of increasing the amount of cooked food in your diet. I'm not going to give you any limits, you can decide that for yourself.

What you want to do is maintain your new weight. If you decide to add a little more cooked food into your diet, do it gradually. You might want to make it two-thirds raw and one-third cooked or even 50/50. Try it for a few days. Monitor your weight. If you start to gain weight, cut back on the cooked food.

Everyone is different. We eat different foods, cooked in different ways. Some people tend to eat cooked foods that are higher in calories than others. These differences will determine how much cooked food you can add to your diet without gaining weight. The only way to find out is to increase your cooked food portion gradually, and at the same time monitor your weight. Some people may be able to maintain their weight with a 25% raw, 75% cooked diet.

Regardless of the exact percentages, this is a very good diet that you can stay on for a lifetime. Because it focuses on fresh fruits and vegetables you receive a high dose of health promoting, natural vitamins and minerals. Not only will you lose excess weight, but you will enjoy a higher level of health and vitality.

Chapter 16

RECIPES ███

In this chapter I offer some suggestions for recipes that fit the Low-Carbohydrate Coconut Diet and the Raw-Foods Coconut Diet. These recipes are provided as examples. You are encouraged to experiment with the foods you like best. Use recipes in cookbooks and adjust them as needed. You can find both low-carb and raw-food recipe books in stores and on the Internet.

Each recipe is marked with one, two, or three stars (☆) or a diamond (❖). Recipes marked with ☆ means it is suitable for Phase I of the Low-Carb Coconut Diet. Those marked with ☆☆ are suitable for Phase II. Those with ☆☆☆ are for Phase III. If you are on Phase I use only those recipes marked with one star. If you are in Phase II you can use recipes marked with either one or two stars. If you are on Phase III you can use any recipe marked with one, two, or three stars. The ❖ signifies that the recipe uses mostly all raw ingredients and is uncooked and, therefore, suitable for the Raw-Foods Coconut Diet. Some recipes are useable in either diet and will have both a diamond and one or more stars.

SALADS AND DRESSINGS
Tossed Green Salad ☆❖

This is the popular lettuce-based salad we generally think of when someone mentions salad. But our version combines a variety of vegetables and toppings to make it into a meal. So many ingredients can go into a tossed salad that you can make a different one every day of the week.

Combine any raw vegetables: lettuce, cucumber, bell peppers, tomato, avocado, parsley, onion, carrots, radishes, and/or jicama. Don't limit yourself to just iceberg lettuce, try other varieties.

Toppings: hard-boiled eggs, bacon, ham, chicken, tuna, salmon, crab, shrimp, nuts, seeds, pork rinds, cheese. Feta cheese is great tasting in salads. You might also try using different hard and soft cheeses, including cottage cheese, for a variety of flavors.

Dressing: any number of dressings. Olive oil, coconut oil, vinegar, or dairy-based. Avoid dressing with processed vegetable oils, sugar, or MSG.

Seasoning: Salt, herbs, and spices can be added to taste.

Creamy Ranch Dressing ☆❖

^{1}/$_3$ cup sour cream
^{1}/$_4$ cup heavy cream
1 teaspoon onion powder
1 teaspoon dried cilantro or dill
salt and pepper to taste

This is an easy ranch dressing for salads and vegetable dips that closely resembles those typically sold in the store. Blend all ingredients together and chill.

Creamy Herb Dressing ☆❖

^{1}/$_3$ cup sour cream
^{1}/$_4$ cup heavy cream
^{1}/$_4$ teaspoon vinegar
^{1}/$_2$ teaspoon celery seed
^{1}/$_4$ teaspoon crumbled dried thyme
salt and pepper to taste

Blend all ingredients together and chill.

Vinaigrette Dressing ☆❖

^{1}/$_4$ cup red or white wine vinegar
^{1}/$_4$ teaspoon salt
^{1}/$_8$ teaspoon white pepper
^{1}/$_3$ cup olive oil
^{1}/$_3$ cup coconut oil

For those readers who are more familiar with the meteric system you can use the following measurements for the recipes in this chapter: ^{1}/$_2$ cup = 175 ml, 1 cup = 250 ml, 2 cups = 500 ml.

In a bowl mix vinegar, salt, and pepper with a fork. Add oil and mix vigorously until well blended.

Lemon Vinaigrette ☆❖

$^1/_2$ cup lemon juice
$^1/_2$ cup olive oil
$^1/_2$ teaspoon dijon mustard
1 tablespoon finely minced shallots
1 tablespoon minced fresh parsley
salt and pepper to taste

Mix all ingredients together and chill. Use as a dressing for tossed salad or pour over cooked vegetables.

Coconut Mayonnaise ☆❖

1 large egg
$1^1/_4$ tablespoons fresh lemon juice or wine vinegar
$^1/_2$ tablespoon prepared mustard
$^1/_4$ teaspoon salt
1 cup coconut oil

Let all ingredients come to room temperature. Coconut oil should be in a liquid state. Combine egg, lemon juice or vinegar, mustard, salt, and 1 tablespoon oil in bowl and mix in food processor or blender for 60 seconds. While machine is running, slowly dribble the remaining oil into the mixture. Mayonnaise will thicken as oil is added. This mayonnaise is best when used immediately because of its soft texture. Store leftover mayonnaise in an air-tight container in the refrigerator. In the refrigerator the mayonnaise will harden. To soften put container in bath of hot water for a few minutes or simply remove from the refrigerator about 30 minutes before using. The warmth of the room will soften it. Even though this recipe uses a raw egg the mayonnaise will stay good for a couple of months.

Coconut-Olive Mayonnaise ☆❖

1 large egg
$1^1/_4$ tablespoons fresh lemon juice or wine vinegar
$^1/_2$ tablespoon prepared mustard
$^1/_4$ teaspoon salt
$^3/_4$ cup coconut oil
$^1/_2$ cup olive oil

Follow the same directions above for making Coconut Mayonnaise. This recipe makes a mayonnaise that is softer when chilled than the Coconut Mayonnaise, and so is a little more convenient to use. The olive oil gives it a slightly different taste.

253

Spicy Coconut Oil Dressing ☆❖

1/2 cup coconut oil
1/4 cup onion, finely diced
2 tablespoons garlic, finely diced
1/2 teaspoon basil
1/2 teaspoon oregano
1/4 teaspoon paprika
1/4 teaspoon salt
1/8 teaspoon black pepper (or cayenne pepper)

Combine all ingredients in a small saucepan. Heat mixture until just before it begins to simmer. Turn off the heat and let sit until cool. Don't over heat, your goal is not to cook it, but just help the flavors blend. You can use this as a seasoning over cooked vegetables or meat, as a dip for raw vegetables, or as a salad dressing.

Easy Tuna Salad ☆

7 ounces of cooked tuna
1/2 minced Bermuda onion
Juice of 1/2 lemon
3/4–1 cup mayonnaise (depending on how creamy a mixture you want)
2 tablespoons minced parsley
Pinch of salt
1/8 teaspoon pepper

Mix all ingredients and chill several hours before serving. Serve on top of sliced tomatoes and crisp lettuce leaves.

Avacado Salad ☆❖

Romaine or loose-leaf lettuce
2 avocados
1 red onion
1 tomato
1 tablespoon fresh lime or lemon juice
salt and pepper to taste

Slice onions and tomatoes and combine with lettuce in a bowl. Toss gently. Sprinkle with lime juice, salt and pepper. Cut avocado into halves and place on top.

Celery Salad ☆❖

1 bunch celery
1 tablespoon tarragon vinegar
1 onion, finely chopped

1 tablespoon cream
2 hard-boiled eggs, finely chopped
2 tomatoes, sliced
1/2 cucumber, sliced
1 tablespoon prepared mustard
1/4 cup olive or coconut oil
salt and pepper

Slice celery into thin strips, mix with chopped onion and set aside. To make the dressing, mix finely chopped eggs with mustard, oil, vinegar, and cream. Add salt and pepper to taste. Pour dressing over the celery and onion mixture and toss. Garnish with sliced tomatoes and cucumber.

Celery Slaw ☆❖

1/2 cup sour cream or kefir cheese
1/2 bunch celery, thinly sliced
1 onion, sliced
1 medium carrot, shredded
2 teaspoons salt
1/2 teaspoon pepper
1 pinch paprika
1/2 cup olive or coconut oil
3 tablespoons vinegar

To make the dressing combine the salt, pepper, paprika, oil, and vinegar. Beat well. Mix in the sour cream. Pour the dressing over the celery and chill for about three hours. Before serving add onion and carrot and mix thoroughly.

Pepper Slaw ☆❖

4 teaspoons white wine vinegar
1/3 cup olive or coconut oil
1 large red bell pepper
1 large yellow bell pepper
1 medium carrot, finely shredded
2 celery ribs
salt and pepper to taste

Cut peppers and celery in 2-inch-long strips. Combine in a bowl with shredded carrot. In a separate bowl combine vinegar, salt, and pepper. Slowly add oil to the vinegar while mixing vigorously with a whisk. Add to vegetables and mix well.

Orange Salad ☆❖
2 cups torn romaine lettuce
1/2 small red onion, thinly sliced
1 fresh orange, peeled and separated into sections
2 tablespoons pecans
2 tablespoons orange juice
2 tablespoons white wine vinegar
3 tablespoons coconut oil (or olive oil)
1 tablespoon chopped fresh cilantro
2 teaspoons dijon mustard
salt and pepper to taste

Toss lettuce, onion, oranges, and nuts together. Whisk together in a separate bowl orange juice, vinegar, oil, cilantro, dijon mustard, salt, and pepper. Pour the dressing over the vegetable fruit mixture.

Jicama Slaw ☆❖
1 medium red onion
1 1/4 teaspoons salt
1 1/2 tablespoons fresh lime juice
1/3 cup coconut oil
1/4 teaspoon black pepper
1 jicama, shredded (9 to 10 cups)
1/3 cup finely chopped fresh cilantro

Finely chop onion and soak in 1 cup of cold water with 1/2 teaspoon salt for 15 minutes (this gives the onion a milder flavor). Put onion in a sieve, rinse, and pat dry. Whisk together lime juice, oil, pepper, and 3/4 teaspoon salt in a large bowl until well mixed. Add onion, jicama, cilantro, and salt to taste, and toss.

Tropical Salad with Mango Dressing ☆❖
1 large ripe mango, peeled and cut (about 1 1/2 cups)
1/4 cup coconut oil
3 tablespoons fresh lime juice
3 tablespoons rice vinegar or 1 tablespoon white wine vinegar
1 teaspoon paprika
1/8 teaspoon cayenne pepper
1/2 cup shredded coconut
1 10-ounce bag mixed baby lettuce
1 cup diced peeled jicama
1/2 cup salted roasted cashews

To make the dressing combine $^1/_2$ cup mango with oil, lime juice, vinegar, paprika, and cayenne pepper in blender. Puree until smooth. Season to taste with salt and pepper. Transfer to small bowl, cover, and let stand at room temperature for about 10 minutes. This allows flavors to blend. Dressing can be made up to 3 hours before serving.

Combine lettuce, jicama, coconut, and remaining 1 cup mango in large bowl. Toss with enough dressing to coat. Sprinkle top with cashews and serve.

Pineapple Delight ☆☆❖

1 cup cottage cheese
1 cup sliced pineapple
1 tablespoon virgin coconut oil (optional)
2 tablespoons shredded coconut (lightly toasted)

Spread the shredded coconut evenly over the bottom of a pie pan or cookie sheet and bake in oven at 350 degrees for about 10 minutes or until lightly toasted. Check the coconut often as it cooks because it can burn quickly. While the coconut is roasting, combine cottage cheese with coconut oil and mix thoroughly. Oil will eventually blend into the cottage cheese. Virgin coconut oil works best because of its coconut flavor. Fold in the pineapple. Sprinkle toasted coconut on top of salad.

The coconut oil can be left out of this recipe, but it provides a good way to incorporate the oil into your diet. This recipe calls for 1 tablespoon of oil but you can use as much or as little as you like.

Waldorf Salad ☆☆❖

4 medium-sized tart red apples, cored and diced
$^3/_4$ cup finely chopped celery
$^1/_3$ cup coarsely chopped walnuts
$^2/_3$–1 cup coconut mayonnaise

Stir all ingredients together, adding just enough mayonnaise for good consistency. Cover and chill 2–3 hours. Stir well and serve on lettuce leaves.

Vegetable Fruit Salad ☆☆❖

2 celery ribs
1 medium carrot
1 cup grated diakon raddish (or jicama)
2 cups grated coconut
2 medium apples, cored and diced
$^1/_2$ cup sweet red pepper

1 cup coarsely chopped pecans
1¹/₂–2 cups plain yogurt (or coconut milk)
Stevia to taste

Stir all ingredients together using just enough yogurt for good con-sistency. Cover and chill for about 1 hour. If desired you can sweeten the salad lightly with a little stevia. This is a great salad that will stay good for a couple of days if stored in the refrigerator.

This recipe makes about 10 servings. It's excellent for breakfast, lunch, or dinner. If you expect to have leftovers while you are making it, do not mix in the yogurt. Put the salad in individual bowls and mix the yogurt separately just before serving. Refrigerate the remaining salad, without the added yogurt. Yogurt mixed into salads has a tendency to become watery if not eaten for several hours.

Variation ☆☆❖

This salad can be made using additional fruits such as pineapple and banana.

EGG DISHES
Basic Stovetop Omelet ☆

2 eggs
2 tablespoons coconut oil or bacon grease
2 tablespoons wheat bran (optional)
salt and pepper

This is a quick and easy way to make an omelet in a fry pan on the stovetop. Heat fry pan with oil to medium heat. In bowl beat together vigorously eggs, bran, salt, and pepper. Pour egg mixture into fry pan, cover and let cook for about 5–7 minutes or until eggs are thoroughly cooked and somewhat fluffy. Serve as is or top with sour cream or salsa.

Variation ☆

There are many variations to the above basic recipe. Adding other ingredients you can create many different omelets. Ideas for ingredients include sausage, bacon, ham, cheese, onions, peppers, zucchini, cottage cheese, cream cheese, asparagus, diced tomatoes, and shrimp. If you're using meats cook them first before combining with the eggs.

Basic Oven Omelet ☆

2 eggs
3 tablespoons coconut oil or bacon grease

258

2 tablespoons wheat bran (optional)
salt and pepper

The recipe for this simple omelet is basically the same as the previous recipe except it is cooked in the oven.

Preheat oven to 400° F (200° C). Heat baking dish with oil until hot. Remove from oven, add egg mixture and bake for 15 minutes. As the omelet cooks it will rise and increase in volume several times developing a light fluffy omelet. Serve warm.

You can use the variations in the previous recipe for variety.

Zucchini Delight ☆

4 eggs
1 small zucchini, sliced
$^1/_2$ cup chopped onion
$^1/_4$ cup chopped bell pepper
$^1/_8$ cup hot pepper (optional)
$^1/_2$ cup cheese
2 tablespoons wheat bran (optional)
$^1/_3$ cup diced tomato
4 tablespoons coconut oil
salt and pepper

This is a great meal for breakfast, lunch, or dinner. Heat oil in fry pan and lightly sauté all vegetables except the tomatoes. In large mixing bowl beat eggs and wheat bran. Add egg mixture to vegetables in fry pan, cover and cook for about 5 minutes or until eggs are about half-way cooked. Remove lid, sprinkle cheese on top, cover and cook until cheese is melted. Uncover, sprinkle top with diced tomato, re-cover, and turn off heat. Let sit for 1–2 minutes to warm the tomato without cooking it.

Variation ☆

Add sausage, ham, bacon, or ground beef to the above recipe.

MAIN DISHES
Chicken Stir Fry ☆

1 pound de-boned chicken
$^1/_2$ cup chopped onion
$^1/_2$ cup snow peas, cut in half
$^1/_2$ cup chopped bok choy
$^1/_2$ cup chopped bell pepper
$^1/_2$ cup mushrooms
1 cup bean sprouts
$^1/_2$ cup water chestnuts

259

$^1/_2$ cup bamboo shoots
$^1/_4$ cup coconut oil
soy sauce
salt and pepper

This makes a great one-dish meal. Cut raw chicken into bite-sized pieces. Sauté chicken and vegetables in coconut oil until cooked and tender. Turn off heat, add soy sauce, salt and pepper to taste, and serve. You may use any combination of vegetables listed and vary the quantities to your own preferences.

Variation ☆

You may substitute the chicken in this recipe with pork or beef.

Chicken-Broccoli Delight ☆

$^1/_2$ cup slivered almonds
1 head broccoli, cut into florets
5 tablespoons butter
5 tablespoons whole wheat flour
1 teaspoon salt
2 cups heavy cream
1 cup water
2 cups grated cheddar cheese
$^1/_2$ teaspoon black pepper
4 cups diced cooked chicken or turkey

Using coconut oil, grease a 9-by-13-inch baking dish. Toast almonds by stirring them in a dry skillet or baking them in a 350° F (175° C) oven for about 10 minutes, until they are golden brown and fragrant. Set aside.

Boil 1 quart water. Cut broccoli florets into smallish pieces, about 1 inch, leaving about 1 inch or so of stem. Dunk in boiling water for 2 minutes, or until they are bright green and barely tender. Drain well, spread on a cloth towel and set aside. (The broccoli will tend to give off a little moisture when you bake the casserole if you don't let it drain on absorbent toweling. Meanwhile, melt butter in a saucepan over medium heat. Add flour and salt and stir to blend. Add cream and water, stirring to prevent lumps (this is easier with a whisk). Bring the mixture to a boil, whisking often, then remove from heat. Add 1 cup cheese and pepper. Stir to melt cheese.

Put broccoli in the bottom of the baking pan and scatter chicken over it. Pour sauce over the top and sprinkle with remaining cheese and almonds.

Bake at 350° F (175° C) for 20 minutes, or until the mixture is heated through and bubbly.

Pork Chops with Creamy Sauce ☆

2 tablespoons coconut oil
4 pork chops
1 14-oz can coconut milk
1 cup water
1–2 tablespoons flour
1 cup chopped mushrooms
1/2 cup diced onion
Salt and pepper

Heat oil in fry pan and brown both sides of pork chops. Reduce heat and cover. Cook chops until nearly done. Add chopped mushrooms and onions. In small mixing bowl combine water, flour, and coconut milk. Mix thoroughly. Add this mixture to the fry pan bathing the pork chops. Stir to keep gravy from scorching bottom of pan. Add more water if gravy becomes too thick. Add salt and pepper to taste.

Serve pork chops with gravy. Goes well with steamed or mashed cauliflower.

Fish Patties ☆

1 6-oz can tuna
2 eggs
1/4 cup diced onion
1/4 cup wheat bran
1/2 teaspoon lemon pepper
1 tablespoon water
coconut oil or bacon grease
salt

Combine tuna, eggs, onion, wheat bran, water, lemon pepper, and salt and mix thoroughly. Heat fry pan to medium heat. Form mixture into patties about 2 1/2 inches in diameter. Put enough oil into pan to cover bottom. Place patties in fry pan and cover. Cook thoroughly, turning once, and browning both sides.

Variation ☆

In place of tuna you can use salmon, halibut, crab, or any other fish. Top it with cocktail sauce.

Beef Patties ☆

1/2 pound ground beef
3 eggs

$^1\!/_2$ cup diced onion
$^1\!/_4$ cup diced bell pepper
$^1\!/_2$ cup wheat bran
2 tablespoons Worcestershire sauce
coconut oil
salt and pepper

Combine ground beef, eggs, onion, wheat bran, Worcestershire sauce, salt, and pepper and mix thoroughly. Heat fry pan to medium heat. Form mixture into patties about $2^1\!/_2$ inches in diameter. Put enough oil into pan to cover bottom. Place patties in fry pan and cover. Cook thoroughly, turning once and browning both sides.

Chicken Coconut Gravy ☆

This recipe makes a wonderful gravy or sauce that tastes great poured over steamed or mashed vegetables, brown rice, or whole grain pasta.
1 14-oz can coconut milk
3 tablespoons whole wheat flour
2 cups chopped chicken
2 tablespoons butter
salt, pepper, spices

Put coconut milk in sauce pan. Mix flour in thoroughly. Add chicken, either cooked or raw. Heat stirring occasionally until it thickens and chicken is thoroughly cooked. Add salt, pepper, spices to taste. Serve over a bed of steamed or mashed vegetables. Vegetables that work well include cauliflower, broccoli, peas, green beans, zucchini, and eggplant.

Variation ☆☆☆

Use the above gravy mixture over brown rice or whole grain pasta.

Chicken Almondine ☆

1 14-oz can coconut milk
3 tablespoons whole wheat flour
2 cups chopped chicken
$^1\!/_2$ cup sliced or slivered almonds
$^1\!/_2$ cup mushrooms
$^1\!/_2$ cup chopped onions
2 tablespoons butter
$^1\!/_4$ cup sour cream
salt and pepper

Toast almonds by stirring them in a dry skillet or baking them in a 350° F (175° C) oven for about 10 minutes, until they are golden brown and fragrant. Set aside. Keep an eye on the almonds while they are toasting because they can burn quickly. Put coconut milk in sauce pan. Mix flour in thoroughly. Add chicken, either cooked or raw. Heat stirring occasionally until it thickens and chicken is thoroughly cooked. Sauté mushrooms and diced onions in butter, then add to gravy mixture and simmer for another 3–5 minutes. Remove from heat and add sour cream, almonds, salt, and pepper to taste. Serve over bed of steamed vegetables. Goes very well over steamed cauliflower.

SOUPS AND CHOWDERS
Clam Chowder ☆
3 cups chopped cauliflower
$^1/_2$ cup chopped onion
3 cloves chopped garlic
1 cup chopped celery
$3^1/_2$ cups coconut milk (28 ounces)
$3^1/_2$ cups water
1 teaspoon salt
$^1/_8$ teaspoon white pepper
$^1/_8$ teaspoon paprika
1 10-oz can chopped or baby clams (do not drain)
1 8-oz bottle clam juice
2 tablespoons wheat bran (optional)
2 tablespoons butter

Sauté vegetables in butter until tender. Combine vegetables with water, salt, pepper, and clam juice; cover and simmer for 30 minutes. Add wheat bran and coconut milk; cover and simmer for 15 minutes. Add clams with juice and simmer for 5–7 minutes.

Variation ☆
Instead of clams you may substitute an equal amount of baby shrimp, oysters, or fish.

Cauliflower Soup ☆
4 cups cauliflower, cut into individual florets
2 cups chopped ham, pork, or chicken
1 medium onion, diced
1 cup sliced mushrooms
1 cup diced celery
2 cups coconut milk

2 cups water
4 cloves garlic, chopped
2 tablespoons wheat bran (optional)
$^1/_8$ teaspoon white pepper
1 teaspoon salt
1 tablespoon butter
2 tablespoons coconut oil
   Stir-fry meat and vegetables in 2 tablespoons coconut oil until tender. Add water, coconut milk, butter, wheat bran, and seasonings; bring to a boil, reduce heat and simmer for 30 minutes.

Creamy Chicken Soup ☆
2 14-oz cans coconut milk
1 cup water
2 cups chopped chicken
$^1/_2$ cup chopped onion
$^1/_2$ cup sliced carrots
1 cup chopped cauliflower
$^1/_2$ cup peas
1 cup celery
2 tablespoons coconut oil
salt and pepper
   Sauté chicken and vegetables in coconut oil until lightly browned. Combine with water, coconut milk and seasonings. Simmer for 30 minutes.

Variation ☆
   You can give this recipe a taste of India by adding 1–2 teaspoons curry powder and thickening with 2–4 tablespoons wheat bran.

Vegetable Beef Chili (without beans)☆
1 pound ground beef
1 cup chopped onion
4 cloves chopped garlic
2 cups chopped cauliflower
1 cup chopped bell pepper
1 cup green beans
1 16-oz can tomato sauce
1 tablespoon chili powder
1 teaspoon paprika
1 teaspoon salt
2–4 tablespoons wheat bran

3 cups water

1/4 cup hot peppers (optional)

Cook ground beef until brown. Add vegetables and sauté until tender. Add water and bring to a boil. Reduce heat, add spices, and simmer for 45 minutes. Add wheat bran to thicken, stir, and simmer 30 minutes.

Variation ☆

You may add other vegetables of your choosing to this recipe. Vegetables you might try include okra, eggplant, carrots, peas, zucchini, and other varieties of squash.

Minestrone ☆☆

1 pound ground beef

4 cups water

1 cup chopped carrots

1/2 cup chopped onion

1 cup chopped celery

1/2 cup peas

1 cup cooked kidney beans

4 cloves chopped garlic

1 28-oz can crushed tomatoes, undrained

1 teaspoon oregano

Salt

In a fry pan brown the ground beef. While the beef is cooking add the carrots, onion, celery, and garlic and sauté until tender. Combine meat mixture with water and all remaining ingredients. Bring to a boil then reduce heat, and simmer for 30 minutes.

Chili with Beans ☆☆

1 pound ground beef

2 cups cooked dried beans (pinto, red, or black)

1 cup chopped onion

4 cloves chopped garlic

1 cup chopped cauliflower

1 cup chopped bell pepper

1 cup green beans

1 16-oz can tomato sauce

1 tablespoon chili powder

1 teaspoon paprika

1 teaspoon salt

2–4 tablespoons wheat bran
3 cups water
¹/₄ cup hot peppers (optional)

Cook ground beef until brown. Add vegetables and sauté until tender. Add water and bring to a boil. Reduce heat, add spices and beans, and simmer for 45 minutes. Add wheat bran to thicken, stir, and simmer 30 minutes.

BREADS AND BAKED GOODS
All-Bran Basic Muffins ☆

3 eggs
1 cup wheat bran
¹/₂ cup gluten
1 teaspoon baking powder
³/₄ cup heavy cream
¹/₄ teaspoon salt
¹/₄ cup coconut oil or butter

All bran muffins are made without any flour so they are low in carbohydrate. You can use them as you would any muffin or as a replacement for bread. A great complement to any meal.

Preheat oven to 400° F (200° C). Mix bran, cream, and eggs together and set aside. In another bowl mix together gluten, baking powder, and salt and set aside.

Using coconut oil or butter generously coat the inside of 12 muffin cups. Pour the remaining oil in the bran mixture and stir in. Add the dry ingredients to the wet and mix thoroughly with a spoon. Fill muffin cups evenly with the mixture. Bake for 15 minutes.

All-Bran Meaty Muffins ☆

¹/₂ pound ground beef or sausage
4 eggs
³/₄ cup wheat bran
¹/₂ cup gluten
1 teaspoon baking powder
³/₄ cup water
³/₄ cup grated cheese
¹/₄ teaspoon salt
¹/₂ cup chopped onion
¹/₂ cup salsa
¹/₄ cup coconut oil

266

All-bran meaty muffins make an excellent breakfast. Leftover muffins provide a quick, tasty lunch.

Preheat oven to 400° F (200° C). Mix bran, water, salsa, eggs, and ¹/₂ cup of grated cheese together in bowl and set aside. In another bowl mix together gluten, baking powder, and salt and put aside. Thoroughly cook meat and chopped onion in fry pan, remove from heat, and let cool.

Using coconut oil generously coat the inside of 12 muffin cups. Add the meat and onion mixture along with meat drippings to the bran and egg mixture and stir together. Now add the gluten mixture and mix thoroughly with a spoon. Fill muffin cups evenly with the mixture. Sprinkle remaining cheese on top. Bake for 15 minutes.

All-Bran Pizza Muffins ☆

¹/₂ pound sausage
4 eggs
³/₄ cup wheat bran
¹/₂ cup gluten
1 teaspoon baking powder
³/₄ cup water
³/₄ cup grated cheese
¹/₄ teaspoon salt
¹/₂ cup chopped onion
³/₄ cup tomato sauce
1 teaspoon oregano
¹/₄ cup chopped bell peppers (optional)
¹/₂ cup sliced black olives
¹/₄ cup coconut oil

Preheat oven to 400° F (200° C). Mix bran, water, eggs, oregano, tomato sauce, and ¹/₂ cup of grated cheese together in bowl and set aside. In another bowl mix together gluten, baking powder, and salt and put aside. Thoroughly cook meat, onion, and bell pepper in fry pan, remove from heat, and let cool.

Using coconut oil generously coat the inside of 12 muffin cups. Add the meat mixture along with meat drippings to the bran and egg mixture and stir together. Now add the gluten mixture and mix thoroughly with a spoon. Fill muffin cups evenly with the mixture. Sprinkle remaining cheese on top. Bake for 15 minutes.

All-Bran Seafood Muffins ☆

1¹/₂ cup cooked fish (your choice of tuna, salmon, halibut, etc.)
4 eggs

1 cup wheat bran
$1/2$ cup gluten
1 teaspoon baking powder
$3/4$ cup water
$3/4$ cup grated cheese
$1/4$ teaspoon salt
$1/2$ tablespoon lemon pepper
$1/2$ cup diced onion
$1/3$ cup coconut oil

Preheat oven to 400° F (200° C). Mix bran, water, eggs, onion, fish, and $1/2$ cup of grated cheese together in bowl and set aside. In another bowl mix together gluten, baking powder, lemon pepper, and salt and put aside.

Heat the coconut oil so it is liquid. Generously coat the inside of 12 muffin cups. Add the remaining oil to the bran mixture and stir in. Now add the gluten mixture and mix thoroughly with a spoon. Fill muffin cups evenly with the mixture. Sprinkle remaining cheese on top. Bake for 15 minutes.

Variation ☆

Use shrimp, crab, or lobster as the fish in the above recipe. Add $1/2$ of cocktail sauce and leave out the lemon pepper and onion.

All-Bran Fruity Muffins ☆☆
$1^1/2$ cup of fresh fruit
4 eggs
1 cup wheat bran
$1/2$ cup gluten
1 teaspoon baking powder
1 cup heavy cream
1 tablespoon vanilla
20–40 drops liquid stevia
$1/8$ teaspoon salt
$1/4$ cup shredded coconut
$1/3$ cup coconut oil

Preheat oven to 400° F (200° C). Mix bran, cream, eggs, vanilla, and stevia together in bowl and set aside; for mildly sweet muffins use 20 drops of liquid stevia, for medium sweetness use 40 drops. In another bowl mix together gluten, baking powder, and salt and put aside.

You can use most any type of fruit you like in this recipe. Fruits that work well include: pineapple, peaches, blueberries, raspberries, blackberries, cherries, and apples.

Heat the coconut oil so it is liquid. Generously coat the inside of 12 muffin cups. Add the remaining oil to the bran mixture and stir in. Combine the fruit with the wet and dry ingredients and mix thoroughly with a spoon. Fill muffin cups evenly with the mixture. Bake for 16-18 minutes.

Whole Wheat Coconut Pancakes ☆☆☆

3/4 cup whole wheat flour
1 teaspoon baking powder
1/8 teaspoon salt
1/4 cup shredded coconut
1 egg
1/4 cup coconut oil
1 tablespoon molasses
2/3 cup lukewarm water

Combine flour, baking soda, salt, and coconut in bowl and mix. In a separate bowl combine egg, molasses, 1/4 cup oil, and lukewarm water and mix. The water is warm so coconut oil remains liquid. If you don't have molasses, honey can be substituted. Heat 2 tablespoons of coconut oil in a skillet. Mix the dry ingredients with the liquids. For thinner pancakes use more water. Spoon batter onto hot skillet making pancake about 3 inches in diameter. Makes about 8 pancakes. Top pancakes with a generous amount of fresh chopped fruit, nuts, and yogurt.

Appendix

RESURCES ■

REBOUNDERS
Top-quality rebounders are available by mail through Piccadilly Books, Ltd. PO Box 25203, Colorado Springs, CO, 80936, 719-550-9887. Write for free brochure.

USEFUL WEB SITES

www.WestonAPrice.org
Web site of The Weston A. Price Foundation, 4200 Wisconsin Ave, NW, Washington, DC 20016. This organization offers information on traditional diets and accurate nutritional information. They also provide resources for natural foods.

www.Price-Pottenger.org
Web site of the Price-Pottenger Nutrition Foundation, 7890 Broadway, Lemon Grove, CA 91945. This organization provides nutritional information reflecting the discoveries of Weston A. Price, D.D.S., and Francis Pottenger, M.D.

www.coconut-info.com
Sponsored by Tropical Traditions, Inc., PMB #120, 337 N. Main Street, West Bend, WI 53095, a company that markets herbs and oils. Web site contains articles and resources, and hosts an open discussion group about the health aspects of coconut products.

www.eatwild.com
This web site lists resources for whole, natural foods. Excellent resources for raw milk, organic eggs, grass-fed beef, etc. Sources are listed state-by-state and includes Canada.

www.realmilk.com
You can learn about the health benefits of raw milk on this web site. Includes sources for raw milk in the US, Canada, UK, Australia, and Belgium.

www.WilsonsThyroidSyndrome.com
Web site devoted to understanding thyroid system dysfunction and its treatment.

www.BrodaBarnes.org
Sponsored by the Broda O. Barnes, M.D. Research Foundation, P.O. Box 110098, Trumbull, CT 06611. This organization is devoted to education and research on hypothyroidism and other metabolic problems.

www.epicurious.com
A gourmet foods web site with many recipes.

www.fabulousfoods.com
Contains many recipes that could be adapted to either a low-carb or raw-food diet.

www.carb-lite.au.com
Contains low-carb recipes, many of which are raw.

BIBLIOGRAPHY
Information on Fats and Oils

The Cholesterol Myths. Uffe Ravnskov, 2000: New Trends Publishing, Inc., Washington, DC.

The Healing Miracles of Coconut Oil. Bruce Fife, 2001: HealthWise Publications, Colorado Springs, CO.

Heart Frauds: Uncovering the Biggest Health Scam in History. Charles T. McGee, 2001: HealthWise Publications, Colorado Springs, CO.

Know Your Fats: The Complete Primer for Understanding the Nutrition of Fats, Oils, and Cholesterol. Mary G. Enig, 2000: Bethesda Press, Silver Spring, MD.

Raw Food Recipe Books

Hooked On Raw. Rhio, 2000: Beso Entertainment, New York, NY.

Living In The Raw. Rose Lee Calabro, 2000: Beso Entertainment, New York, NY.

RAW: The Uncook Book. Juliano, 1999: HarperCollins Publishers, New York, NY.

Raw Gourmet. Nomi Shannon, 1999: Alive Books, Vancouver, Canada.

Sunfood Cuisine. Frederic Patenaude, 2002: Genesis 1:29, San Diego, CA.

Stevia Recipe Books

Baking with Stevia. Rita DePuydt, 1998: Sun Coast Enterprises, Oak View, CA.

The Stevia Cookbook. Donna Gates, 1999: Avery Publishing Group, Garden City Park, NY.

Stevia: Nature's Sweetener. Rita Elkins, 1997: Woodland Publishing, Pleasant Grove, UT.

Health, Nutrition, and Diet

Excitotoxins: The Taste That Kills. Russell L. Blaylock, 1994: Health Press, Santa Fe, NM.

Health and Light. John N. Ott, 1973: Ariel Press, Columbus, OH.

Hypothyroidism: The Unsuspected Illness. Broda O. Barnes, 1976: Harper & Row, New York, NY.

Nourishing Traditions: The Cookbook that Challenges Politically Correct Nutrition and the Diet Dictocrats. Sally Fallon and Mary G. Enig, 1999: New Trends Publishing, Inc., Washington, DC.

Nutrition and Physical Degeneration. Weston A. Price, 1997: Keats Publishing, Los Angeles, CA.

Your Body's Many Cries for Water. F. Batmanghelidj, 1997: Global Health Solutions, Falls Church, VA.

REFERENCES ■

Chapter 1—Eat Fat and Lose Weight

1. McGee, C.T. 2001. *Heart Frauds: Uncovering the Biggest Health Scam in History*. Colorado Springs, CO: HealthWise Publications.
2. Prior, I.A., et al. 1981. Cholesterol, coconuts, and diet on Polynesian atolls: a natural experiment: the Pukapuka and Tokelau Island studies. *Am. J. of Clin. Nutr.* 34:1552.

Chapter 2—Big Fat Lies

1. Kekwick, A. and Pawan, G.L.S. 1956. Calorie intake in relation to body weight changes in the obese. *Lancet* 2:155.
2. Kekwick, A. and Pawan, G.L.S. 1957. Metabolic study in human obesity with isocaloric diets high in fat, protein or carbohydrate. *Metabolism* 6:447-460.
3. Vigilante, K. and Flynn, M. 1999. *Low-Fat Lies: High-Fat Frauds and the Healthiest Diet in the World*. Washington, DC: Life Line Press.
4. Ibid.
5. McManus, K, et al. 2001. A randomized controlled trial of a moderate-fat, low-energy diet compared with a low-fat, low-energy diet for weight loss in overweight adults. *Int. J. Obes. Relat. Metab. Disord.* 25(10):1503-11.
6. Vigilante, K. and Flynn, M. 1999. *Low-Fat Lies: High-Fat Frauds and the Healthiest Diet in the World*. Washington, DC: Life Line Press.
7. Fuller, R. and Moore, J.H. 1967. The inhibition of the growth of clostridium welchii by lipids isolated from the contents of the small intestine of the pig. *J. Gen. Microbiol.* 46:23.

Chapter 3—Are You In Need of An Oil Change?

1. Cleave, T.L. 1973 *The Saccharine Disease*. New Canaan, CT: Keats Publishing.
2. Raloff, J. 1996. Unusual fats lose heart-friendly image. *Science News*. 150(6):87.
3. Kummerow, F.A. 1975. *Federation Proceedings* 33:235.
4. Mensink, R.P. and Katan, M.B. 1990. Effect of dietary trans fatty acids on high-density and low-density lipoprotein cholesterol levels in healthy subjects. *N. Eng. J. Med.* 323(7):439.
5. *Science News*. 1990. Trans fats: worse than saturated? 138(8):126.

6. Willett, W.C., et al. 1993. Intake of trans fatty acids and risk of coronary heart disease among women. *Lancet* 341(8845):581.

7. Thampan, P.K. 1994. *Facts and Fallacies About Coconut Oil.* Jakarta: Asian and Pacific Coconut Community.

8. Booyens, J. and Louwrens, C.C. 1986. The Eskimo diet. Prophylactic effects ascribed to the balanced presence of natural cis unsaturated fatty acids and to the absence of unnatural trans and cis isomers of unsaturated fatty acids. *Med. Hypoth.* 21:387.

9. Kritchevsky, D., et al. 1967. *Journal of Atherosclerosis Research* 7:643.

10. Gutteridge, J.M.C. and Halliwell, B. 1994. *Antioxidants in Nutrition, Health, and Disease.* Oxford: Oxford University Press.

11. Ibid.

12. Addis, P.B. and Warner, G.J. 1991. *Free Radicals and Food Additives.* Aruoma, O.I. and Halliwell, B. eds. London: Taylor and Francis.

13. Loliger, J. 1991. *Free Radicals and Food Additives.* Aruoma, O.I. and Halliwell, B. eds. London: Taylor and Francis.

14. Liebman, B. and Hurley, J. 1993. The heart of the matter. *Nutrition Action Healthletter.* 20(8).

15. Carroll, K.K. and Khor, H.T. 1971. *Lipids.* 6:415.

16. Mascioli, E.A., et al. 1987. *Lipids.* 22(6):421.

17. C.J. Meade and J. Martin. 1978. *Adv. Lipd. Res.* 127. Cited by Ray Peat, *Ray Peat's Newsletter.* 1997 Issue, p 3.

18. Ip, C., et al. 1985. *Cancer Res.* 45.

19. Naji and French. 1989. *Life Sciences.* 44.

20. Kramer, J.K.G., et al. 1983. *Lipids.* 17:372. Cited by Ray Peat, *Ray Peat's Newsletter,* 1997 Issue, p 3.

21. Davis, G.P. and Park, E. 1984. *The Heart: The Living Pump.* New York: Torstar Books.

22. Kramer, J.K.G., et al. 1983. *Lipids.* 17:372. Cited by Ray Peat, *Ray Peat's Newsletter,* 1997 Issue, p 3.

23. Harman, D., et al. 1976. Free radical theory of aging: effect of dietary fat on central nervous system function. *Journal of the American Geriatrics Society* 24(7): 301.

24. Lea, C.H. 1962. The oxidative deterioration of food lipids, in *Symposium on Foods: Lipids and Their Oxidation,* ed. by H.W. Schultz, E.A. Day and R.O. Sinnhuber. Westport, CT: Avi Publ. Co.

25. Harman, D., et al. 1976. Free radical theory of aging: effect of dietary fat on central nervous system function. *Journal of the American Geriatrics Society.* 24(7): 301.

Chapter 4—What You Should Know About Cholesterol

1. White, P.D. 1971. *Prog. Cardiovascular Dis.* 14:249.

2. *Statistical Abstracts of the United States.* United States Department of Commerce. Cited by McGee, C.T. 2001. *Heart Frauds: Uncovering the Biggest Health Scam in History.* Colorado Springs, CO: HealthWise Publications.

3. McCully, K.S. 1997. *The Homocysteine Revolution*. New Canaan, CT: Keats Publishing.

4. McGee, C.T. 2001. *Heart Frauds: Uncovering the Biggest Health Scam in History*. Colorado Springs, CO: HealthWise Publications.

5. Liebman, B. 1999. Solving the diet-and-disease puzzle. *Nutrition Action Health Letter* 26(4):6.

6. Rosenberg, H. *The Doctor's Book on Vitamin Therapy*. New York: Putnam.

7. Krumholz, H.M. 1994. Lack of association between cholesterol and coronary heart disease and morbidity and all-cause mortality in persons older than 70 years. *JAMA* 272:1335.

8. Addis, P.B. and Warner, G.J. 1991. *Free Radicals and Food Additives*. Aruoma, O.I. and Halliwell, B. eds. London: Taylor and Francis.

9. Gutteridge, J.M.C. and Halliwell, B. 1994. *Antioxidants in Nutrition, Health, and Disease*. Oxford: Oxford University Press.

10. Ibid.

11. McCully, K.S. 1997. *The Homocysteine Revolution*. New Canaan, CT: Keats Publishing.

12. Napier, K.1995. Partial absolution. *Harvard Health Letter*. 20(10):1.

13. Biss, K., et al. 1971. Some unique biologic characteristics of the Masai of East Africa. *New England Journal of Medicine* 284(13):694.

14. Leaf, A. 1975. *Youth in Old Age*. New York: McGraw Hill.

15. Benet, Sula. 1976. *How to Live to Be 100*. New York: Dial Press.

16. Smith, et al. 1976. Autopsy analysis of disease frequency in Kinshasa, Republic of Zaire *Am. J. Trop. Med. Hyg.* 25(4):637.

17. Biss, K, et al. 1971. Some unique biologic characteristics of the Masai of East Africa. *New England Journal of Medicine* 284:694.

18. Marmot, M.G. 1975. Epidemiologic studies of coronary heart disease and stroke in Japanese men. *American Journal of Epidemiology* 102:511.

19. Davis, G.P. and Park, E. 1984. *The Heart: The Living Pump*. New York: Torstar Books.

20. *The Colorado Springs Gazette*. Heart disease the leading cause of death worldwide, study finds. May 3, 1997.

21. Cathcart, M.K., et al. 1985. Monocytes and neutrophils oxidize low-density lipoprotein making it cytotoxic. *Journal of Leukocyte Biology* 38:341.

22. Passwater, R. 1992. *The New Superantioxidant—Plus*. New Canaan CT: Keats Publishing.

23. Imai, H., et al. 1976. Angiotoxicity and atherosclerosis due to contaminants of USP-grade cholesterol, *Archives of Pathology and Laboratory Medicine* 100:565.

24. Steinberg, D., et al. 1989. Beyond Cholesterol. *N. Engl. J. of Medicine* 320:915.

25. Addis, P.B. and Warner, G.J. 1991. *Free Radicals and Food Additives*. Aruoma, O.I. and Halliwell, B. eds. London: Taylor and Francis.

26. Steinberg, D., et al. 1989. Beyond cholesterol: modifications of low-density lipoprotein that increase its atherogenicity. *N. Engl. J. of Medicine* 320:915.

27. Addis, P.B. and Warner, G.J. 1991. *Free Radicals and Food Additives*. Aruoma, O.I. and Halliwell, B. eds. London: Taylor and Francis.

28. McGee, C.T. 2001. *Heart Frauds: Uncovering the Biggest Health Scam in History*. Colorado Springs, CO: HealthWise Publications.

29. Addis, P.B. and Park, S.W. 1989. *Food Toxicology. A Perspective on the Relative Risks*. Taylor, S.L. and Scanlan, R.A. eds. New York: Marcel Dekker.

30. McGee, C.T. 2001. *Heart Frauds: Uncovering the Biggest Health Scam in History*. Colorado Springs, CO: HealthWise Publications.

31. McCully, K.S. 1997. *The Homocysteine Revolution*. New Canaan, CT: Keats Publishing.

32. Sampsidis, N. 1983. *Homogenized!* Glenwood Landing, NY: Sunflower Publishing.

33. Spencer, P.L. 1995. Fat faddists. *Consumers' Research* 78(5):43.

34. Fallon, S. 1996. Why cholesterol is good for you. *Consumers' Research* 79(3):13.

35. Oster, K.A. 1973. St. Vincent Park City Hospitals Medical Bulletin March 1973. Cited by Sampsidis, N. 1983. *Homogenized!* Glenwood Landing, NY: Sunflower Publishing.

36. Sander, B.D., et al. 1989. *Journal of Food Protection*. 52:109.

37. Park, S.W. and Addis, P.B. 1987. *Journal of Food Science*, 52:1500.

38. Addis, P.B. and Park, S.W. 1989. *Food Toxicology. A Perspective on the Relative Risks*. Taylor, S.L. and Scanlan, R.A. eds. New York: Marcel Dekker.

Chapter 5—The Truth About Saturated Fat

1. Rose, G.A. 1965. *British Medical Journal* 1:1531.

2. Simon, H. 1990. The scales of evidence: eating fish cuts heart attacks, but fish oils may not, *American Health* 9(6):91.

3. Ravnskou, U. 1998. The questionable role of saturated and polyunsaturated fatty acids in cardiovascular disease. *J Clin Epidemiol* 51(6):443-60.

4. Watkins, B.A. and Seifert, M.F. 1996 Food lipids and bone health *Food Lipids and Health*, R.E. McDonald and D.B. Min (eds). New York, NY: Marcel Dekker, Inc.

5. Corliss, R. Should you be a vegetarian? *Time Magazine*, July 15, 2002.

6. Kabara, J.J. 1978. *The Pharmacological Effects of Lipids*. Champaign, IL: The American Oil Chemist's Society.

7. Cohen, L.A., et al. 1986. Dietary fat and mammary cancer. II. Modulation of serum and tumor lipid composition and tumor prostaglandins by different dietary fats: association with tumor incidence patterns. *J. Natl . Cancer Inst.* 77:43.

8. Nanji, A.A., et al. 1995. Dietary saturated fatty acids: a novel treatment for alcoholic liver disease. *Gastroenterology* 109(2):547-54.

9. Cha, Y.S. and Sachan, D.S. 1994. Opposite effects of dietary saturated and unsaturated fatty acids on ethanol-pharmacokinetics, triglycerides and carnitines. *J. Am. Coll. Nutr.* 13(4):338-43.

10. Dahlen, G.H. et al., 1998. The importance of serum lipoprotein(a) as an independent risk factor for premature coronary artery disease in middle-aged black and white women from the United States. *J Intern Med* 244(5):417-24.

11. Khosla, P and Hayes, K.C. 1996. Dietary trans-monounsaturated fatty acids negatively impact plasma lipids in humans: critical review of the evidence. *J. Am. Coll. Nutr.* 15:325-339.

12. Clevidence, B.A., et al. 1997. Plasma lipoprotein (a) levels in men and women consuming diets enriched in saturated, cis-, or trans-monounsaturated fatty acids. *Arterioscler Thromb Vasc Biol* 17:1657-1661.

13. Carroll, K.K. and Khor, H.T. 1971. Effects of level and type of dietary fat on incidence of mammary tumors induced in female sprague-dawley rats by 7, 12-dimethylbenzanthracene. *Lipids* 6:415.

14. Yamori, Y., et al. 1987. Pathogenesis and dietary prevention of cerebrovascular diseases in animal models and epidemiological evidence for the applicability in man. In: Yamori Y., Lenfant C. (eds.) *Prevention of Cardiovascular Diseases: An Approach to Active Long Life.* Amsterdam, the Netherlands: Elsevier Science Publishers.

15. Ikeda, K., et al. 1987. Effect of milk protein and fat intake on blood pressure and incidence of cerebrovascular disease in stroke-prone spontaneously hypertensive rats (SHRSP). *J. Nutr. Sci. Vitaminol.* 33:31.

16. Kimura, N. 1985. Changing patterns of coronary heart disease, stroke, and nutrient intake in Japan. *Prev. Med.* 12:222.

17. Omura, T., et al. 1987. Geographical distribution of cerebrovascular disease mortality and food intakes in Japan. *Soc Sci Med.* 24:40.

18. McGee, D., et al. 1985. The relationship of dietary fat and cholesterol to mortality in 10 years. *Int. J. Epidemiol.* 14:97.

19. Gillman, M. W., et al. 1997. Inverse association of dietary fat with development of ischemic stroke in men. *JAMA* 278(24):2145.

20. Prior, I.A. 1981. Cholesterol, coconuts, and diet on Polynesian atolls: a natural experiment: the Pukapuka and Tokelau island studies. *Am. J. of Clin. Nutr.* 34(8):1552-61.

21. Ibid.

22. Stanhope, J.M., et al. 1981. The Tokelau Island migrant study. Serum lipid concentrations in two environments. *J. Chron. Dis.* 34:45.

23. Prior, I.A.M., 1971. The price of civilization. *Nutrition Today.* July/Aug p. 2-11.

24. Kabara, J.J. 1978. *The Pharmacological Effects of Lipids.* Champaign, IL: The American Oil Chemist's Society.

25. Ibid.

26. Ibid.

27. Ibid.

28. Applegate, L. 1996. Nutrition. *Runner's World.* 31:26.

29. Garfinkel, M., et al. 1992. Insulinotropic potency of lauric acid; a metabolic rationale for medium chain fatty acids (MCF) in TPN formulation. *Journal of Surgical Research* 52:328.

30. Kabara, J.J. 1978. *The Pharmacological Effects of Lipids.* Champaign, IL: The American Oil Chemist's Society.

31. Tantibhedhyangkul, P. and Hashim, S.A. 1978. Medium-chain triglyceride feeding in premature infants: effects on calcium and magnesium absorption. *Pediatrics*, 61(4):537.

32. Kabara, J.J. 1978. *The Pharmacological Effects of Lipids*. Champaign, IL: The American Oil Chemist's Society.

33. Sadeghi, S, et al. 1999. Dietary lipids modify the cytokine response to bacterial lipopolysaccharide in mice. *Immunology* 96(3):404.

34. Kabara, J.J. 1978. *The Pharmacological Effects of Lipids*. Champaign, IL: The American Oil Chemist's Society.

35. Cohen, L.A. and Thompson, D.O. 1987. The influence of dietary medium chain triglycerides on rat mammary tumor development. *Lipids*. 22(6):455.

36. Reddy, B.S. 1992. Dietary fat and colon cancer: animal model studies. *Lipids*. 27(10):807.

37. Hopkins, G.J., et al. 1981. Polyunsaturated fatty acids as promoters of mammary carcinogenesis induced in Sprague-Dawley rats by 7, 12-dimethylbenz[a]lanthracene. *J. Natl. Cancer Inst.* 66(3):517

38. Cohen, L.A. 1988. Medium chain triglycerides lack tumor-promoting effects in the n-methynitrosourea-induced mammary tumor model. In *The Pharmacological Effects of Lipids vol III*. Jon J. Kabara editor. The American Oil Chemist's Society.

39. Hegsted, D.M., et al. 1965. Qualitative effects of dietary fat on serum cholesterol in man. *Am. J. of Clin. Nutrition* 17:281.

40. Hashim, S.A., et al. 1959. Effect of mixed fat formula feeding on serum cholesterol level in man. *Am. J. of Clin. Nutr.* 1:30.

41. Bray, G.A., et al. 1980. Weight gain of rats fed medium-chain triglycerides is less than rats fed long-chain triglycerides. *Int. J. Obes.* 4:27-32.

42. Geliebter, A. 1983. Overfeeding with medium-chain triglycerides diet results in diminished deposition of fat. *Am. J. of Clin. Nutr.* 37:104.

43. Baba, N. 1982. Enhanced thermogenesis and diminished deposition of fat in response to overfeeding with a diet containing medium chain triglycerides. *Am. J. of Clin. Nutr.* 35:678.

44. Greenberger, N.J. and Skillman, T.G. 1969. Medium-chain triglycerides: physiologic considerations and clinical implications. *N. Engl. J. Med.* 280:1045-58.

45. Fino, J.H. 1973. Effect of dietary triglyceride chain length on energy utilized and obesity in rats fed high fat diets. *Fed. Proc.* 32:993.

46. Dahlen, G.H. et al., 1998. The importance of serum lipoprotein(a) as an independent risk factor for premature coronary artery disease in middle-aged black and white women from the United States. *J Intern Med* 244(5):417-24.

47. Clevidence, B.A. et al., 1997. Plasma lipoprotein (a) levels in men and women consuming diets enriched in saturated, cis-, or trans-monounsaturated fatty acids. *Arterioscler Thromb Vasc Biol* 17:1657-1661.

48. Nanji, A.A., et al. 1995. Dietary saturated fatty acids: a novel treatment for alcoholic liver disease. *Gastroenterology* 109(2):547 .

49. Manuel-y-Keenoy, B., et al. 2002. Effects of intravenous supplementation with alpha-tocopherol in patients receiving total parenteral nutrition containing medium- and long-chain triglycerides. *Eur. J. Clin. Nutr.* 56(2):121-8.

50. Fichter, S.A. and Mitchell, G.E, Jr. 1997. Coconut oil as a protective carrier of dietary vitamin A fed to ruminants. *Int. J. Vitam. Nutr. Res.* 67(6):403-6.

51. Henry, G.E., et al. 2002. Antioxidant and cyclooxygenase activities of fatty acids found in food. *J. Agric. Food Chem.* 50(8):2231-4.

52. Fife, B. 2001. *The Healing Miracles of Coconut Oil.* Colorado Springs, CO: HealthWise Publications.

53. Ross, D.L., et al. 1985. Early biochemical and EEG correlates of the ketogenic diet in children with atypical absence epilepsy. *Pediatr Neurol* 1(2):104.

54. Monserrat, A.J., et al. 1995. Protective effects of coconut oil on renal necrosis occurring in rats fed a methyl-deficient diet. *Ren Fail* 17(5):525.

55. Nanji, A.A., et al. 1995. Dietary saturated fatty acids: a novel treatment for alcoholic liver disease. *Gastroenterology* 109(2):547.

56. Cha, Y.S. and Sachan, D.S. 1994. Opposite effects of dietary saturated and unsaturated fatty acids on ethanol-pharmacokinetics, triglycerides and carnitines. *J. Am. Coll. Nutr.* 13(4):338.

57. Enig, M.G. 2000. *Know Your Fats.* Silver Spring, MD: Bethesda Press.

58. Baba, N. 1982. Enhanced thermogenesis and diminished deposition of fat in response to overfeeding with diet containing medium chain triglyceride. *Am. J. of Clin. Nutr.* 35:678-82.

59. Ibid.

60. Kiyasu G.Y., et al. 1952. The portal transport of absorbed fatty acids. *Journal of Biological Chemistry* 199:415-19.

61. Geliebter, A. 1980. Overfeeding with a diet containing medium chain triglyceride impedes accumulation of body fat. *Clinical Research* 28:595A.

62. Bray, G.A., et al. 1980. Weight gain of rats fed medium-chain triglycerides is less than rats fed long-chain triglycerides. *Int. J. Obes.* 4:27-32.

63. Geliebter, A., et al. 1983. Overfeeding with medium-chain triglycerides diet results in diminished deposition of fat. *Am. J. Clin. Nutr.* 37:1-4.

64. Geliebter, A. 1980. Overfeeding with a diet containing medium chain triglyceride impedes accumulation of body fat. *Clinical Research* 28:595A.

65. Bray, G.A., et al. 1980. Weight gain of rats fed medium-chain triglycerides is less than rats fed long-chain triglycerides. *Int. J. Obes.* 4:27-32.

66. Geliebter, A., et al. 1983. Overfeeding with medium-chain triglycerides diet results in diminished deposition of fat. *Am. J. Clin. Nutr.* 37:1-4.

67. Fife, B. 2001. *The Healing Miracles of Coconut Oil.* Colorado Springs, CO: HealthWise Publications.

68. Thampan, P.K. 1994. *Facts and Fallacies About Coconut Oil.* Jakarta: Asian and Pacific Coconut Community.

69. Kabara, J.J. 1978. *The Pharmacological Effects of Lipids.* Champaign, IL: The American Oil Chemist's Society.

Chapter 6—Carbohydrates: Friend or Foe?

1. Reiser, S., et al. 1985. Indices of copper status in humans consuming a typical American diet containing either fructose or starch. *Am. J. Clin. Nutr.* 42(2):242-251.

2. Forristal, LJ. 2001. The murky world of high fructose corn syrup. *Wise Traditions* 2(3):60-61.

3. Stoddard, M.N. *The Deadly Deception*. Dallas, TX: Aspartame Consumer Safety Network.

4. Roberts, J.J. *Aspartame (NutraSweet), Is it Safe?* Dallas, Texas: Aspartame Consumer Safety Network.

Chapter 7—Calories and Appetite

1. Whitney, E.N., et al. 1991. *Understanding Normal and Clinical Nutrition* 3rd ed. St. Paul, MN: West Publishing Company.

Chapter 8—Malnutrition Can Make You Fat

1. Senate Document #264, published by the 2nd session of the 74th Congress 1936

2. Wright, J.V., 1990. *Dr. Wright's Guide to Healing with Nutrition*. New Canaan, CT: Keats Publishing.

3. Ibid.

4. Binnert, C., et al. 1998. Influence of human obesity on the metabolic fate of dietary long- and medium-chain triacylglycerols. *Am. J. Clin. Nutr.* 67(4):595-601.

5. Tantibhedhyangkul, P. and Hashim, S.A. 1978. Medium-chain triglyceride feeding in premature infants: effects on calcium and magnesium absorption. *Pediatrics*, 61(4):537.

6. Gerster, H. 19989. Can adults adequately convert alpha-linolenic acid (18:3n-3) to eicosapentaenoic acid (20:5n-3) and docosahexaenoic acid (22:6n-3)? *Int. J. Vitam. Nutr. Res.* 68(3):159.

Chapter 9—How to Supercharge Your Metabolism

1. Kimura, S., et al. 1976. Development of malignant goiter by defatted soybean with iodine-free diet in rats. *Gann* 67:763-765.

2. Chorazy, P.A., et al. 1995. Persistent hypothyroidism in an infant receiving a soy formula: Case report and review of the literature. *Pediatrics*, 96(1)Pt1:148-150.

3. Pinchers, A., et al. 1965. Thyroid refractoriness in an athyreotic cretin fed soybean formula, *New Eng. J. Med.* 265:83-87.

4. Ishizuki, Y., et al. 1991. The effects on the thyroid gland of soybeans administered experimentally to healthy subjects. *Nippon Naibunpi Gakkai Zasshi* 67:622-629.

5. Divi, R. L., et al. 1997. Identification, characterization and mechanisms of anti-thyroid activity of isoflavones from soybean. *Biochem. Pharmacol.* 54:1087-1096.

6. Fort, P., et al. 1990. Breast and soy-formula feedings in early infancy and the prevalence of autoimmune thyroid disease in children. *J. Am. Clin. Nutr.* 9:164-167.

7. Nagata, C. et al. 1998. Decreased serum total cholesterol concentration is associated with high intake of soy products in Japanese men and women. *J. Nutr.* 128:209-13

8. Fushiki, T. and Matsumoto, K. 1995, Swimming endurance capacity of mice is increased by chronic consumption of medium-chain triglycerides. *Journal of Nutrition* 125:531.

9. Applegate, L. 1996. Nutrition. *Runner's World* 31:26.

10. Thampan, P.K. 1994. *Facts and Fallacies About Coconut Oil.* Jakarta: Asian and Pacific Coconut Community.

11. Baba, N. 1982. Enhanced thermogenesis and diminished deposition of fat in response to overfeeding with diet containing medium-chain triglyceride. *Am. J. Clin. Nutr.* 35:678.

12. Bach, A.C., et al. 1989. Clinical and experimental effects of medium chain triglyceride based fat emulsions-a review. *Clin. Nutr.* 8:223.

13. Hill, J.O., et al. 1989. Thermogenesis in humans during overfeeding with medium-chain triglycerides. *Metabolism* 38:641.

14. Hasihim, S.A. and Tantibhedyangkul, P. 1987. Medium chain triglyceride in early life: Effects on growth of adipose tissue. *Lipids* 22:429.

15. Geliebter, A. 1980. Overfeeding with a diet containing medium chain triglyceride impedes accumulation of body fat. *Clinical Research* 28:595A.

16. Baba, N. 1982. Enhanced thermogenesis and diminished deposition of fat in response to overfeeding with diet containing medium chain triglyceride. *Am. J. of Clin. Nutr.* 35:678-82.

17. Murray, M. T. 1996. *American Journal of Natural Medicine* 3(3):7.

18. Hill, J.O., et al. 1989. Thermogenesis in man during overfeeding with medium chain triglycerides. *Metabolism* 38:641-8.

19. Seaton, T.B., et al. 1986. Thermic effect of medium-chain and long-chain triglycerides in man. *Am. J. of Clin. Nutr.* 44:630.

20. Seaton, T.B., et al. 1986. Thermic effect of medium-chain and long-chain triglycerides in man. *Am. J. Clin. Nutr.* 44:630-634.

22. Geliebter, A., et al. 1983. Overfeeding with medium-chain triglyceride diet results in diminished deposition of fat. *Am. J. Clin. Nutr.* 37:1-4.

23. Crozier, G., et al. 1987. Metabolic effects induced by long-term feeding of medium-chain triglycerides in the rat. *Metabolism* 36:807-814.

24. Lavau, M.M. and Hashim, S.A. 1978. Effect of medium chain triglyceride on lipogenesis and body fat in the rat. *J. Nutr.* 108:613-620.

25. Lasekan, J.B., et al. 1992. Energy expenditure in rats maintained with intravenous or intragastric infusion of total parenteral nutrition solutions containing medium- or long-chain triglyceride emulsions. *J. Nutr.* 122:1483-1492.

26. Seaton, T.B., et al. 1986. Thermic effect of medium-chain and long-chain triglycerides in man. *Am. J. Clin. Nutr.* 44:630-634.

27. Dulloo, A.G., et al. 1996. Twenty-four hour energy expenditure and urinary catecholamines of humans consuming low to moderate amounts of medium-chain triglycerides; a dose-response study in human respiratory chamber. *Eur. J. Clin. Nutr.* 50:152-158.

28. Scalfi, L., et al. 1991. Postprandial thermogenesis in lean and obese subjects after meals supplemented with medium-chain and long-chain triglycerides. *Am. J. Clin. Nutr.* 53:1130-1133.

29. Crozier, G., et al. 1987. Metabolic effects induced by long-term feeding of medium-chain triglycerides in the rat. *Metabolism* 36:807-814.

30. Lavau, M.M. and Hashim, S.A. 1978. Effect of medium chain triglycende on lipogenesis and body fat in the rat. *J. Nutr.* 108:613-620.

31. St.-Onge, M. and Jones, P. 2002. Physiological effects of medium-chain triglycerides: potential agents in the prevention of obesity. *J. Nutr.* 132:329-332.

32. Peat, R. *Ray Peat's Newsletter* 1997 Issue, p.2-3.

33. *Encyclopedia Britanica Book of the Year*, 1946. Cited by Ray Peat, *Ray Peat's Newsletter*, 1997 Issue, p.4.

34. Roos, P.A. 1991. Light and electromagnetic waves: the health implications. *Journal of the Bio-Electro-Magnetics Institute.* 3(2):7-12.

35.Garland, F.C., et al. 1990. Occupational sunlight exposure and melanoma in the U.S. Navy. *Archives of Environmental Health.* 45:261-267.

36. Editorial. 1991. Excessive sunlight exposure, skin melanoma, linked to vitamin D. *International Journal of Biosocial and Medical Research.* 13(1):13-14.

37. Garland, F.C., et al. 1990. Occupational sunlight exposure and melanoma in the U.S. Navy. *Archives of Environmental Health.* 45:261-267.

Chapter 10—Satisfy Your Hunger Longer

1. Eyton, A. 1983. *The F-Plan Diet.* New York, NY: Crown Publishers, Inc.

2. Vigilante, K. and Flynn, M. 1999. *Low-Fat Lies: High-Fat Frauds and the Healthiest Diet in the World.* Washington, DC: Life Line Press.

3. Rolls, B.J. and Miller, D.L. 1997. Is the low-fat message giving people a license to eat more? *Journal of the American College of Nutrition*, 16:535.

4. Furuse, M., et al. 1992. Feeding behavior in rats fed diets containing medium chain triglyceride. *Physiol. Behav.* 52(4):815.

5. Rolls, B.J., et al. 1988. Food intake in dieters and nondieters after a liquid meal containing medium-chain triglycerides. *Am. J. Clin. Nutr.* 48(1):66.

6. Stubbs, R.J. and Harbron, C.G. 1996. Covert manipulation of the ration of medium- to long-chain triglycerides in isoenergetically dense diets: effect on food intake in ad libitum feeding men. *Int. J. Obes.* 20:435-444.

7. Van Wymelbeke, V., et al. 1998. Influence of medium-chain and long-chain triacylglycerols on the control of food intake in men. *Am. J. Clin. Nutr.* 68:226-234.

8. Rolls, B. and Barnett, R.A., 2000. *Volumetrics: Feel Full on Fewer Calories.* HarperCollins Publishers.

Chapter 11—Drink More, Weigh Less

1. Kleiner, S.M. 1999. Water: an essential but overlooked nutrient, *American Dietetic Association Journal* 99(2):200-206.

2. Dauterman, K.W., et al. 1995. Plasma specific gravity for identifying hypovolemia. *J Diarrhoeal Dis. Res.* 13:33-38.

3. Ershow, A.G., et al. 1991. Intake of tapwater and total water by pregnant and lactating women. *Am. J. Public Health* 81:328-334.

4. Dauterman, K.W., et al. 1995. Plasma specific gravity for identifying hypovolaemia. *J Diarrhoeal Dis. Res.* 13:33-38.

5. Torranin, C., et al. 1979. The effects of acute thermal dehydration and rapid rehydration on isometric and isotonic endurance. *J. Sports Med. Phys. Fitness* 19:1-9.

6. Armstrong, L.E., et al. 1985. Influence of diuretic-induced dehydration on competitive running performance. *Med. Sci. Sports Exerc.* 17:456-461.

7. Sawka, M.N. and Pandolf, KR 1990. Effects of body water loss on physiological function and exercise performance. In : Gisolfi C.V. and Lamb, D.R. eds. *Fluid Homeostasis During Exercise.* Carmel, Ind: Benchmark Press.

8. Sansevero, A.C. 1997. Dehydration in the elderly: strategies for prevention and management. *Nurse Pract.* 22:41-42, 51-57, 63-72.

9. Sagawa, S., et al. 1992. Effect of dehydration on thirst and drinking during immersion in men. *J. Appl. Physiol.* 72:128-134.

10. Gopinathan, P.M., et al. 1988. Role of dehydration in heat stress-induced variations in mental performance. *Arch. Environ. Health* 43:15-17.

11. Torranin, C., et al. 1979. The effects of acute thermal dehydration and rapid rehydration on isometric and isotonic endurance. *J. Sports Med. Phys. Fitness* 19:1-9.

12. Armstrong, L.E., et al. 1985. Influence of diuretic-induced dehydration on competitive running performance. *Med. Sci. Sports Exerc.* 17:456-461.

13. Sagawa, S., et al. 1992. Effect of dehydration on thirst and drinking during immersion in men. *J. Appl. Physiol.* 72:128-134.

14. Curhan, G.C. and Curhan, S.G. 1994. Dietary factors and kidney stone formation. *Comp. Ther.* 20:485-489.

15. Goldfarb, S. 1990. The role of diet in the pathogenesis and therapy of nephrolithiasis. *Endocrinol .Metab. Clin. North Am.* 19:805-820.

16. Bitterman, W.A., et al. 1991. Environmental and nutritional factors significantly associated with cancer of the urinary tract among different ethnic groups. *Urologic Clin. North Am.* 18:501-508.

17. Shannon, J., et al. 1996. Relationship of food groups and water intake to colon cancer risk. *Cancer Epidemiol. Biomarkers Prev.* 5:495-502.

18. Stookey, J.D., et al. 1997. Relationship of food groups and water intake to colon cancer risk. *Cancer Epidemiol. Biomarkers Prev.* 6:657-658.

19. Wilkens, L.R., et al. 1996. Risk factors for lower urinary tract cancer: the role of total fluid consumption, nitrites and nitrosamines, and selected foods. *Cancer Epidemiol. Biomarkers Prev.* 5:161-166.

20. Bitterman, W.A., et al. 1991. Environmental and nutritional factors significantly associated with cancer of the urinary tract among different ethnic groups. *Urologic. Clin. North Am.* 18:501-508.

21. Wilkens, L.R., et al. 1996. Risk factors for lower urinary tract cancer: the role of total fluid consumption, nitrites and nitrosamines, and selected foods. *Cancer Epidemiol. Biomarkers Prev.* 5:161-166.

22. Shannon, J., et al. 1996. Relationship of food groups and water intake to colon cancer risk. *Cancer Epidemiol. Biomarkers Prev.* 5:495-502.

23. Stookey, J.D., et al. 1997. Relationship of food groups and water intake to colon cancer risk. *Cancer Epidemiol .Biomarkers Prev.* 6:657-658.

24. Stamford, B.1993. Muscle cramps: untying the knots. *Phys. Sportsmed.* 21:115-116.

INDEX

Acesulfame K, 92, 93
Addis, Paul, 54
Alcohol, 182
Allergies, 121-122
Alpha-linolenic acid, 213
Amylase, 119
Antihistamines, 152, 157
Appetite, 106-108
Armour, 153, 157
Artificial fats. *See* Fake fats
Artificial sweeteners, 90-94, 208
Aspartame, 91
Atherosclerosis, 50, 53-54, 58-63, 65, 67, 71, 77
Ayurvedic medicine, 75

Baby formula, 8, 123
Basal metabolic rate (BMR), 102
Batmanghelidj, Fereydoon, 170-172, 173-174
Benefat, 41
Behavior, 106-108
Ben Joseph, Eliezer, 79
Beta-carotene, 26, 85
Betaine HCL, 122
Bile, 123-124
Bitterman, W.A., 177
Body temperature, 127, 134, 136-138, 139-142, 149, 153-154, 155
Blaylock, Russell L., 94
Butter, 36, 66, 129, 209

Cabbage, 130
Caffeine, 179, 181
Calcium, 27, 72, 86, 115, 153
Calories, 19-20, 25, 101-106, 145, 180, 219-220
Cancer, 44, 73, 177
Carbohydrates, 82-100, 114
    complex, 83
    simple, 83

Cardiovascular disease. *See* Heart disease
Castelli, William, 7
Cayenne pepper, 124
Cell membrane, 23-24, 62, 70, 71
Childbirth, 138
Cholesterol, 30, 47, 52-63, 69, 155
Cholesterol hypothesis. *See* Cholesterol theory
Cholesterol-lowering drugs, 53
Cholesterol regulation, 54-56
Cholesterol theory, 49, 51, 52-58
Chronic dehydration, 169-170, 172-173, 174-178
Coconut, 245-246
Coconut diet, 8-10
Coconut milk, 246
Coconut oil,
    daily use, 210-211
    diet, 8-10
    digestion, 122-123
    energy, 143-145
    EFA, 214
    health aspects, 74-81
    history, 12-13
    low-calorie fat, 145-146
    metabolism, 146-148, 157, 220
    recommendations, 209
    satiety, 164-165
    sunscreen, 216
    virgin, 210
    WTS, 148-149
Coconut water, 246
Collagen, 90
Cooking, 61, 67
Copper deficiency, 90
Coronary heart disease, 50. *See also* Heart disease
Cortisone, 138, 152
Crisco, 36
Cruciferous vegetables, 130, 157, 208

Cyclamate, 92-93
Cytomel, 157

Dayrit, Conrado, 80
DeBakey, Michael, 53
Dehydration, 174-178. *See also* Chronic
    dehydration
Diet-induced obesity, 106
Digestion, 83-85, 118-123
Digestive aids, 124-125
Digestive enzymes, 119
Disaccharide, 83

Eggs, 62, 67-68
Energy, 143-145
Enig, Mary, 38, 81
Essential fatty acids (EFA), 25, 213-214
Excitotoxins: The Taste That Kills, 94
Exercise, 189-199, 214-215

Fake fats, 39-41, 208
Fat
    building block, 23-24
    digestion, 115, 123
    energy source, 24-25
    nutritional source, 25-27
    protection from disease, 28-29
    satiety, 163-165
Fatty acids, 25, 28, 31
Field, Meira, 90
Fiber, 83, 84, 161-162
Flynn, Mary, 22, 27
Food cravings, 111-115
Food quality, 116, 209
Food sensitivities, 121-122
Framingham study, 7, 53, 74
Frankenfoods, 86-87, 91, 92, 208
Free radicals, 26, 42-46, 52, 59-63
Fructose, 51, 83, 88-89
Fruit smoothie, 249

Gallbladder, 123-124
Genetics, 56-58
Germs, 28
Gillman, Matthew, 73

Glucose, 83, 89, 90
Glutamic HCL, 122
Gluten, 223, 239
Goat milk, 66
Goiter, 128
    simple, 128
    toxic, 130
Goitrogens, 130-131

Hardening of the arteries. *See*
    Atherosclerosis
Healing Miracles of Coconut Oil, The,
    12, 14, 81
Healthy Lifestyle Plan, 9-10, 203-221
Heartburn, 120
Heart disease, 37-38, 44, 50, 52, 61, 65,
    70, 72, 73
Heart Frauds, 27, 53, 62
Heidelberg capsule, 122
Hippocrates, 176
Homocysteine, 61
Homogenized milk, 61, 64-65
Hormones, 24
Hot baths, 153-154, 157
Hunger, 106-108
Hydrochloric acid, 120
Hydrogenated oil, 36-38, 208
Hypothyroidism, 127-131

Ice cream, 68
Iodine, 128-129
Irish study, 57-58
Iron, 61

Japanese study, 57
Jialal, Ishwarlal, 58

Kabara, Jon J., 80
Kefir, 65
Kekwick, Alan, 21
Krumholz, Harlan, 53

Lard, 36, 209
Lee, Lita, 79
Lipase, 119

Lipid, 30
Lipoprotein, 58, 70, 143
Linoleic acid, 52, 213
Liquid candy, 182, 183
Long-chain fatty acid (LCFA), 77, 122-123, 143, 147, 165
Low-carbohydrate coconut diet, 222-240
Low-carbohydrate diet, 179, 222-240
Low-fat diets, 7-8, 19-23
Low-Fat Lies, 22
Low-refined-carbohydrate diet, 100, 204-205
Lp(a), 72
lycopene, 86

Magnesium, 50
Malnutrition, 109-125, 137-136. *See also* Subclinical malnutrition
Margarine, 36-38, 129, 208
Masai, 56
Melanoma, 157-158
Monosaccharide, 83
Mattson, Fred, 36
McCully, Kilmer, 55, 62
McGee, Charles, 27, 53, 62
Medium-chain fatty acid (MCFA), 77-78, 122-123, 143-145, 147, 165
Medium-chain triglyceride (MCT), 77, 144
Mental ability, 46
Metabolism, 105, 126-149, 152-158, 179, 194, 219-221
Milk, 51, 56, 63-68, 208, 209, 211. *See also* Raw milk
Minerals, 50, 113-115, 116-118, 121, 211-213
Monounsaturated fatty acids, 31, 39
Multiple enzyme dysfunction (MED), 134-136, 141-142, 155
Murray, Michael, 80

Nutrient deficiency, 50-52, 88. *See also* Malnutrition *and* Subclinical malnutrition

Obesity, 19
Olean, 40
Olestra, 39-40
Omega-3, 25, 213-214
Omega-6, 25, 213-214
Organic foods, 116, 209-210
Osteoporosis, 72, 86, 153
Oster, Kurt, 65
Oxidation, 33, 43, 52, 58-63, 90
Oxidized cholesterol, 58-63

Pasteurization, 51, 65-66
Pawan, Gaston, 21
Peat, Ray, 79, 148
Phospholipids, 30
Pica, 112
Polysaccharide, 83
Polyunsaturated fatty acids, 31, 69-70, 73-74, 157
Powdered milk, 63, 67-68, 208
Powdered eggs, 63, 67-68, 208
Pregnancy, 138
Prior, Ian, 76-77
Pritikin, Nathan, 27
Processed meats, 63, 67
Prostaglandins, 24, 52
Protein, 162-163, 179
Protease, 119
Pukapuka, 75-77

Raw-foods coconut diet, 241-250
Raw milk, 56, 64, 65-66, 209
Rebound exercise, 199-202, 215
Reduced cholesterol, 58-63

Saccharide, 83
Saccharin, 92-93
Salatrim, 41
Salt, 113-115, 173-174, 207, 244-245
Sampsidis, Nicholas, 62
Satiety, 160-161
Saturated fat, 18019, 31, 39, 52, 54, 69-78
Saunas, 153-154, 157
Seasonal affective disorder (SAD), 156

Schroeder, Henry, 64
Shortening, 36-37, 208
Soybean oil, 36
Soybeans, 130-131, 157, 208
Splenda, 93
Sri Lanka, 12-13
Sterols, 30
Stevia, 94-95, 209
Stomach acid, 115, 120-122
Stookey, J.D., 177
Stress, 121, 137-138
Stroke, 73-74
Subclinical malnutrition, 52, 88, 111, 138. *See also* Malnutrition
Sucralose, 92
Sucrose, 51, 87-88, 89
Sugar, 50-51, 82-100, 110, 114, 204, 207, 209, 223
Sugar addiction, 96-99
Sulfa drugs, 152, 157
Sunlight, 155-158, 215-216
Synthroid, 132, 133, 153, 157

T3, 133-142
T4, 133-142
Tallow, 209
Tokelau, 75-77
Tonga, 217
Thirst, 175, 181, 184-186
Thyroid gland, 127-131, 133, 142, 155
Thyroid system, 133-142
Trace minerals, 112-115, 173-174, 212, 213
Trans fatty acid, 37-38

Tree of life, 12
Triglycerides, 30

Ulcers, 121
US senate document, 117

Vegetable juice, 206, 248
Vegetable oil, 31-39, 52, 61, 63, 67, 69-70, 73, 208
Vigilante, Kevin, 22
Vitamin and mineral deficiency, 50-52
Vitamin D, 24, 50, 155, 158
Vitamins, 26, 40, 50-52, 109-111, 116-118, 123, 211-212

Warner, Gregory, 54
Water, 165-167, 168-188, 206, 218
Wheat bran, 223
Whitaker, Julian, 147
White bread, 83, 207, 223
Whole wheat, 83, 208, 209, 238-239
Wickremasinghe, Robert, 79
Wilkens, L.R., 177
Willet, Walter, 21, 37
Wilson, Denis, 133, 139, 142
Wilson's thyroid syndrome (WTS), 131-142
Wright, Jonathan, 121

Xanthine oxidase, 61, 64-65

Yogurt, 65
Your Body's Many Cries for Water, 121
Yo-yo effect, 106

A HEALING MIRACLE

If there was an oil you could use for your daily cooking needs that helped protect you from heart disease, cancer, and other degenerative conditions, improved your digestion, strengthened your immune system, protected you from infectious illnesses, and helped you lose excess weight, would you be interested? This is what coconut oil can do for you.

Coconut oil has been called the "healthiest dietary oil on earth." If you're not using coconut oil for your daily cooking and body care needs you're missing out on one of nature's most amazing health foods.

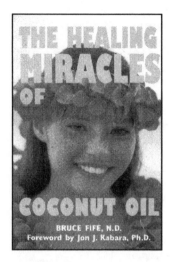